D1447582

The Tobacco Epidemic

2nd, revised and extended edition

Progress in Respiratory Research

Vol. 42

Series Editor

Felix J.F. Herth Heidelberg

The Tobacco Epidemic

2nd, revised and extended edition

Volume Editors

Robert Loddenkemper Berlin

Michael Kreuter Heidelberg

85 figures, 31 in color, 29 tables, 2015

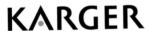

Basel · Freiburg · Paris · London · New York · Chennai · New Delhi ·
Bangkok · Beijing · Shanghai · Tokyo · Kuala Lumpur · Singapore · Sydney

Prof. Dr. Robert Loddenkemper
Hertastrasse 3
D-14169 Berlin
Germany

Ass. Prof. Dr. Michael Kreuter
Department of Pneumology and Respiratory Critical Care Medicine
Thoraxklinik, University of Heidelberg
Amalienstrasse 5
D-69126 Heidelberg
Germany

Library of Congress Cataloging-in-Publication Data

The tobacco epidemic / volume editors, Robert Loddenkemper, Michael Kreuter.
-- 2nd, revised and extended edition.
 p. ; cm. -- (Progress in respiratory research, ISSN 1422-2140 ; vol. 42)
 Includes bibliographical references and indexes.
 ISBN 978-3-318-02656-6 (hard cover : alk. paper) -- ISBN 978-3-318-02657-3 (electronic version)
 I. Loddenkemper, Robert, editor. II. Kreuter, Michael, editor. III. Series: Progress in respiratory research ; v. 42. 1422-2140
 [DNLM: 1. Smoking. 2. Smoking Cessation--methods. 3. Tobacco Products. 4. Tobacco Smoke Pollution. 5. Tobacco Use Disorder. W1 PR681DM / QV 137]
 RC567
 616.86'5--dc23
 2015000956

Bibliographic Indices. This publication is listed in bibliographic services, including Book Citation Index in Web of Science™.

1st edition published in 1997 and edited by C.T. Bolliger and K.O. Fagerström as *The Tobacco Epidemic* (Progress in Respiratory Research, Vol. 28)

2nd edition © Copyright 2015 by S. Karger AG, P.O. Box, CH-4009 Basel (Switzerland)
www.karger.com
Printed in Germany on acid-free and non-aging paper (ISO 9706) by Kraft Druck GmbH, Ettlingen
ISSN 1422–2140
e-ISSN 1662–3932
ISBN 978–3–318–02656–6
e-ISBN 978–3–318–02657–3

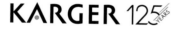

Contents

Foreword

Tobacco entered America long before the Europeans arrived. A Spanish crew member of the Santa Maria, the flagship of Christopher Columbus's first expedition, is credited with being the first European smoker. In Japan, tobacco was introduced by Portuguese sailors in the middle of the 16th century. In Australia, smoking started when it was introduced to northern-dwelling communities by visiting Indonesian fishermen in the early 18th century.

The world was conquered by tobacco and the disaster started.

The 42nd volume of *Progress in Respiratory Research* presents an updated edition of this topic. In this revised and extended version, all actual aspects of the epidemic are covered. In 23 chapters, the complete tobacco story is considered, starting with its history and ending with an emerging problem: electronic cigarettes.

The editors were able to motivate the 'who is who' in the field, and, true to the heart of the series, the book concentrated on an ongoing problem in the world, and all authors included the latest relevant references.

My congratulations to the editors and the authors for this great volume.

Enjoy reading

Felix J.F. Herth, Heidelberg

Preface

Tobacco use causes one of the world's deadliest epidemics ever. It killed 100 million people in the 20th century and, if trends do not change, will be responsible for the deaths of 1 billion people in this century. Most of those projected deaths will occur in low- and middle-income countries, where the tobacco industry has shifted its efforts to recruit new smokers (Framework Convention Alliance, Moscow, October 13–18, 2014).

In 1997, our friend Chris Bolliger – who sadly died in 2012 – wrote in his preface to the 1st volume of the book series *Progress in Respiratory Research* under his editorship: 'For this first volume "*The Tobacco Epidemic*" to appear under my editorship I have chosen the area of smoking, which is more than just "timely" considering the current legal developments on everything concerning smoking in the USA. It further represents a topic which should appeal to a large readership across many medical specialities, but also to non-medical people interested in tobacco'.

We, the editors of this 2nd edition of 'The Tobacco Epidemic', have to acknowledge the progress meanwhile achieved in many areas against this deadly tobacco epidemic; however, as outlined in several chapters, recent data show that the global problem has even been aggravated since 1997.

In their foreword to the book the two editors Chris Bolliger and Karl Olov Fagerström stated: 'In the summer of 1997, American tobacco companies were pushed against the wall and agreed to: (a) pay well over USD 300 billion to smokers and health care givers; (b) restrict their marketing, and (c) make sure that smoking in adolescence declines'. The contributions in this 2015 edition reveal that this has not been implemented; on the contrary, the predictions of the former editors have unfortunately come true: 'The to-bacco industry is now likely to be "rolled back" on other fronts, too. Actions are now also mounting in Europe. Cigarette smoking will most likely not be exempt from regulations as in the past. However, smoking may still grow in the developing world and make up for the sales lost in the USA and other developed countries'.

However, in the past 18 years, some essential progress has been made in the fight against the deadly epidemic, the most important being certainly the WHO Framework Convention on Tobacco Control, approved in 2006, which changed the landscape of public health being one of the most widely adopted treaties in the history of the United Nations, with 179 Parties to the Convention covering over 85% of the world's population. This was followed in 2008 by the introduction of six WHO MPOWER measures, a policy package intended to assist implementation of effective interventions to reduce tobacco use worldwide at the country level. The first Tobacco Atlas was released in 2002 and the editors of the 4th edition in 2012 stated rightly that the last 10 years had likely been the most productive period in the history of tobacco control, but that far too much remains to be done. The regular US Surgeon General's Reports – last year under the heading *The Health Consequences of Smoking – 50 Years of Progress* – helped essentially to raise the awareness about the dangers related to tobacco and its industry. In several countries, strict regulations with smoking bans were introduced, 'smoke free' – the first complete ban on workplace smoking – in Ireland in 2004. Seventeen European Union (EU) countries have introduced comprehensive laws since then and more than 60 countries worldwide and 28 US states have comprehensive smoke-free laws. In the EU, the first Tobacco Product Directive of 2001 was comprehensively revised in 2014, thus strengthening the

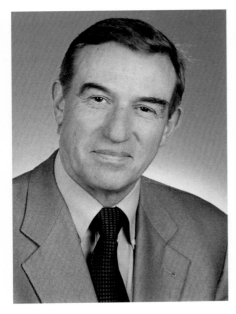 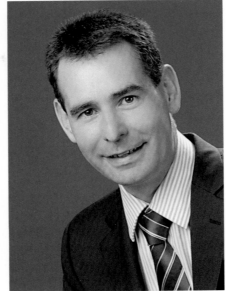

Robert Loddenkemper   Michael Kreuter

rules on how tobacco products are manufactured, produced and presented in the EU and introducing specific rules for certain tobacco-related products.

The scientific knowledge on the health hazards of tobacco – almost all organs of the body are now found to be affected – and on nicotine addiction has enlarged considerably since the 1st edition. This 2nd edition with its 23 chapters written by outstanding experts covers all clinical, public health and political aspects on tobacco smoking. The book is illustrated with 85 figures and 29 tables and contains a broad range of the most recent literature. The reader can learn about the long history of tobacco production and use, about the economical aspects of tobacco use and control as well as the health consequences of voluntary and involuntary smoking, both in adults and in children. Special chapters depict the impact of media, movies and TV on tobacco use in the youth, the most relevant target of the cigarette industry. The patterns and predictors of smoking cessation in the general population as well as in different social subgroups are described. The reader will further be updated on the development and features of nicotine dependence, how it can be treated with nicotine replacement medications and other drugs, the role of general practitioners, nurses and pharmacists in aiding smokers to quit, what effects smoke-free environments, advertising bans and price increases have on smoking prevalence, and, of course, what smoking prevalence looks like worldwide. Besides chapters on smoke-less and waterpipe tobacco smoking, the final chapter analyses the potential harms and benefits of e-cigarettes and other electronic nicotine-delivering devices, a topic which has recently achieved high public attention and which – on one side – may help smokers to quit but entails – on the other side – the danger of renormalization of smoking, in particular appealing to the youth.

We are convinced that the request of Chris Bolliger that 'Individual contributions should be a mix of highly scientific but also easy-to-read writing…' has been fulfilled in this extended and completely revised 2nd edition. We are grateful to all authors representing so many countries and organisations for their dedicated contributions. We hope that this book will be helpful not only to medical doctors, medical trainees and nurses from various fields who witness the burden of smoking-related diseases in their daily practice (e.g. public health, respiratory medicine, thoracic surgery, cardiology, internal medicine, paediatric medicine, psychiatry, psychology, occupational medicine and obstetrics) but also to interested journalists and politicians/legislators.

As an outlook to a potential 3rd edition, we express the hope that the fight against the tobacco epidemic will move on successfully to stop the epidemic and that this 2nd edition will contribute to the success and assist those engaged in this fight.

Robert Loddenkemper, Berlin
Michael Kreuter, Heidelberg

Chapter 1

Loddenkemper R, Kreuter M (eds): The Tobacco Epidemic, ed 2, rev. and ext.
Prog Respir Res. Basel, Karger, 2015, vol 42, pp 1–18 (DOI: 10.1159/000369289)

History of Tobacco Production and Use

Joan Hanafin · Luke Clancy

TobaccoFree Research Institute Ireland, Dublin, Ireland

Abstract

Tobacco has been in use for over 10,000 years and worldwide for over 500 years, but its use was limited by the intensity of time and labour involved in producing, preparing and using it. From the late 1800s, developments in mechanisation, transport and technology led to greater ease of production and use. Marketing, advertising and promotion by tobacco companies led to tobacco use on such a scale as to be called an epidemic. Tobacco regulation has existed since at least 1500. Growing scientific evidence based on tobacco-related mortality and morbidity, notably since the early 20th century, and public health interventions in place since the mid-20th century, led to a decrease in tobacco use amongst better-off, industrialised, western populations. There has been a concomitant increase in tobacco use among middle- and lower-income countries. As tobacco is a main risk factor for chronic diseases, including cancer, lung diseases and cardiovascular diseases, the late 20th and early 21st century have been characterised by public health campaigns to regulate tobacco. Many countries have enacted legislation in conformity with the WHO Framework Convention on Tobacco Control, but the number of smokers continues to rise, and tobacco-related disease and death continue to increase. © 2015 S. Karger AG, Basel

This chapter provides an overview of the history of tobacco: its early agricultural and ceremonial origins; the globalization of tobacco cultivation and use; changes in tobacco production and use that occurred with industrialisation and mass production; the development of an empirical, epidemiological, scientific evidence base regarding the health effects of tobacco use; historic and current initiatives in regulating and controlling tobacco, and the evolving strategies of the tobacco industry in combatting tobacco control and increasing the number of users of its products, leading to the current global state of play regarding tobacco production, use and control.

The chapter is divided into three sections. Firstly, a brief history of tobacco cultivation, production, preparation and use throughout the ages is presented; secondly, a historical account of beliefs and knowledge about the health effects of tobacco are described, and, thirdly, the history of tobacco control and regulation and of the responses of the tobacco industry are summarised. The chapter concludes with a brief account, within the foregoing historic context, of current global trends and issues in tobacco use and control.

Tobacco Cultivation, Production, Preparation and Use

This section gives an account of tobacco from its earliest cultivation and use in agricultural societies for religious, creative and social purposes through the globalization of tobacco cultivation and use following the creation of new trade routes in the 1500s, to its greatly increased use following industrialisation, peaking in developed countries in the mid-20th century, and the pattern of socially unequal use in the early decades of the 21st century, characterised by differentiated patterns of use by age, gender, material resources and geography.

Early Tobacco Cultivation

The oldest record of tobacco, dating to the Pleistocene Era 2.5 million years ago, is a small cluster of fossilised tobacco leaves reported to have been found in 2010 by palaeontologists in northeastern Peru [1]. There is no indication of habitual use of tobacco by humans in the Ancient World on any continent except the tropical Americas, and it is thought that the tobacco plant began growing there about 6000 BCE

[1]. By 1 CE, tobacco was 'nearly everywhere' in the Americas and ways of using tobacco included various smoking methods, chewing and probably hallucinogenic enemas [1].

The tobacco plant refers to any of various members of the genus *Nicotiana* in the nightshade (Solanaceae) family, which includes also the potato, tomato, garden pepper and many garden ornamental flowers. The plant genus *Nicotiana* was named in 1756 by the Swedish botanist Carolus Linnaeus; he described two species: *Nicotiana rustica* (fig. 1) and *Nicotiana tabacum* (fig. 2). Within the *Nicotiana* genus, there are about seventy species. *N. tabacum* does not occur naturally but is a product of human cultivation, a hybrid of *Nicotiana sylvestris* and Nicotiana *tomentosiformis* [2]. Native Americans used several species, the most popular of which was *N. tabacum*, thought to have been first cultivated in the highlands of Peru and Ecuador [3]. Tobacco can grow in any warm, moist environment, which means it can be farmed on all continents except Antarctica.

From its origins in tropical America, tobacco spread northwards during prehistoric times [4]. *N. rustica* (developed later in Russia as *machorka*) was the variety cultivated in North America and has higher nicotine content than the other tobacco plants [2]. Tobacco plants are cultivated for their leaves, which are dried and processed, mainly for smoking in cigarettes, cigars and pipes; it is also cut to form chewing tobacco or ground to make snuff or dipping tobacco, as well as other less common preparations [2]. Amerindians, in cultivating tobacco, developed the major ways of consuming the herb that are in use today [5]. All tobacco products deliver nicotine, a highly addictive ingredient to the central nervous system, with a confirmed risk of dependence [6, 7] (see also chapter 5).

Unlike every other crop cultivated by indigenous peoples during prehistoric times, tobacco was not cultivated for nutritional purposes. According to many accounts, tobacco played a critical role in religious and healing practices. Due to its high nicotine content, as well as the manner in which it was used, early tobacco use could produce hallucinogenic experiences [4]. Tobacco became a sacred plant and 10,000 years ago, Mayan priests lit sacred fires for ceremonial religious purposes, blowing repeatedly on the embers to kindle them into life, inhaling the smoke and thus experiencing the effects of the ingredients of the plant [2, p. 1]. The tobacco plant also attained a ceremonial religious status in the context of bringing a sacrificial offering to the gods [2] although other mixtures of sacred herbs were also common. Between 470 and 630 CE as the Mayas migrated and the Toltecs created the Aztec Empire, two 'castes of smokers emerged ... Those ... who mingled tobacco with the resin of other leaves and smoked pipes with great cer-

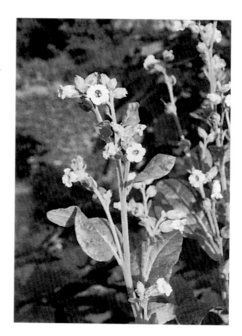

Fig. 1. *N. rustica.*

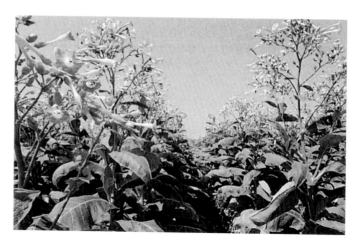

Fig. 2. Field of flowering *N. tabacum.*

emony ... and the lesser Indians, who rolled tobacco leaves together to form a crude cigar' [1]. The first pictorial record (fig. 3) of tobacco being smoked was found on Guatemalan pottery dating from around 600–1000 CE, on which a Maya is depicted smoking a roll of tobacco leaves tied with a string and a more than 1,300-year-old Mayan vessel decorated with hieroglyphics and containing tobacco was discovered by Dmitri Zagorevski, director of the Proteomics Core in the Center for Biotechnology and Interdisciplinary Studies at Rensselaer, and Jennifer Loughmiller-Newman, a doctoral candidate at the University at Albany in 2012.

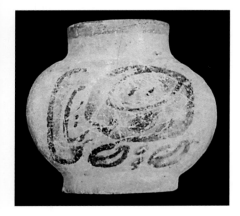
Fig. 3. Guatemalian pottery dating from around 600–1000 CE [53].

The Language of Smoking
The language of smoking has its origins mainly in this place and time. In 1870, Brewer [8, p. 5] wrote that the word tobacco was 'probably derived from Tabac, an instrument used by the Americans in smoking the herb'; others say it derived from the islands of Tobago or Tabasco; others again from 'the circumstances that the herb is wrapped up for use in a dry leaf which forms a sheath or envelope, and this kind of sheath is always called Tabacos by the Carribeans' [8, p. 6]. The Mayan term for smoking is sikar, from which the word cigar and subsequently the word cigarette (derived from the French *cigarette* meaning small cigar) most likely derives.

The Globalization of Tobacco
Europe
From these origins in the Americas, tobacco grew to become, in the 16th and 17th centuries, a global commodity. There is general agreement that tobacco was unknown to Europeans prior to the 15th century and that it was introduced to Europe from the Americas as a result of the increase in naval exploration. Many sources note Columbus's 'voyage of discovery' as the moment of introduction and various individuals are said to have been responsible for the introduction of different uses of tobacco to different European countries. For example, Christopher Columbus is said to have recorded, in 1492, having been offered certain dried leaves; the Spanish explorers Luis de Torres and Rodrigo de Jerez are credited with first observing smoking; Jerez was said to have become a smoker and brought the habit to Spain; the French ambassador to Portugal, Jean Nicot (after whom nicotine was named) sent the tobacco plant to France in 1560; Sir Francis Drake is said to have brought pipe smoking to England in 1572, and so on [9].

In his wide-ranging early history of tobacco, Comptom Mackenzie [10, p. 71] wrote that there was 'not a tittle of evidence' that Columbus brought back any of those dry tobacco leaves; that the two members of Columbus's crew who saw the first cigars being smoked near Havana 'vanished forthwith from recorded history', and that it is 'impossible to find any evidence to justify the de Torres/de Jerez claims'. Rather, Mackenzie [10, p. 73] claimed that a French Franciscan – Frère André Thévet – was the first person to bring tobacco seeds to Europe and that he was growing it in his garden in Angoulême several years before Nicot was given the credit for sending seeds to France from Lisbon. In short, while Columbus may have brought a few tobacco leaves and seeds with him back to Europe at the end of the 15th century, it is likely that most Europeans did not get their first taste of tobacco until around the mid- to late 1550s when adventurers and diplomats began to popularise its use.

When tobacco was first introduced into Europe from the Americas, it was regarded as a medicinal plant, included in the descriptions of plants and their properties known as *Herbals*, and was widely used for medicinal purposes. When Nicot presented the tobacco plant *N. rustica* (fig. 1) to the queen mother Catherine de Medici for the royal herb garden around 1560, it was as a wonderful medicinal herb from the New World [5]. A highly influential treatise on the medicinal uses of tobacco written in 1571 by a Spanish physician was so successful that it was translated into English, Latin, French and Italian [11].

Africa
Tobacco was introduced to Africa in the 17th century by the Ottoman conquests in the north and the slave trade, and cultivation spread rapidly throughout the continent [12]. The first major tobacco manufacturing group was set up in the late 1880s in South Africa, and over time all of the major tobacco trading companies came to be represented there. By 1993, there were 33 African countries growing tobacco with only 2 exporting more than they imported as a combination of urbanization, westernization and increased disposable income together with increased promotion and marketing by the tobacco industry led to increases in smoking [12].

Asia
In the late 16th century, tobacco 'swept into China on the same crest of global mobility that carried it to Africa and other parts of Eurasia' [13, p. 5] although when tobacco first entered China is undocumented. It was introduced by Spanish and Portuguese traders along the maritime coast, by Korean merchants over land and along Central Asian cara-

van routes. Even earlier, prior to the 1560s, before the Ming Dynasty lifted official bans on overseas trade, Chinese merchants and sailors carried out clandestine commerce with neighbours in Japan and Southeast Asia and, by the second half of the 16th century, the habit of tobacco smoking was 'readily appropriated by Chinese, Japanese, and Southeast Asian merchants and sailors' [13, p. 5]. By the late 1630s, tobacco was being commercially grown and traded in China. Snuff and waterpipe tobacco became popular with Chinese elites in the 18th century [13, p. 6]. Unlike in Europe, there was little concern regarding tobacco as a 'foreign' or 'barbaric' product and no concern or restriction of women smoking. By contrast, tobacco consumption placed health at risk by 'crossing moral boundaries of frugality and abstinence into the hedonism of overindulgence' [13, p. 97].

Commercial Production of Tobacco
Europe
By the early decades of the 16th century, Europeans had begun cultivating tobacco in the Americas, and, thanks to Spanish and other European sailors who took the tobacco plant with them on voyages of exploration and trade, tobacco was being grown around the world well before 1700 [5]. Around 1614, Seville was established as a world centre for the production of cigars, and European cigarette use also began here as beggars patched together tobacco from used cigars and rolled them in paper [9]. Slade [5] described many aspects of the economics of tobacco production during this period. European governments set up lucrative state-run monopolies to manage tobacco. The wealthy French monopoly helped to finance the American Revolution. In England, the tobacco trade was organised as a private enterprise, with the government receiving income from excise taxes. British farmers were not permitted to grow tobacco because their produce could not be taxed.

North America
Historically, tobacco is one of the half-dozen most important crops grown by American farmers [2]. In 1612, the tobacco plant *N. tabacum* (fig. 2) was introduced to Virginia and the crop became the economic base for Britain's southern colonies in North America and has remained a major cash crop. Early trade agreements took place around this time and, in 1620, an agreement between the British Crown and the Virginia Tobacco Company banned commercial tobacco growing in England, in return for a duty on Virginia tobacco.

The first successful commercial tobacco crop was cultivated in Virginia in 1621 by Englishman John Rolfe, and,

within 7 years, it was the colony's largest export and remained until 1793 the most valuable staple export from the English American mainland colonies and the United States. Tobacco as a cash crop grew over the next 2 centuries, fuelling the demand in North America for slave labour. By the middle of the 1800s, the tobacco plant was being cultivated throughout 'the whole extent of the United States, Canada, New Brunswick, Mexico, the Western Coast, the Spanish main, Brazil, Cuba, St. Domingo, Trinidad, Turkey, Persia, India, China, Australia, the Philippine Islands, Japan, Egypt, Algeria, the Canary Islands, and the Cape of Good Hope' [14, p. 2].

The latter half of the 19th century was a key period in the increased production and use of tobacco and tobacco products. Developments during this period included new methods of curing tobacco, credited to tobacco farmers in North Carolina, which made smoke easier to inhale, and the discovery by 'a slave named Bill' that intense heat during curing would produce a golden leaf [15]. Other late 19th-century developments included the invention of the Bonsack machine that transformed the labour-intensive cigarette manufacturing industry, being capable of making 120,000 cigarettes in a day; the development and spread of the safety match (for which mass production was refined by 1900) that obviated the need for a burning flame and allowed tobacco to be smoked anywhere, and the development of efficient rail transportation, making it possible to distribute rapidly throughout the nation a perishable product and making it easier for factories to utilize raw materials from distant locations in greater quantity [5] (fig. 4).

Most of the tobacco smoked prior to the 20th century used air-cured rather than flue-cured tobacco, which when burned produced a non-inhalable smoke [3]. Flue curing (the process by which tobacco plants are heated soon after harvest) as a method of tobacco production made cigarettes unique among all forms of tobacco by producing an inhalable smoke, thus making it the single most important manufacturing process responsible for the global lung cancer epidemic [3]. Until the 1960s, the United States not only grew but also manufactured and exported more tobacco than any other country. The publication of conclusive epidemiological evidence in the mid-20th century of tobacco-related disease, disability and death led to a decline in official support for producers and manufacturers of tobacco as an agricultural commodity.

Tobacco Use throughout the Centuries
Various forms of tobacco use developed at different times in different countries between the late 1500s and the early 1900s, until cigarette smoking became the norm in most of the developed world by the mid-20th century [16]. Tobacco

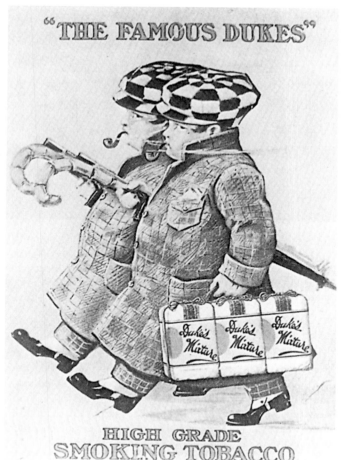

Fig. 4. The Dukes of Durham, Washington Duke and his son, James Buchanan 'Buck' Duke, were the first to recognize fully and develop machine-made commercial tobacco cigarettes. They built the great American Tobacco Company empire, which dominated about 90% of the tobacco market, until it was broken through antitrust action in 1907–1911 [18].

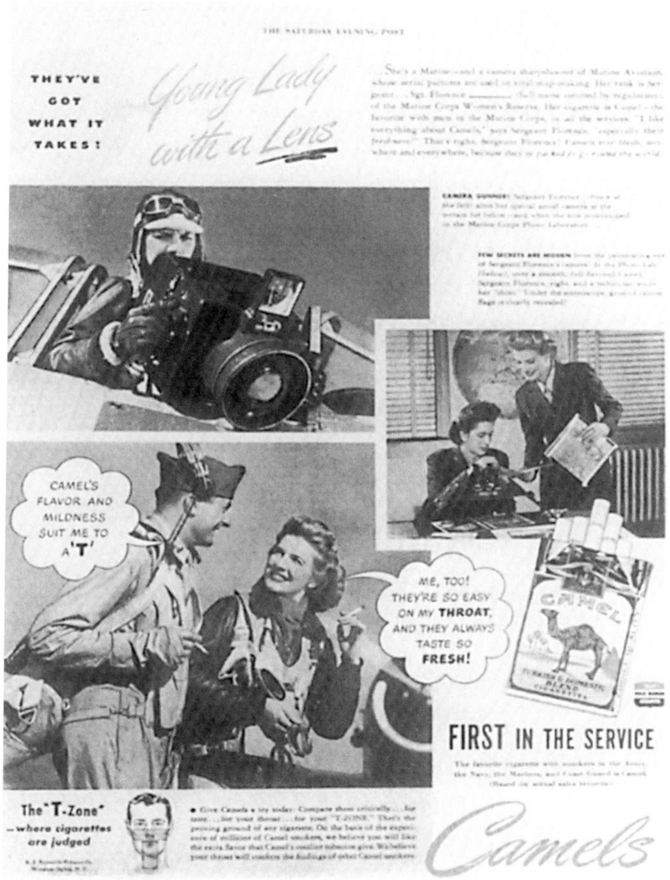

Fig. 5. The advertising of tobacco cigarettes with military personnel, often combined with some representation of women back home, was widely employed during World War II and helped sustain the continued increases in cigarette use by advancing the 'acceptability' of the female smoker. World Wars I and II both helped make cigarette smoking, practiced a century ago almost entirely by women, a 'manly behavior' [18].

use changed and grew over time until, by the mid-20th century, its use was so widespread that it came to be known as the 'tobacco epidemic' [4], so called because of the scale of current and predicted morbidity and mortality caused by its use. The biggest increases in prevalence coincided with the liberal supply of cigarettes to men in both World Wars (promoted by advertisements as in fig. 5) and the post-war targeting by the tobacco industry of smoking by women as an equality and freedom issue (fig. 6) [4].

Within a hundred years of its introduction into Europe, tobacco was being burnt in pipes for pleasure, at first in England, then in Europe and throughout the world [16]. Initially, tobacco was used mainly for pipe smoking, chewing and snuff. Pipe smoking spread quickly throughout the English society in the latter half of the 16th century. Snuff was widely used in the French court, and, in England, it became an aristocratic form of tobacco use. Russia's Peter the Great encouraged tobacco use in his court [17]. Pipe smoking was popular at the Prussian Court: figure 7 depicts the 'Tobacco Council' at the court of the Prussian King Frederick William I (about 1737).

In the early 1800s, cigars became popular, and until the mid- to late 19th century, tobacco was consumed almost entirely by pipe smoking and snuff, with other lesser amounts acquired through cigars, smokeless tobacco plugs and by other means [18].

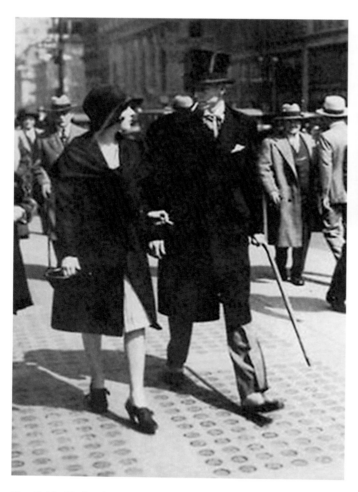

Fig. 6. Mrs Taylor-Scott Hardin parades down New York's Fifth Avenue with her husband while smoking 'torches of freedom', a gesture of protest for absolute equality with men [4]. Courtesy of The Museum of Public Relations, New York, NY.

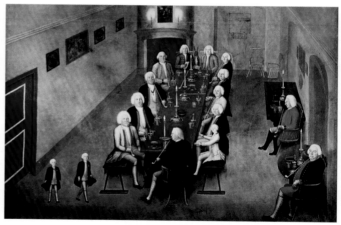

Fig. 7. The Tobacco Council of Frederick William I, King of Prussia (1713–1740). Painting of Georg von Lisiewski (about 1737)/Tabaks-kollegium Friedrich Wilhelms I., GK I 2873/Stiftung Preussische Schlösser und Gärten Berlin-Brandenburg, photographer: Daniel Lindner (reproduced with permission).

Histories of tobacco suggest that by the 1800s, tobacco use by women, men and children was widespread worldwide. The following account by Trall [14, pp 8–9] is from 1855:

'In some countries, men, women, and even children are addicted to smoking. In Campeachy … it is common for children two and three years of age to smoke cigars… in the Sandwich Islands children often smoke before they learn to walk … adults frequently fall down senseless from excessive indulgence in this habit. In India, all classes and both sexes smoke. In Hindostan, boys of fourteen and fifteen use tobacco excessively. In the Burman Empire, both males and females smoke incessantly; even nursing infants have the lighted pipe put in their mouths occasionally by their smoking mothers. In China, young girls wear … a silken pocket to carry a pipe and tobacco. In South America, both sexes use tobacco. In Lima, women are daily seen puffing cigars in the streets; and in Paraguay the 'fair sex' befoul their mouths every day by chewing… The Germans smoke a large portion of their time. The French and Spanish smoke to great excess. The English consume immense quantities of Tobacco, and take the lead in snuffing. And … in the United States more tobacco is raised and consumed in proportion to the population than in any other country.'

Cigarette Smoking

Cigarettes – made from finely cut tobacco leaves, shaped in a small cylinder, rolled in thin paper, lit at one end and allowed to smoulder, and smoke inhaled through the mouth at the other end – were available in crude form since the 1600s. They did not become widely popular in the US until after the civil war with the spread of the cultivation of 'Bright' tobacco, a uniquely cured yellow leaf grown in Virginia and North Carolina and with the mechanisation and industrialisation in the late 1880s that began with the invention of the Bonsack machine, described earlier. As John Slade [19] pointed out in 1997, 19th-century production developments, particularly mechanisation, also led to excess manufacturing capacity. This, in turn, put pressure on manufacturers to expand the market for cigarettes. An identical 21st-century need for market expansion exists for American cigarette manufacturers, although this time excess capacity has resulted from declining cigarette consumption.

From being a relatively luxury pursuit in the Victorian era, cigarette smoking rates grew rapidly in the early decades of the 20th century; cigarettes were heavily promoted by advertisements (fig. 8–10) and following increasing cigarette

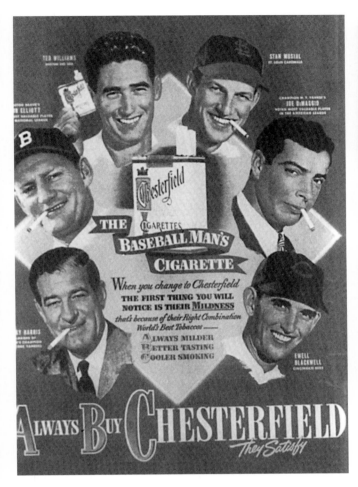

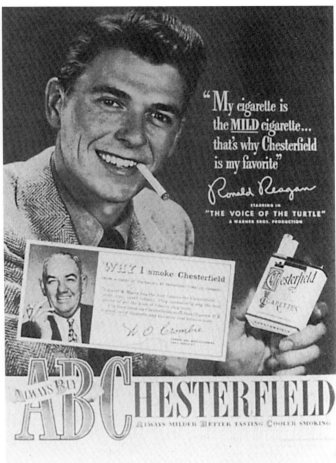

Fig. 8. Popular sports heroes and radio personalities of different eras were used to endorse cigarettes through broader avenues of advertising. Sports heroes were particularly attractive to the children and adolescents who idolized them [18].

Fig. 9. Cinema stars widely endorsed tobacco cigarette use, carrying the positive image of smoking onto the 'silver screen'. One such tobacco-endorsing movie star, Ronald Reagan, was to become the future President of the United States [18].

consumption during World Wars I and II, smoking became more popular ('glamorizing'), especially in the poor and lower classes, and also in women [18]. By the late 1940s, some 82% of British men smoked some form of tobacco and 65% were cigarette smokers, and rates for women rose to just under 50% in the late 1960s [20]. Overall, worldwide cigarette consumption doubled between 1960 and 1986 [19].

Following the 1964 publication of the first US Surgeon General's Report Smoking and Health, the prevalence of cigarette smoking among US adults fell steadily and substantially [21]. From 42.4% in 1965, prevalence rates fell to 18% in 2012, representing about 42 million American smokers [22]. Among British men, rates of cigarette smoking fell rapidly from the 1960s to the 1990s and have continued to

decline slowly since then. An estimated 20% of adults now smoke in England, with rates slightly higher among men than women [20].

Prevalence rates differ by gender, age, ethnicity and education. Men smoke more than women and prevalence rates are much higher among poorer people. For example, in 2012, in the US 20.5% of adult men and 15.8% of adult women smoked, and 27.9% of adults who lived below the poverty line smoked compared with 17% of adults who lived at or above the poverty level [22]. The leading causes of death in most South Asian countries are cancer and heart disease [23], trends that continue to amplify (see chapter 2). Slade's [5] prediction in 1989 that despite declines in the United States and Northern Europe, the tobacco industry is still growing overall thanks to markets in developing countries

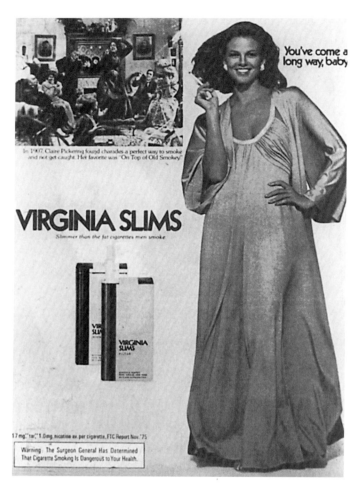

Fig. 10. In the 1960s, the socially emerging 'women's liberation movement' was exploited to capture more female smokers as a large reservoir to be specifically targeted. Even the brand names were chosen to appeal to feminine desires, such as 'thinness' and female independence with 'You've come a long way, baby' [18].

ensuring that tobacco continues to be a profitable investment was correct.

'As the tobacco epidemic comes somewhat under control in the United States, that victory will only have been worthwhile if the epidemic is not merely transferred to other parts of the world. Unfortunately, tobacco use continues to rise elsewhere, aided and abetted by a sophisticated, wealthy and powerful drug cartel based in New York and London' [5, p. 10] (see also chapter 3).

Types of Tobacco Preparation and Use other than Cigarettes
Today, preparations for tobacco use are classified as smoking materials, including cigarettes, cigars, pipes and narghiles, and as smokeless tobacco, including chewing, absorbing by nasal and oral mucosa (snuff), and electronic or

e-cigarettes [6]. While cigarettes are by far the most commonly used means of using tobacco worldwide, other preparations and usage have grown and declined and sometimes grown again during hundreds, even thousands, of years of use. In this section, the types of tobacco preparation and use other than cigarettes are considered [6].

Pipe smoking is one of the oldest forms of smoking. Pipe smokers taste or inhale smoke produced by burning tobacco in a pipe, made from an assortment of natural and manufactured materials. Pipe smoking in the US has declined since the mid-1960s among men and is rare among women. It remains common among men and women in Amerindian populations and also in China [24].

Cigars differ in design from cigarettes, typically being composed entirely of whole-leaf tobacco, wrapped in leaf tobacco and usually smoked without a filter. The prevalence of cigar smoking has been progressively decreasing worldwide. There are distinct differences in mortality patterns between cigar smokers and cigarette smokers, largely explained by differences in smoke exposure by different tissues [6].

Narghiles are waterpipes, known also as gozas, hookahs, hubble-bubble, shishas and bongs. There is a separate chamber for water, a bowl in which the tobacco is placed, and an attached tube and mouthpiece through which the pipe is smoked (see chapter 22). Thought to have originated in India and Asia, narghiles have been widely used for over 400 years. During those centuries, it has come to be commonly used in countries of the Arabian Peninsula as well as in Turkey, Bangladesh and Pakistan. Prevalence of its use varies widely among regions, with an estimated 100 million people worldwide currently using a narghile on a daily basis [6]. There has been a resurgence of its use principally among young people and in some European countries and in the United States, where there are bars specialising in its use, particularly in New York and Los Angeles [6].

Chewing tobacco is one of the oldest modalities of consumption of tobacco leaves, having been used by the Indians who lived in the Americas prior to the 1500s. The use of chewing tobacco peaked at the end of the 19th century and the beginning of the 20th century, after which its use decreased. It continues to be used, however, principally in the southern region of the US and in the interior regions of Latin-American countries. Its use is also prevalent in India, Sri Lanka and Brazil, especially in rural areas [6]. Gutka – a combination of tobacco and betel quid – is widely used on the Indian subcontinent as well as throughout Asia and the Pacific region with global estimates reporting that up to 600 million men and women use some variety [6]. Chewing tobacco has been supplanted by other forms of oral use, a re-surgence of which has been seen in the US, probably influenced by advertising, divulgation and increased regulation of smoking in public places [6].

Snuff consists of finely ground tobacco, sold as a dry or moist powder and placed between the cheek and the gum in the lower part of the mouth. Known as rapé in Brazil, a moist form marketed in Sweden and Norway is known as snus (see chapter 21).

Electronic Cigarettes

Electronic cigarettes or e-cigarettes are battery-operated, nicotine delivery devices that mimic the look and feel of smoking by vaporising a liquid solution such as propylene glycol [25] (for details see chapter 23). Less than a decade on the market and still only a small fraction of traditional cigarette sales, they have garnered such attention that it has been predicted they may eventually eclipse tobacco cigarettes. There is some evidence that they are being used as a 'smoking cessation' aid but also that they are acting as a 'gateway' [26] or 'bridge' product for underage smoking and that they are being promoted for dual usage with cigarette smoking. They are becoming a topic of intense public health debate (see chapter 23), mirroring earlier ones, about harm reduction and abstinence. Concerns are being expressed that marketing campaigns for e-cigarettes are leading to the re-normalization of smoking in the form of 'vaping' after decades of successful, public health campaigns to denormalise smoking [25].

Health and Harmful Effects of Tobacco: From Belief to Knowledge

Many histories of tobacco and smoking trace knowledge of the dangers of tobacco and smoking from the 1600s. One of the most quoted examples of the known damaging effects of tobacco comes from 1604, *The Counterblaste to Tobacco*, written by King James I of England who wrote that smoking is a 'custome lothesome to the eye, hateful to the nose, harmful to the brain, dangerous to the lungs, and in the black and stinking fume thereof resembling the horrible stygian smoke of the pit that is bottomless' [27]. In 1610, Sir Francis Bacon wrote that it was a custom hard to quit [9]. Clinical reports as early as 1795 linked pipe smoking with carcinoma of the lip and tongue [24]. By the mid-1800s, more than 100 books had been written to 'put down the detestable habit of using Tobacco as a luxury' but this was no impediment to its 'for nearly four hundred years, constantly extending the area of its most abominable and relentless slavery' [14, p. 3].

Tobacco as Medicine

The first widespread formal knowledge disseminated about tobacco, however, was in the medicinal *Herbals* and, in these 16th-century health manuals, much was made of the wonders of the tobacco plant as a cure for all manner of maladies and ills, and prescriptions were often dispensed through apothecaries [18]. In the 17th-century Herbals, illustrations of the tobacco plant appeared under the name of *Nicotiana major,* such was the belief in tobacco's healing properties [2]. Among tobacco's medicinal properties, according to Jean Nicot in 1560, were included cures for toothache, worms, halitosis, lockjaw and cancer. Most early European physicians subscribed to the Amerindian belief that tobacco can be an effective medicine and, in many European countries, tobacco came to be seen as a panacea, a situation which lasted about 2 hundred years [10].

Discourses

The discourse surrounding tobacco was at this time as much a matter of moral correctness, anti-paganism, godliness and cleanliness as it was about health-related harms. Tobacco was condemned as the 'pagan herb' or the 'heathen plant' [18]. While the unpleasant effects of second-hand smoke (SHS) did not go unnoticed: in the US 'the whole atmosphere of our cities – glorious Boston excepted – is stifling and pestiferous with Tobacco fumigation; and the country air is far from being clear of it' [14, p. 5], the emphasis generally was not on the associated health harms.

Recent historical analyses of discourses of cleanliness shed light on 19th-century attitudes to tobacco. Suggesting that a nation's standards of private cleanliness reveal much about its ideals of civilization, fears of disease and expectations for public life, Brown [28] shows that by the 1840s, the concept of cleanliness was endowed with a moral force; attention to cleanliness signified not only health and refinement but empowerment and responsibility for oneself. In the absence of scientific evidence on tobacco-related harm, 19th-century Anglo-American attitudes to tobacco are embedded more in a discourse of cleanliness than of health. Tobacco chewing and snuff taking were particularly implicated in the cleanliness discourse: 'all places, public or private, where it is desirable to preserve the external forms of decency, have to be provided with special reservoirs to collect the foul and sickening spittle constantly ejected from the ever-working mouths of the Tobacco-chewers. And in churches, halls, stage-coaches, and other places where spittoons are not furnished, the attendant or passenger is in constant danger of having his clothes besmeared with the vile nuisance' [14, p. 5].

Universality of Knowledge

Although as early as 1761, John Hill had warned of the carcinogenic effects of tobacco use, it is difficult to know at what point knowledge of the disease consequences of tobacco was accepted by the global health community [17]. The idea that knowledge of the fatal harm caused by smoking was widespread before the second half of the 20th century, however, is incorrect, and from the perspective of the 21 century, it may be easy to forget how very recently smoking was an ubiquitous and unobjectionable part of everyday life – in hospitals, classrooms, airplanes, buses, cinemas, theatres, restaurants and courtrooms. 'For the first six or seven decades of the twentieth century, tobacco was a respectable commodity, a dignified habit. Etiquette guides as late as the 1970s recommended that the polite hostess offer cigars to the men and cigarettes to the women. And it was not at all unusual for physicians to smoke … One in ten reported actually having advised their patients to smoke' [29, p. 8]. Advertisement for Lucky Strike cigarettes in the 1950s used even the medical professionals' images for promotion (fig. 11).

Beginning of Scientific Knowledge

By the early 20th century, as cigarette smoking increased, articles on the health effects of smoking appeared in scientific and medical journals. In the 1930s, researchers in Germany made a statistical correlation between cancer and smoking, and in the US scientists reported that smokers do not live as long as non-smokers do [22]. Still, no definitive links were shown. In the 1950s, four new types of scientific evidence marked the turning point for the Anglo-American world: epidemiological studies showing smokers were far more likely to contract lung cancer than were non-smokers; animal experiments showing that tobacco tars could produce tumours; studies of human lungs at autopsy showing that smokers were far more likely to have precancerous lesions than were non-smokers, and chemists both inside and outside the tobacco industry showing that cigarette smoke contains carcinogens [29, pp. 8–9].

Key Moments

The seminal moment in the history of tobacco harm came in 1950 when two papers, carried out independently by two groups of researchers [30, 31], reporting innovative case-control studies showing the association between smoking and lung cancer in the US, were published in the *Journal of the American Medical Association* and similarly in the *British Medical Journal* [32]. Subsequent cohort studies from the 1950s showed links between smoking and the development of other diseases, too [16].

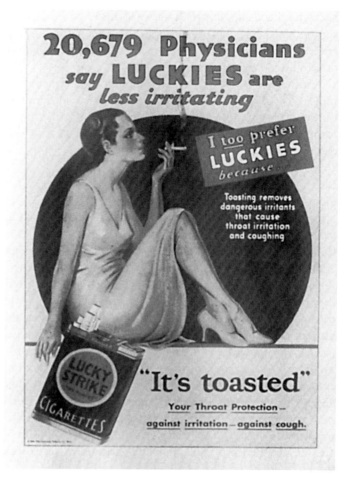

Fig. 11. 1950s style of advertisement for Lucky Strike cigarettes using endorsements of the medical profession for promotion [54].

In the late 1980s, Doll [16], one of the authors of the seminal studies, suggested that, in retrospect, it could be seen that medical evidence of the harm done by smoking had been accumulating for 200 years, at first in relation to cancers of the lip and mouth, and then in relation to vascular disease and cancer of the lung. The evidence was generally ignored until case-control studies relating smoking to the development of lung cancer were published in 1950. Links had now been established between smoking and cancer, but no causal relationship had yet been shown. At this time, however, the general public knew little of the growing scientific evidence on tobacco harm.

In the US, two publications were key in informing the general public on tobacco harm. The first was an article that appeared in the popular magazine *Reader's Digest* in 1952 detailing dangers of smoking, entitled Cancer by the Carton. Similar articles followed and, the following year, cigarette

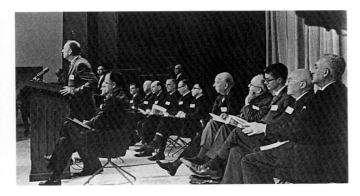

Fig. 12. US Surgeon General Luther Terry addressing press conference at the release of the 1964 Report on Smoking and Health. The Advisory Committee which compiled the report is seated behind the podium [33].

sales declined for the first time in over 2 decades. The second was the report of the US Surgeon General's Advisory Committee on Smoking and Health detailing the growing scientific evidence on tobacco harm and related unequivocally the causal link between smoking and lung cancer in men. Figure 12 shows US Surgeon General Luther Terry at the release of this historic report at the press conference 1964, which was published in 1964 and entitled Smoking and Health [33].

The Ostrich/Hermit Fallacy
The idea that knowledge of the harm caused by smoking was widespread before the second half of the 20th century is incorrect. Yet this idea was used by the tobacco industry to refute responsibility for tobacco harm and implicate individual agency. Proctor [3] calls this the ostrich/hermit argument: not to have known about tobacco harm, a person would have to have either deliberately ignored the evidence or been shut away from society and knowledge of such evidence. From these beginnings, scientific research on tobacco harm has investigated and demonstrated many other damaging effects of smoking on health and life. These include vascular diseases, particularly heart attacks and strokes, and chronic diseases, such as ischaemic heart disease, and the damage to respiratory health in terms of asthma, chronic obstructive pulmonary disease, tuberculosis, HIV and other infections, such as pneumonia, as well as effects on fertility and reproduction (see chapters 7 and 8). The were also effects of SHS or environmental tobacco smoke (ETS) on the health of smokers and non-smokers (see chapter 10), the effects of SHS on infant and child mortality and morbidity (see chapter 9), the importance of monitoring and surveillance, the effects of advertising, sponsorship and marketing on tobacco sales, the roles of taxation and illicit trade, the use of cigarette packaging (see chapters 12 and 13) and the use of tobacco in film, video and pop culture to attract young people (see chapter 15).

Such knowledge notwithstanding, tobacco use increased to such proportions as to create an epidemic. We summarise here from the US Surgeon General's 2014 Report that many factors were responsible for this increase in smoking, but the tobacco industry was the central driver through these three modalities:

(1) The development of industrial technology enabling cigarette mass production, packaging and distribution.

(2) Aggressive pricing and marketing combined with positive portrayals in films, and endorsements by film stars, sports idols and even physicians, and including cigarettes in daily rations for soldiers in World Wars I and II.

(3) Widespread industry actions throughout society to advance its interests, including lobbying and using tactics later found to constitute fraud and racketeering, such as misleading the public about the risks of smoking [34, p. 846].

Tobacco Regulation, Legislation and Control and the Counter-Efforts of the Tobacco Industry

Tobacco control refers to a range of comprehensive measures to protect people from the effects of tobacco consumption and SHS, and has constituted an important and long-standing element of the history of tobacco. Tobacco control actions are intended to prevent young people from starting to use tobacco (see chapter 14), help current tobacco users to quit and protect non-smokers from SHS exposure [35] (see chapters 12 and 13). These measures have been resisted everywhere in the world by the tobacco industry, viz. people, organisations and companies involved in the growth, preparation for sale, shipment, advertisement, and distribution of tobacco and tobacco-related products, cigarettes, cigars, snuff, and chewing and pipe tobacco (see chapter 3). By the early decades of the 21st century, following extensive merger and acquisition activity in the 1990s and 2000s, the international tobacco market was dominated by five firms. The tobacco industry is one of the largest, most profitable industries in the world (see chapter 11).

Early Tobacco Regulation
Early examples of tobacco regulation and prohibition exist in many countries, mainly outside of the Americas [14]. In Persia, in 1593, tobacco use was forbidden by penal statutes.

In England, King James I, and his successor Charles, prohibited the use of tobacco under severe penalties; James was the first to impose a heavy tax on tobacco, and Queen Elizabeth I published an edict against its use [14] (see also chapter 19). In 1693, smoking was banned in the chamber of the House of Commons in the UK [9]. In 1653, a severe punishment was decreed against all who smoked in the canton of Appenzell while in Russia, at about the same time, the penalty of death was proclaimed against the offence of tobacco chewing, and those who smoked 'were condemned to have their noses cut off' [14, p. 3]. The Qing Dynasty of China decreed death for violators of a smoking ban [17]. In Constantinople, about 1690, every Turk caught smoking was conducted in ridicule through the streets 'seated on an ass, his face directed toward the animal's tail, and a pipe transfixed through his nose' [14, p. 3].

The Catholic Church, prominent in histories of tobacco, regulated tobacco use in churches in Mexico and Peru from the late 1500s and in Rome from the early 1600s. Papal bulls remain among the earliest instances of tobacco regulation. While many objections to tobacco use were based on cleanliness and fear of the foreign, the bulls were issued as a rejection of non-Christian spirituality on the altar and interference with religious ceremonies. In 1642, Urban VIII issued a bull declaring that anyone taking tobacco in any form – smoking, chewing or snuffing – would be penalised by excommunication. Similar bulls later were issued by Innocent X and XI. In 1725, Pope Benedict XIII, himself a snuff taker, revoked the penalty of excommunication. Tobacco remained subject to further regulation by the church and was also the subject of popular discussion in the day, giving rise to a belief in the 1800s that Bracci's famous funerary monument (fig. 13) commemorating Benedict XIV depicts him holding a snuff box in his left hand and shaking off snuff with his right [36].

For the majority of the last half millennium, however, tobacco regulation has been based on a request model rather than on a rights model. In the 1800s, in the US, signs requesting people ('Gentlemen are requested not to smoke in this room') not to smoke appeared where people travelled although these seem to have been mainly ignored [14]. If rights existed, they lay with the rights of the person who smoked to exercise personal freedom rather than with the rights of non-smokers to protection from ETS.

Early 20th-Century Policies of Restriction
The early 20th century saw a gradual move towards restrictive smoking policies in many parts of the developed world. Societies were formed to discourage smoking in several

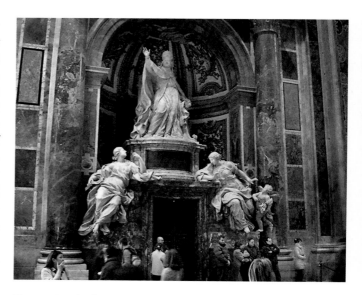

Fig. 13. Tomb of Pope Benedict XIV, St. Peter's Basilica, Vatican. Wikimedia commons.

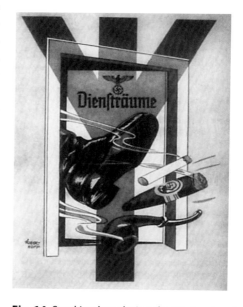

Fig. 14. Smoking ban during the Nazi regime in German public places and, amongst others, in duty rooms (Diensträume) [37].

countries, but they had little success except in Germany where they were officially supported by the Nazi party after they seized power (fig. 14) [16, 29]. After World War II and the end of the Nazi regime, the cigarette industry used this psychologically in a clever way to propagate cigarette smoking as symbol of freedom/liberty ('European and American tobacco companies have both tried to play the Nazi card, associating smoking restrictions with Nazi-like policing' [37]).

In the UK, bans on the sale of tobacco to children were introduced in 1908 and extended in 1933; the first smoking withdrawal clinic was established in 1958; cigarette advertising on TV was banned in 1965; the first voluntary agreement with the tobacco industry on advertising and health warnings on packs was introduced in 1971; in the 1970s, smoking was phased out in public transport and cinemas, and tax increases on tobacco were justified on health grounds [38, pp. 2–3].

Tobacco Control and Public Health Policy

With the scientific debate about the link between tobacco and disease conclusively established, a new phase began, which was the public health response to what was now recognised as an epidemic [17] (see chapters 1 and 12). The decades between the 1940s and early 2000s revealed an array of policy and legislative responses to the growing scientific evidence of tobacco-related harms, and the counter-efforts of the tobacco industry (see chapter 3). In first-world countries, although responses have varied according to the 'vested economic interests, cultural practices, and political factors' of each country [39, p. 215], broad trends include advertising bans on TV and radio, warning labels and graphic images on cigarette packs, health education campaigns since the 1960s, higher taxation levels since the 1980s, and, in recent decades, full bans on advertising and a prohibition on smoking in public places [38, 39].

Between the 1950s and the 1970s, health education in the UK about tobacco changed from giving information about tobacco harm and letting people choose, to harm reduction approaches in the 1960s, to absolutism in the 1970s, educating that there is no safe level of tobacco smoking [38, p. 48].

Tobacco control came to be seen by some as an example of the potentially positive influence of public health evidence on policy, and has increasingly been positioned as a case study from which other areas of public policy, including food, alcohol and transport policy, might learn [20, p. 64]. Indeed, both Allan Brandt's [4] 2007 history of the cigarette ('The Cigarette Century') as a cultural icon and a public health nightmare and Virginia Berridge's [40] history of smoking ('Marketing Health') and the discourse of public health in the UK illuminate a scientific revolution in how people have come to think about disease. Brandt showed that proving the connection between smoking and disease required 'a fundamental transformation in medical ways of knowing in the mid-twentieth century' and 'the integration

of methods and approaches across the biomedical sciences' [4].

Tobacco control was also a key agent in relation to other legislative changes, contributing to changes in product liability law in the 1980s and public interest law in the 1990s [4].

A timeline of key evidence concerning tobacco-related harms and the implementation of major tobacco control interventions in the UK [20] suggests strong links between emerging evidence and policy and legislative change, often, however, with a considerable time lag. Smith [20] draws attention to this lag, seeking to explain it. Links between lung cancer and smoking from case-control studies in the 1940s and 1950s were followed by the banning of TV advertising for cigarettes (although not for cigars) in the UK in 1965. The 1964 Surgeon General's Report in the US confirming smoking was a cause of lung cancer and bronchitis preceded the introduction of health warnings on cigarette packs in the USA in 1967.

Berridge's [40] analysis of tobacco debates in Britain in the 1950s and 1960s suggests that policy makers understood the main messages emerging from research and that resistance to 'taking policy action was only partially related to the extent to which individuals were persuaded by this evidence' [20, p. 65]. Significant delays between recognition of tobacco-related harm and policy interventions to reduce those harms were accompanied by politicians variously arguing for and against tobacco control interventions, a situation explained by Berridge [40] as being about differences in values, family background and election strategies as much, if not more than, differences in interpretations of evidence.

Differences between the US and British responses to the growing scientific evidence base of tobacco health harm have been noted [40]. Berridge writes that the initial response in Britain in the 1950s was in part conditioned by the role of the tobacco industry and the financial importance of tobacco: the British tobacco industry had closer relationships with government than the American one, and did not rely on public relations; rather public health interests in Britain worked with the industry. Further, she argues that politicians in Britain were concerned about the fluidity of epidemiological evidence, fall-out from increased attention to air pollution, financial and ideological implications of health education, and electoral dangers of intervening in a popular mass habit. This led to stability in post-war tobacco policy that stemmed from an 'insulated industry-government relationship underpinned by socio-economic conditions' [38, p. 47]. A policy monopoly by the tobacco industry emerged during the following decades, a result of an anti-tobacco campaign that was underfunded and only in its infancy, a medical association that was not well organised, and a tobacco industry that set the agenda by calling in public debates on organisations representing tobacco workers, retailers and consumers giving the appearance of a 'broad constituency of support' [38, p. 48]. In short, tobacco companies controlled the policy image of tobacco framing as an economic issue (thus gaining continued government support) and as a matter of individual choice and agency.

Not everyone agrees that this 'dominance narrative' explains the rapid change in UK tobacco policy following long periods of stability; an alternative 'incremental narrative' suggests that the exclusion of science and medicine was exaggerated and that policy change was incremental but on a clear path towards tobacco control, where limited tobacco control initiatives 'signalled that legislation would follow if self-regulation failed' [38, p. 64].

Tobacco Industry Strategy of Manufacturing Doubt
A somewhat contrasting picture emerged in the US, with the tobacco industry adopting both a defensive and offensive approach to the early case-control studies in the US and UK linking lung cancer and smoking [4]. By late 1953, when smoking was categorically linked to the dramatic rise in lung cancer, the industry faced 'a crisis of cataclysmic proportions' [41, p. 63]. Central to their strategy was 'manufacturing doubt'. Detailing the protracted campaign of the tobacco industry to create uncertainty about smoking being harmful to health, Brandt [4] describes the late 1950s as a time when 'Just as the tobacco industry in the late nineteenth century had developed the technology for mass production of cigarettes, so now it developed techniques for the mass production of controversy and doubt'. Confronted by compelling scientific evidence of the harms of smoking, the tobacco industry used sophisticated public relations approaches to undermine and distort the emerging science. Industry-academic conflicts of interest were created for the creation of a scientific controversy. These deliberate attempts to disrupt science are now well known, largely as a result of whistle-blowers and legislation that led to the revelation of millions of pages of internal tobacco documents that articulated this strategy and that documented its implementation [41, p. 70], which documents are now in the public domain [42] and the subject of ongoing research and analysis [3].

Defensive and Offensive Strategies of the Tobacco Industry
Cigarette manufacturers used two complementary strategies – one defensive, one offensive – to deal with the public relations problems resulting from the massive evidence that their products are highly addictive and fatal to their customers [5]. The defensive strategy constituted the development of an aggressive lobbying organisation, epitomized by the Tobacco Institute (formed in the mid-1950s on the advice of the public relations firm Hill and Knowlton), and the support of research on health effects through an industry-controlled committee formed in 1954. The offensive strategy used to combat its public relations problem was the production and marketing of products designed to appear safe. These included filter cigarette brands heavily promoted during the 1950s, 'low-poison'/'low-tar' cigarettes introduced in the 1960s, the so-called 'smokeless cigarette' in the 1980s, cigarettes that produced less sidestream smoke and cigarettes with a built-in air freshener aimed at promoting acceptance of smoking by non-smokers. All of these offensive strategies encountered difficulties on varying grounds of health, safety, use and accuracy.

General Strategies of the Tobacco Industry
Recent accounts by historians have identified the massive political, social and economic power of the tobacco industry characterised by features that include: a decade-long conspiracy, revealed through analysis of the formerly secret internal documents of the industry, to downplay the dangers of smoking by blocking the recognition of tobacco/cancer hazards; the use of multiple means by cigarette makers to reassure smokers about their tobacco use, including the marketing of filter, low-tar, light, menthol and mild products; the deliberate marketing to children; a denialist campaign that co-opted scientists and politicians to the extent of being able to influence peer-reviewed scientific literature, congressional and parliamentary deliberations, positions taken by professional medical associations, the drafting of bills and legislation, the content of popular media and popular attitudes towards smoking [3] (for details see chapter 3).

The need to measure tobacco industry counter-efforts and their effects constitutes a major challenge in evaluating tobacco control efforts. An overarching conceptual model that analyses the tactics of the tobacco industry includes what the industry says and what the industry does, and examines tactics, both covert and public in nature [43]. These tactics include messages the tobacco industry issues or tries to control – undermining science and legitimate messages from scientific quarters; the manipulation of the media; public relations efforts, and gaining control of the public agenda and also the actions of the industry – lobbying and legislative strategy, the use of front groups and artificially created 'grass-roots' movements that create the illusion of support; legal and economic intimidation, and harassment of tobacco control professionals. Such a conceptual model suggests a possible hierarchy for measures than can be used to understand tobacco industry strategies and also allow predictions to be made of likely progression of industry reactions as public health programmes become more successful and therefore more threatening to industry profits (see also chapter 3).

Responses to the Tobacco Epidemic
As evidence about tobacco harm accumulated, calls for policy responses grew louder; advocacy for public policy interventions to address what had become known as the 'tobacco epidemic' increased, including the setting up of the Action on Smoking and Health [9] in 1971. An emerging consensus in the 1990s that ETS or SHS was associated with carcinogen exposure led to a series of public policy efforts to reduce tobacco harm [20]. These included health warning on packs, bans on tobacco advertising, tax-funded smoking cessation services and bans on smoking in indoor public places [20, 38].

Demarcation of Public Space/Denormalisation of Smoking/ Environmental Tobacco Smoke
The demarcation of public spaces where smoking is allowed or prohibited has been a key battleground in tobacco control efforts to protect non-smokers, encourage smokers to quit and, increasingly, to denormalise the act of smoking. From the 1970s, restrictions were introduced in enclosed spaces where non-smokers faced prolonged exposure to SHS, such as on aeroplanes, public transport and restaurants. In 1973, the Civil Aeronautics Board required airlines to designate non-smoking sections of airlines for domestic flights. Some early restrictions preceded epidemiologic and scientific evidence on SHS-related harms and were introduced on grounds of nuisance rather than health. It was not until 1993 that the Environmental Protection Agency in the US classified SHS as a class A carcinogen. The number and variety of locations that were protected from SHS grew as evidence of the links between exposure to SHS and elevated risks of many diseases, including lung cancer, cardiovascular disease or asthma, became proven. Smoke free – the first complete ban on workplace smoking – was introduced in Ireland in 2004 [44]. Seventeen EU countries have since introduced comprehensive laws and more than 60 countries worldwide and 28 US states have comprehensive smoke-free laws. In many countries, educational establishments, sports stadiums and private workplaces, for example, implement smoking bans. Most recently, tobacco control efforts on the creation of safe smoke-free public spaces have centred on the consideration of the elimination of smoking from outdoor areas such as parks, beaches, playgrounds and so on.

Global Tobacco Control in the 21st Century

21st-Century Momentum
In the history of tobacco control, the early years of the 21st century have been characterised by an unprecedented momentum in implementing effective and far-reaching interventions, most of which could not have been anticipated a mere 50 years ago. A number of measures stand out [45]. In 2001, Canada introduced large pictorial health warnings on all tobacco packaging, and almost 60 countries have since joined them. In 2004, Ireland became the first country to introduce a ban on smoking in all indoor and public workplaces, and more than 60 countries have followed suit. In 2009, Ireland removed point-of-sale tobacco advertising and displays becoming the first country in the European Union to do so, but following similar legislation in Iceland, Thailand, and some provinces and territories in Canada. In 2010, Mauritius banned 'corporate social responsibility' marketing (which had included university scholarships, and entrepreneurship and environmental programmes) from the tobacco industry. In 2010, Norway announced that it had fully divested its government pension fund – a divestment of over USD 2 billion – from tobacco. In 2012, Australia mandated 'plain packaging' for tobacco products, closing off the last marketing space available to the tobacco industry [45].

The World Health Organisation Framework Convention on Tobacco Control (FCTC) [46] is an indicator of the widespread support that exists for tobacco control measures. This global tobacco control treaty entered into force in 2005 committing its over 170 Parties to reducing demand and supply of tobacco products. It is unique in being the only internationally binding treaty focusing on health, and the only one focusing on a particular product. It has become one of the most widely embraced treaties of the United Nations covering 88% of the world's population (for details see chapter 13). It was the first legal instrument designed to reduce tobacco-related deaths and disease around the world and includes a specific Article (5.3) that recognises the various strategies of the tobacco industry to undermine and subvert tobacco control efforts, and requires Parties to protect public health policies with respect to tobacco control from commercial and vested interests of the tobacco industry. It set international standards and guidelines for tobacco control in the following areas: tobacco price and tax increases, sales to and by minors, tobacco advertising and sponsorship, labelling, illicit trade and SHS.

In 2008, a number of specific measures were identified that would support improved implementation of the provisions of the FCTC. Known as MPOWER (see also chapters 2 and 12), each measure corresponds to at least one provision of the Convention [35]:
- Monitoring tobacco use and prevention policies
- Protecting people from tobacco use
- Offering help to quit tobacco use
- Warning about the dangers of tobacco
- Enforcing bans on tobacco advertising, promotion and sponsorship
- Raising taxes on tobacco

That these types of policy interventions can reduce tobacco use is clear from the differences observed in the past decades in the US where some states such as California and New York have done better than other states, and indeed, through well-funded, long-running tobacco control programmes that raise taxes on tobacco, countries ban smoking in public places, promote free nicotine replacement therapy and run large media campaigns emphasising 'the immorality of marketing a deadly product and the unacceptability of smoking around others'; likewise, there are different results depending on the intensity of the different interventions in Australian states [47].

Challenges for the 21st Century

In the context of the history of the globalization of tobacco over the last 500 years and the relatively short history of the public health response to the tobacco epidemic over the last 50 years, Glynn et al. [17, p 52] name 21 challenges for the 21st century.

Challenges to increase
- Support for and adherence to the WHO FCTC
- Tobacco excise taxes and unit price of tobacco
- Access to comprehensive treatment for tobacco dependence
- Media-based tobacco counter-marketing campaigns
- Regulation of all tobacco products
- Health warnings on tobacco packaging
- Availability of tobacco health/economic information to the general public
- Primacy of health over commerce in trade agreements
- Basic and applied tobacco control research
- Extent and accuracy of tobacco epidemiologic data
- Litigation aimed at the tobacco industry

Challenges to decrease
- Physician and other health care provider tobacco use
- Targeting of women for increased tobacco use

- Exposure to SHS
- Illicit trade and smuggling of tobacco
- Duty-free and reduced-cost sales of tobacco
- Tobacco advertising, promotion and sponsorship
- Misleading tobacco product claims/descriptors
- Targeting of youth for increased tobacco use
- Subsidies for tobacco production and sales
- Youth access to tobacco

The authors draw particular additional attention to the need to develop a new generation of tobacco control leaders encompassing a wide range of disciplines, skills and professionals [17, p. 59].

Lessons from Tobacco History

As certain population markets decline, so others will be targeted for tobacco consumption. Young people, poor people, women, and people in middle- and low-income countries are now key targets, and already stepped into the gap [48, 49]. It is likely that tobacco use will continue to decline in well-educated, better-off populations worldwide. Globally, the data are very clear that the tobacco epidemic has now expanded to, and become more focused on, the world's low- and middle-income countries, due largely to the expansion of marketing efforts of the tobacco industry in Eastern Europe, Asia, Africa and Latin America [17]. History also shows that smoking in the population as a whole will not reduce without vigorous and consistent actions by governments and health organisations [47–50]. In Australia, after an initial decline in the 1960s, smoking increased again in the early 1970s in response to more aggressive marketing by tobacco companies, especially advertising aimed at young women [47]. Finally, although tobacco as a product is unique, many other industries have studied the tobacco industry strategy of manufactured controversy [41] and:

'As a result, they have come to better understand the fundamentals of influence within the sciences and the value of uncertainty and scepticism in deflecting regulation, defending against litigation, and maintaining credibility despite the marketing of products that are known to be harmful to public health. Also, they have come to understand that the invention of scientific controversy undermines notions of the common good by emphasizing individual assessment, responsibility, and judgment' [41, p. 70].

Conclusion

The tobacco epidemic that has taken place over the last 100 years has been identified as one of the biggest public health threats the world has ever faced [35] and the favourable impact of increasingly intense tobacco control efforts in the last 30 years have been considered one of the top public health achievements of this time [34]. Myriad changes in tobacco use and production during the half millennium of global tobacco presence have been detailed. Notwithstanding the extent of regulation described above, the epidemic of tobacco-related disease, disability and death has only begun. Tobacco use continues to increase. There are now, in the second decade of the 21st century, an estimated 1 billion smokers worldwide. The WHO has estimated that 100 million people were killed by tobacco in the 20th century and that figure will rise to 1 billion people in the 21st century if the current trend continues. There are currently about 6 million deaths each year from tobacco-related illnesses. Unchecked, by 2030, that figure will rise to 8 million each year, more than 80% of them in low- and middle-income countries (see also chapter 2).

Nevertheless, a discussion has begun within the field of tobacco control of what has come to be called the tobacco 'endgame'. The US Surgeon General's 2014 Report [34, p. 853] summarises strategies discussed in the scientific literature in the recent past: reducing nicotine yields, reducing product toxicity, gradual supply reduction, prohibiting sales to future generations, banning cigarettes and/or cigarettes plus additional tobacco products and selling tobacco through a not-for-profit agency. Some of these interventions are more applicable in the USA rather than elsewhere the authors concede. In the European Union recommendations in the PPACTE project [51] and the Tobacco Products Directive [52] offer further prospects for advancement of tobacco control. While Australia has recommended similar interventions, and some more geared towards their own situation [47], for most of the world the FCTC offers the best chance of progress in the medium term.

Key Points

- Tobacco has been used for over 10,000 years and has been smoked for at least 2,000 years.
- Uniquely among crops, tobacco was cultivated by indigenous populations, not for nutritional but for religious and healing purposes, and was at first introduced to Europe as a medicinal plant.
- The first successful commercial crop was cultivated in Virginia in 1621 and was the colony's largest export until 1793.
- Bosnack's machine in 1880 led to mass production and vastly increased capacity and was accompanied by dedicated marketing and promotion. Flue curing in the 20th century enabled the production of an inhalable smoke and with that a multitude of diseases in man.
- There was knowledge of harmful effects of tobacco from the 1700s, but the 1964 US Surgeon General's Report was crucial in getting the world to accept the importance of the detrimental effects of smoking.
- The repeated use by the Tobacco industry of a plethora of strategies to oppose tobacco control is widely recognised, including in Article 5.3 of the FCTC. The Framework Convention for Tobacco Control encapsulates the efforts of 176 countries to control tobacco usage in the 21st century.

References

1 Borio G: The Tobacco Timeline. TOBACCO.ORG. archive.tobacco.org/resources/history/tobacco_history.html (accessed June 12, 2014).
2 Haustein KO, Groneberg D: Tobacco or Health? Physiological and Social Damages Caused by Smoking, ed 2. Berlin, Springer, 2010.
3 Proctor R: Golden Holocaust: Origins of the Cigarette Catastrophe and the Case for Abolition. Oakland, University of California Press, 2012.
4 Brandt A: The Cigarette Century. The Rise, Fall, and Deadly Persistence of the Product That Defined America. New York, Basic Books, 2007.
5 Slade J: The tobacco epidemic: lessons from history. J Psychoactive Drugs 1989;21:281–291.
6 Viegas CA: Noncigarette forms of tobacco use. J Bras Pneumol 2008;34:1069–1073.
7 Benowitz NL: Nicotine addiction. N Engl J Med 2010;362:2295–2303.
8 Brewer H: Revelations about Tobacco. A Prize Essay on the History of Tobacco, and Its Physical Action on the Human Body, through Its Various Modes of Employment. London, Pitman, 1870.

9 ASH (Action on Smoking and Health UK): Key Dates in the History of Anti-Tobacco Campaigning. http://www.ash.org.uk/files/documents/ASH_741.pdf (accessed February 28, 2014).
10 Mackenzie C: Sublime Tobacco. London, Chatto & Windus, 1957.
11 Monardes N: Joyful Newes out of the Newe Founde Worlde. 1577. Amsterdam, Da Capo Press, 1970 (reprint).
12 Yach D: Tobacco in Africa. Tobacco or Health. World Health Forum 1996;17:29–36.
13 Benedict C: Golden-Silk Smoke. A History of Tobacco in China, 1550–2010. Oakland, University of California Press, 2011.
14 Trall RT: Tobacco: Its History, Nature, and Effects with Facts and Figures for Tobacco-Users. New York, Fowlers & Wells, 1855.
15 Tilley NM: The Bright-Tobacco Industry 1860–1929. Chapel Hill, University of North Carolina Press, 1948.
16 Doll R: Uncovering the effects of smoking: historical perspective. Stat Methods Med Res 1988;7:87–117.

17 Glynn T, Seffrin JR, Brawley OW, Grey N, Ross H: The Globalization of Tobacco Use: 21 challenges for the 21st century. CA Cancer J Clin 2010;60:50–61.
18 Huber GL, Pandina RJ: The economics of tobacco use; in Bolliger CT, Fagerström KO (eds): The Tobacco Epidemic. Prog Respir Res. Basel, Karger, 1997, vol 28, pp 12–63.
19 Slade J: Historical notes on tobacco; in Bolliger CT, Fagerström KO (eds): The Tobacco Epidemic. Prog Respir Res. Basel, Karger, 1997, vol 28, pp 1–11.
20 Smith K: Beyond Evidence-Based Policy in Public Health: The Interplay of Ideas. London, Palgrave Macmillan, 2013.
21 Mendez D, Warner KE, Courant PN: Has smoking cessation ceased? Expected trends in the prevalence of smoking in the United States. Am J Epidemiol 1998;147:249–258.

22 Centers for Disease Control and Prevention: Cigarette Smoking in the United States. Atlanta, Centers for Disease Control and Prevention, 2014, http://www.cdc.gov/tobacco/campaign/tips/resources/data/cigarette-smoking-in-united-states.html#lgbt (accessed February 28, 2014).

23 Mackay J, Eriksen M, Shafey O: The Tobacco Atlas. Atlanta, American Cancer Society, 2006.

24 Henley SJ, Thun MJ, Chao A, Calle EE: Association between exclusive pipe smoking and mortality from cancer and other diseases. J Natl Cancer Inst 2004;96:853–861.

25 Fairchild A, Bayer R, Colgrove J: The renormalization of smoking? E-cigarettes and the tobacco 'endgame'. N Engl J Med 2014;370:293–295.

26 Kandel ER, Kandel DB: A molecular basis for nicotine as a gateway drug. N Engl J Med 2014;371:932–943.

27 King James I: A Counter-Blaste to Tobacco. London, Bibliotheca Curiosa, 1604/Edinburgh, Goldsmid, 1884.

28 Brown KM: Foul Bodies Cleanliness in Early America. New Haven, Yale University Press, 2009.

29 Proctor R: History of the Knowledge – and Ignorance – of Harms from Cigarettes in Canada, 1950–2000. Expert Report submitted by Robert N. Proctor, Stanford University, for Letourneau vs Imperial Tobacco Canada Ltd., et al. and Conseil Québécois sur le Tabac et la Santé vs. JTI-Macdonald Corp. et al., Aug. 19, 2011. http://www.nsra-adnf.ca/cms/file/files/pdf/110819_robert_proctor_expert_report.pdf (accessed June 12, 2014).

30 Levin M, Goldstein H, Gerhardt P: Cancer and tobacco smoking: a preliminary report. JAMA 1950;143:336–338.

31 Wynder EL, Graham EA: Tobacco smoking as a possible etiologic factor in bronchogenic carcinoma: a study of six hundred and eighty-four proved cases. JAMA 1950;143:329–336.

32 Doll R, Hill AB: Smoking and carcinoma of the lung: preliminary report. Br Med J 1950;ii:739–748.

33 US Department of Health, Education and Welfare, Public Health Service: Smoking and Health: Report of the Advisory Committee to the Surgeon General of the Public Health Service. Public Health Service Publ No 1103. Washington, Government Printing Office, 1964, http://profiles.nlm.nih.gov/ps/access/NNBBMQ.pdf.

34 US Department of Health and Human Services: The Health Consequences of Smoking – 50 Years of Progress. A Report of the Surgeon General; chapt 15: The Changing Landscape of Tobacco Control – Current Status and Future Directions. Atlanta, US Department of Health and Human Services, Centers for Disease Control and Prevention, National Center for Chronic Disease Prevention and Health Promotion, Office on Smoking and Health, 2014, pp 845–864.

35 World Health Organisation (WHO): Tobacco. Geneva, World Health Organisation, 2014. http://www.who.int/gho/tobacco/en/ (accessed June 10, 2014).

36 Maes C: Tabaco in chiesa proibito. II Cracas 1893;VI(268):786–792.

37 Proctor RN: Nazi War on Cancer. Princeton, Princeton University Press, 1999.

38 Cairney P: A 'multiple lenses' approach to policy change: the case of tobacco policy in the UK. British Politics 2007;2:45–68.

39 Studlar DT: Tobacco control policy in a shrinking world: how much policy learning; in Vogoda-Gadot E, Levi-Faur D (eds): International Public Policy and Management: Policy Learning and Policy beyond Regional, Cultural and Political Boundaries. New York, Dekker, 2004.

40 Berridge V: Marketing Health. Smoking and the Discourse of Public Health in Britain, 1945–2000. Oxford, Oxford University Press, 2007.

41 Brandt AM: Inventing conflicts of interest: a history of tobacco industry tactics. Am J Public Health 2012;102:63–71.

42 Legacy Tobacco Documents Library (LTDF). San Francisco, University of California, 2014. http://legacy.library.ucsf.edu/ (accessed June 10, 2014).

43 Trochim, WMK, Stillman FA, Clark PI, Schmitt CL: Developments of a model of the tobacco industry's interference with tobacco control programmes. Tob Control 2003;12:140–147.

44 Currie LM, Clancy L: The road to smoke-free legislation in Ireland. Addiction 2011;106:15–24.

45 ASH (Action on Smoking and Health UK): A Half Century of Avoidable Death. A Global Perspective on Tobacco in America. http://ash.org/wp-content/uploads/2014/06/US-TOBACCO-REPORT_FNL-WEB.pdf (accessed June 10, 2014).

46 World Health Organisation Framework Convention on Tobacco Control. Geneva, WHO, 2003 (updated reprint 2004, 2005).

47 Commonwealth of Australia: Australia: The Healthiest Country by 2020. Technical Report 2. Tobacco Control in Australia: Making Smoking History. 2009. http://www.health.gov.au/internet/preventativehealth/publishing.nsf/Content/96CAC56D5328E3D0CA2574DD0081E5C0/$File/tobacco-jul09.pdf (accessed June 12, 2014).

48 Jha P, Chaloupka FJ: Tobacco Control in Developing Countries. Oxford, Oxford University Press, 2000.

49 Warren CW, Jones NR, Peruga A, Chauvin J, Baptiste J-P, de Silva VC, el Awa F, Tsouros A, Rahman K, Fishburn B, Betcher DW, Asma S; Centers for Disease Control and Prevention (CDC): Global youth tobacco surveillance, 2000–2007. MMWR Surveill Summ 2008;57:1–28.

50 Cairney P, Studlar DT, Mamudu HM: Global Tobacco Control. Power, Policy, Governance and Transfer. London, Palgrave Macmillan, 2012.

51 Currie L, Townsend J, Leon Roux M, Godfrey F, Gallus S, Gilmore AB, Levy D, Nguyen L, Rosenqvist G, Clancy L: Policy Recommendations for Tobacco Taxation in the European Union Integrated Findings from the PPACTE project (Health-F2-2009-223323). Dublin, TobaccoFree Research Institute Ireland, 2012, www.ppacte.eu.

52 Directive 2014/40/EU of the European Parliament and of the Council of 3 April 2014. http://ec.europa.eu/health/tobacco/docs/dir_201440_en.pdf (accessed June 23, 2014).

53 Scientists discover the first physical evidence of tobacco in a Mayan container. Rensselaer Res Rev 2011–2012, http://www.rpi.edu/dept/metasite/research/magazine/winter12/tobacco-1.html.

54 Wyser C, Bolliger CT: Smoking-related disorders; in Bolliger CT, Fagerström KO (eds): The Tobacco Epidemic. Prog Respir Res. Basel, Karger, 1997, vol 28, pp 78–106.

Prof. Luke Clancy, BSc, MB, MD, PhD, FRCPI, FRCP (Edin), FFOMRCPI, Director General
TobaccoFree Research Institute Ireland
PO Box 12489, DIT Focas Building, 8 Camden Row
Dublin 8 (Ireland)
E-Mail lclancy@tri.ie

Loddenkemper R, Kreuter M (eds): The Tobacco Epidemic, ed 2, rev. and ext.
Prog Respir Res. Basel, Karger, 2015, vol 42, pp 19–26 (DOI: 10.1159/000369320)

Global Tobacco Epidemic

Judith Mackay[a] · Neil Schluger[b]

[a]World Lung Foundation, Kowloon, Hong Kong, SAR, China; [b]World Lung Foundation, New York, N.Y., USA

Abstract

This review covers global deaths, prevalence, consumption, tobacco economics, obstacles to tobacco control and tobacco control action in the tobacco epidemic. It highlights that 80% of smokers now live in low- and middle-income countries, and addresses the economic drain of tobacco on both national economies and smokers and their families. The tobacco epidemic, in spite of different populations and stages of development and different economic systems among countries, is comparable globally, with the same products, similar harm, identical obstacles and intervention measures needing to be taken. It shows that much progress has been made over the last half century, especially with the adoption of the World Health Organisation Framework Convention on Tobacco Control. Many millions are now covered by the WHO MPOWER measures, yet less than one in five of the world's population are covered by smoke-free areas, bans on all forms of advertising, promotion and sponsorship, optimum tobacco taxation, packet warning labels and cessation programmes at the highest, optimal level. There has been an increase in global funding for tobacco control, yet national funding remains woefully inadequate. © 2015 S. Karger AG, Basel

The level of development, systems of government and population size is very different between countries in the world (the latter ranging from about 1,000 to over 1.3 billion), but there is a shared similarity of the tobacco epidemic, including the products, harm caused, obstacles faced and tobacco control actions needed [1].

In general, the high-income countries were the first to recognize the tobacco epidemic and take action, but some low- and middle-income countries have a long history of tobacco control activities since the 1970s, and even today the Western Pacific Region remains the only World Health Organisation (WHO) region where all countries have ratified the WHO Framework Convention on Tobacco Control (FCTC) (see chapter 13) [1].

Global Deaths

Tobacco use in any form is dangerous and is the single greatest preventable cause of death. In 2014, tobacco use killed almost 6 million people, with nearly 80% of these deaths occurring in low- and middle-income countries [2]. This number of deaths includes 600,000 deaths from secondhand smoking (fig. 1).

More than half of all tobacco users will ultimately die of a tobacco-related illness, and men and women with comparable smoking patterns exhibit similar rates of tobacco-related death.

Unless urgent action is taken, more than 8 million people will die annually from tobacco by the year 2030 [2]. Tobacco caused 100 million deaths during the 20th century, and if current trends continue, about 1 billion people will die during the 21st century from tobacco. Yet, tobacco-related deaths are entirely preventable.

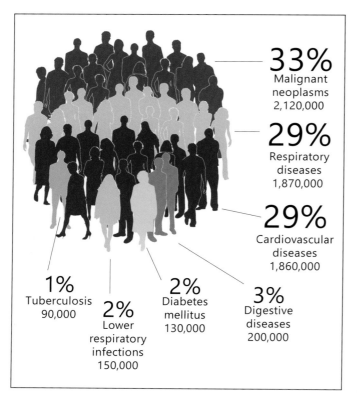

33%
Malignant
neoplasms
2,120,000

29%
Respiratory
diseases
1,870,000

29%
Cardiovascular
diseases
1,860,000

1%
Tuberculosis
90,000

2%
Lower
respiratory
infections
150,000

2%
Diabetes
mellitus
130,000

3%
Digestive
diseases
200,000

Fig. 1. Projected global tobacco-caused deaths by cause (2015 baseline scenario). Totals might not sum due to rounding [5].

Second-Hand Smoke

Globally, latest WHO estimates are that 40% of children, 33% of non-smoking adult males and 35% of non-smoking adult females are exposed to second-hand smoke. Of the 600,000 global deaths attributable to second-hand smoke, 28% occur in children and 47% in women [2, 3] (see chapters 9 and 10).

Exposure to second-hand smoke most commonly occurs in the home, workplace and public areas. Infants, children, pregnant women and foetuses are at a particularly high risk from second-hand smoke exposure.

Prevalence and Consumption

Research undertaken by the Institute for Health Metrics and Evaluation at the University of Washington (USA) is the first research to track prevalence and consumption from 1980 to 2012 in 187 countries. Overall, age-standardized smoking prevalence decreased by 42% for women and 25% for men between 1980 and 2012. Four countries –

Canada, Iceland, Mexico and Norway – have reduced smoking by more than half in both men and women since 1980 [4].

Consumption

Approximately 18% of the world's population smokes. Smoking is decreasing in high-income countries, but increasing in the low- and middle-income countries. Smokers consumed 5.8 trillion cigarettes in 2009, representing a 13% increase in cigarette consumption in the past decade. More than half the tobacco consumed in the world today is consumed in Asia [1].

The pattern of nicotine consumption may shift in the future as people seek alternative nicotine delivery systems, such as smokeless tobacco and electronic cigarettes (see chapters 21–23).

Prevalence

Men
More than 1 billion men throughout the world are smokers. Almost 20% of the world's adult male smokers live in high-income countries, while over 80% are in low- and middle-income countries [2]. Among the top 14 countries where more than 50% of men smoke, all but 1 (Greece) is classified as a low- or middle-income country [5].

The stages of the tobacco epidemic are seen in all countries: first, a dramatic increase in smoking, followed by a decline and then, several decades later, an increase in smoking-related illnesses and disease (fig. 2). In general, individuals who begin smoking in the first stage are usually males who are wealthier and more educated. These individuals quit sooner, but their smoking behaviour is imitated by lower-income, lower-educated groups who find it more difficult to quit and are less able to deal with the harm that smoking causes. While countries may have similar prevalence rates, each country's location on the curve is important to guide appropriate interventions.

Women
Approximately 240 million women throughout the world smoke cigarettes. In 2010, 50% of the world's female smokers were in high-income countries, 46% in middle-income countries and 4% in low-income countries [5]. The overwhelming use of tobacco by women in low- and middle-income countries is of smokeless tobacco in India and Bangladesh [6].

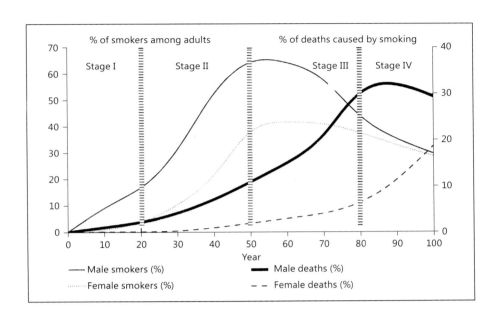

Fig. 2. A model of the cigarette epidemic [37].

If women in low- and middle-income countries begin smoking at rates equivalent to men, the world will face a public health disaster of enormous proportions (see the predictions on fig. 4 in chapter 7).

Youth Smoking
While there are large differences in smoking rates among adults by gender, smoking rates among boys and girls (aged 13–15 years) vary minimally in many regions of the world. In 47% of countries, smoking rates among boys and girls differ by less than 5%. Girls even smoked more than boys in at least 25 countries [5]. This similarity of today's boys' and girls' smoking rates suggests that, in the future, there may be an increase in female smoking rates.

The majority of smokers around the world begin smoking in their youth (see also chapter 14). For example, in every one of the first 22 GATS (Global Adult Tobacco Survey) countries surveyed (covering 61% of the world's adult population and conducted principally in the low- and middle-income countries), the average age of initiation was under 20 years [7]. Youth begin smoking in response to peer pressure, misconceptions that smoking is cool or enhances popularity, easy access to tobacco products, cigarette pricing and tobacco marketing (see chapter 15). Tobacco marketing associates male smoking with masculinity, happiness, wealth, virility and power, and female smoking by creating an association between smoking and gender equality, slimness, popularity and glamour. Women often choose 'light' and 'low-tar' cigarettes because of the false assumption that the products are less harmful than full-flavour cigarettes.

Smoking has an immediate harmful impact on health during youth, such as causing a reduction in stamina and an increase in respiratory symptoms. Even in youth, smoking causes genetic changes that predispose to cancer, heart disease and other problems later in life. Recent work demonstrates structural changes in the brain tissue of smokers as young as 16 years [8]. Youth smokers are entering into an addiction that shortens their lifespan and increases the likelihood they will die early from tobacco-related diseases. A person who becomes addicted to smoking at a young age shortens his or her life by at least 10 years [9–12].

Health Professionals
Worldwide, health professionals are respected and trusted as opinion leaders, with an ability to impact social norms and assist in cessation. Globally, as high as 40% of health profession students still smoke, and health professionals who are smokers are less likely to advise their patients to quit smoking. Few receive formal training in cessation assistance in medical and allied health schools [13].

Other Forms of Nicotine Use

Cigarette smoking is the most common form of tobacco use in the world, but there is a wide range of different products, ranging from smokeless tobacco and moist snuff to the newer electronic cigarettes, most of which contain nicotine.

Smokeless tobacco accounts for a significant and growing portion of tobacco use throughout the world, especially in South Asia, where a large majority of the world's smoke-less tobacco is consumed. In some countries, there is a 'dual-use' consumption pattern of both smoking and using smokeless tobacco. The highest percentage of men using both smoked and smokeless tobacco products in the 22 GATS countries is in Bangladesh, India and Egypt [14].

Global patterns of smokeless tobacco use vary widely. The import and sale of smokeless tobacco products are banned in 40 countries and areas. In some countries, men use smokeless tobacco products in much greater numbers than women because such products are perceived as mascu-line. Elsewhere – for example in South Africa, Thailand and Bangladesh – women use smokeless tobacco products more than men because smokeless tobacco is seen to be a more discreet way to consume tobacco [5].

Economics

Costs to Society

Direct costs are the medical costs of treating tobacco-related illnesses, which is only a portion of the total cost of tobacco to society. Indirect costs include losses in labour productivity; cigarette butt, matches, packet littering; fire damage and dam-age to property; environmental harm from destructive farm-ing practices; the intangible suffering of the victims and fam-ilies, and the costs of life lost. The burden of death, disease and disability caused by the use of tobacco products more than outweighs any economic benefit from their manufacture and sale (see also chapter 11). Research has long demonstrated the link between tobacco and poverty [15]. Between 2003 and 2008, about 3% of total health care expenditures in China was used to treat tobacco-related illnesses [16]. As economies im-prove, and their health systems develop further, the medical costs of tobacco-related disease will continue to grow.

Costs to the Smoker

The market price of a cigarette does not reflect the true eco-nomic cost that the product inflicts on society. When the costs of lost life, lost labour productivity and medical costs of treating tobacco-related diseases are taken into account, the true price of a cigarette is many times greater than its market price. Since the market does not correct for these external costs, people consume more cigarettes than they would if the price reflected the true costs.

Money spent on tobacco is diverted from resources needed for necessities such as nutrition, health care, education, cloth-ing, shelter and transportation. These opportunity costs im-pose a significant burden on tobacco users and their families,

burying many of them in a vicious circle of poverty that spans generations. Expenditures on tobacco inhibit progress toward Millennium Development Goals to eradicate extreme poverty.

Over 60 min of work are required to purchase a pack of cigarettes in Venezuela and Singapore, and more than 45 min in Kenya, India and Romania [5]. For the cost of a packet of Marlboro, a person could buy 81 servings of rice in Cambodia or over 40 servings in China, Indonesia, Thailand and Vietnam [5].

'Affordability' is the percentage of a worker's income or duration of work time required to buy that product. The more income is required to purchase cigarettes or the longer one must work to earn enough money for cigarettes, the less affordable cigarettes are. Despite cigarette prices being much higher in high-income countries, cigarettes are on av-erage more affordable in those countries. Between 2000 and 2010, cigarettes became 10% less affordable in the high-in-come countries, and 22% more affordable in the low- and middle-income countries, with the highest increase in af-fordability observed in the Eastern Mediterranean and South-East Asia [5].

In China in 2000, nearly 14% of the average per capita income was needed to buy 100 packs of the cheapest ciga-rettes; in 2010, this number dropped to less than 3% [5].

Growing Tobacco

Tobacco is grown in 124 mainly low- and middle-income countries, occupying 3.8 million hectares of agricultural land and diverting land from growing food. China is in a league of its own, producing 43% of the world's tobacco, more than the other top nine tobacco-producing countries combined [5]. In 2009, six of the top ten tobacco-producing countries had undernourishment rates between 5 and 28% [5].

Tobacco farming negatively affects the environment. Each year, 20,000 hectares of forests are cleared to cure to-bacco. Tobacco leaches the soil of many nutrients, so fertilis-ers and pesticides are heavily used in tobacco production. These chemicals endanger workers and create run-off that pollutes the environment.

No matter in which country tobacco farmers work, these individuals experience illnesses through their exposure to pesticides and nicotine. In addition to health impacts, many tobacco farmers are trapped in a cycle of poverty, as they are required to purchase high-cost equipment and infrastruc-ture, with little profit remaining.

The WHO FCTC calls for financial and technical assis-tance to tobacco growers to shift from growing tobacco to growing economically and environmentally viable alternatives, but the 2010 Global Progress Report indicated that few countries have implemented such measures. An exception is the landmark Yuxi pilot project in the Yunnan Province in China. The annual income in 458 farm families (involving 1,200 acres) quickly increased between 21 and 110% per acre when farmers' switched from growing tobacco to growing vegetables, flowers and other products [17].

Obstacles to Tobacco Control

Obstacles to tobacco control are similar around the world (see also chapter 12). These include a focus on curative not preventive medicine; tobacco tax revenue but not the debit is seen; misperceived concerns about economic losses if tobacco control measures are taken, and governments preoccupied with other events or diseases that cause far fewer deaths than tobacco, such as SARS, avian flu or financial crises [1].

By far the biggest obstacle is the tobacco industry (for details see chapter 3). Both national monopolies and commercial transnational tobacco companies operate around the world, often side by side. They have denied the health evidence, promoted smoking, established pro-tobacco institutes, challenged tobacco control legislation, attacked individuals, organisations and the WHO, and even secretly employed scientists such as in the infamous Asian 'Whitecoat Project' to work undercover to slant the science on secondhand smoke [1, 18–20].

The tobacco industry and its allies have launched legal challenges to government tobacco control action in all six WHO regions [21], obstructing and delaying tobacco control, including the triad of legal challenges to block the Australian law on plain packaging, invoking internal constitutional, bilateral investment treaties and World Trade Organization challenges [1]. In almost all cases, these challenges have been dismissed by the courts. In Article 5.3, the WHO FCTC requires party governments to protect their public health policies from commercial and other vested interests of the tobacco industry, recognizing the fundamental and irreconcilable conflict between the tobacco industry's interests and public health [22, 23].

Action

As of going to print, there are 180 parties to the 2005 WHO FCTC, making it one of the fastest-track United Nations treaties of all time [24].

Although tobacco control legislation is often thought more advanced in high-income countries, many tobacco control measures were pioneered by the low- and middle-income countries. Singapore banned tobacco advertising and smoking in the auditoria of cinemas and theatres and on public buses in 1970, 3 years ahead of any western nation; in 1991, Singapore was also the first country to ban incoming duty-free cigarettes. Several countries have demonstrated that tobacco control is not the prerogative of high-income countries, and that low- and middle-income countries can grasp the political nettle of tobacco control, and can do so effectively [1].

Many countries started tobacco control measures during the 1970s and 1980s, most beginning with health education in schools or textual health warnings on cigarette packs. Commensurate with the global experience of that time, most of the early laws were neither sufficiently specific nor comprehensive, or they contained loopholes. For example, many early bans on promotion only specified tobacco advertising and not the full range of marketing, such as sponsorship; these laws had to be progressively revised and strengthened. Early educational messages were underfunded (in comparison with the slick advertisements of the tobacco industry), clumsy, technical and difficult for the general public to understand [1].

In 2008, WHO packaged and promoted six proven measures to reduce tobacco use worldwide. Known as MPOWER, the measures support scale-up of specific provisions of the WHO FCTC on the ground (see fig. 1and 2 in chapter 12):

Monitoring tobacco use and prevention policies

Protecting people from tobacco smoke

Offering help to quit tobacco use

Warning about the dangers of tobacco

Enforcing bans on tobacco advertising, promotion and sponsorship

Raising taxes on tobacco

Today, only one country, Turkey, now protects its entire population of 75 million people with all MPOWER measures at the highest level [25] (see also chapter 12).

Monitoring Tobacco Use and Prevention Policies
Until recently, the bulk of monitoring and research on tobacco was undertaken in the high-income countries. One notable early exception was in 1981, when the late Takeshi Hirayama [26] in Japan published the first major global cohort study on passive smoking among 91,000 non-smoking married Japanese women, showing that the wives of heavy smokers had a higher risk of lung cancer.

National governments, university departments and other health organisations have increasingly conducted high-quality research on prevalence and consumption; adverse health effects of active and second-hand smoking [27, 28]; public opinion; effective tobacco control interventions; the behaviour of the tobacco companies, and the economic costs and trade aspects of tobacco [1].

Research has been sometimes supported technically and financially by international organisations, e.g. WHO (Global Tobacco Control Reports and the tracking of progress by the WHO FCTC), the US CDC Global Tobacco Surveillance System [29], the Clinical Trial Service Unit at the University of Oxford, the International Tobacco Control Project [30], the US National Institutes of Health and the Institute for Health Metrics and Evaluation at the University of Washington. It is important to note that the tobacco industry itself tried to influence research efforts by funding biased and flawed studies which minimized the harm that cigarettes do. As a result, many scientific journals now prohibit publication of work funded by the industry [31].

Translating research into policy is a particular challenge in every country, as many governments do not instinctively reach for data when designing government policy, and few policy makers have the scientific background to interpret the validity of the evidence, especially in low- and middle-income countries.

Protecting People from Tobacco Smoke
More than 1 billion people are now protected from second-hand smoke by comprehensive national smoke-free laws in 43 countries [22].

Offering Help to Quit Tobacco Use
In general, low- and middle-income countries have few comprehensive, available and affordable cessation services. This is now beginning to change: more than half a billion people in nine countries gained access to appropriate cessation services between 2007 and 2012. However, there has been little progress since 2010, as only four additional countries with a combined population of 85 million were newly provided access to cost-covered services including a toll-free national quit line [25]; 60% of countries operating toll-free national quit lines are in high-income countries [32].

mHealth for Tobacco Control. According to the International Telecommunication Union, there are now close to 5 billion mobile phone subscriptions in the world, over 70% of them residing in low- and middle-income countries. Over 85% of the world's population is now covered by a commercial wireless signal, dwarfing fixed internet deployment. The use of mHealth in tobacco control is largely limited to smoking cessation in the high-income countries, particularly in New Zealand, Norway, the United Kingdom and the United States. In 2011, the WHO launched an initiative to promote the use of mHealth for tobacco control in low- and middle-income countries [33].

Warning about the Dangers of Tobacco
National mass media campaigns were conducted between 2011 and 2013 by about one fifth of countries, housing more than half the world's population [25].

Pioneered by Canada, as of 2012, over 60 countries or jurisdictions, covering 40% of the world's population, have implemented pictorial packet warnings, a rapid increase from the 34 that had implemented by 2010. Several have already introduced new sets of warnings. Forty-seven countries or jurisdictions have warnings covering at least 50% of the package front and back. Australia now has the largest warnings in the world at 82.5% of the package front and back. Australia also implemented plain packaging to prohibit tobacco company colours, logos and design elements on the brand part of the package [34].

Enforcing Bans on Tobacco Advertising, Promotion and Sponsorship
According to WHO in 2013, one third of youth experimentation with tobacco occurs as a result of exposure to tobacco advertising, promotion and sponsorship [25].

Only 10% of the world's population is covered by a complete tobacco advertising, promotion and sponsorship ban. The population covered by this ban is increasing, with 99% of the people newly covered living in low- and middle-income countries [25].

Raising Taxes on Tobacco
Only 530 million people (8% of the world's population in 32 countries) are now living in countries with the recommended minimum tobacco taxes [22]. Low-income countries, which are in greater need of government funding for tobacco control programmes, are the least likely to have sufficiently high tax rates [22].

Research on the effectiveness of tobacco tax is recognised by all international economic institutions to be an essential component of tobacco control. In 2012, the Asian Development Bank estimated that raising tax would not only reduce the number of smokers and the number of smoking-related deaths, but also generate substantial new revenues. The Bank noted that the poorest socio-economic groups in each country would bear only a relatively small part of the extra tax burdens, but reap a substantial proportion of the health benefits of reduced smoking [35].

Few countries utilise a proportion of the tobacco tax to fund tobacco control activities or even public health, so tobacco control remains seriously underfunded. In the United States, for example, it is estimated that of the roughly USD 25 billion collected in cigarette taxes annually, only 1.9% are spent on tobacco control activities. The tobacco industry spends USD 18 on advertising for every USD 1 the country spends to reduce tobacco use [36]. The Bloomberg Philanthropies and the Bill and Melinda Gates Foundation have recently donated significant global funding for tobacco control in the low- and middle-income countries, but national funding commensurate with the magnitude of the epidemic is mostly lacking.

The Global Future

Even if prevalence is reduced, there will be more smokers in the world for several decades to come, due to increases in population mainly in the low- and middle-income countries, and increasing longevity.

An 'endgame' target of a prevalence rate of 5% or below has been announced by a few countries, such as New Zealand, Ireland, Finland and Scotland – a target unthinkable even at the Millennium. This will be first achieved in higher-income jurisdictions where the current prevalence rate is below 15%. There are many advantages for countries to announce an endgame date: confidence in the belief that the epidemic can be beaten; the focus of government strategy to achieve that goal with an orderly plan of action, and the end of the need for tobacco control advocates to continually fight for annual action, e.g. tax increases. There is uncertainty as to how much the growing popularity of electronic cigarettes will affect the endgame scenario (for details see chapter 23).

In May 2013, the World Health Assembly adopted the WHO global action plan for the prevention and control of non-communicable diseases (NCDs) 2013–2020, in which reducing tobacco use is identified as one of the critical elements of effective NCD control. The global action plan comprises a set of actions which – when performed collectively by Member States, WHO and international partners – will set the world on a new course to achieve nine globally agreed targets for NCDs; these include a reduction in premature mortality from NCDs by 25% in 2025 and a 30% relative reduction in the prevalence of current tobacco use in persons aged 15 years and older [25]. To achieve this, all countries will need to put much greater and immediate emphasis on price policies and smoking cessation.

Key Points

- Tobacco use in any form is dangerous and is the single greatest preventable cause of death in the world.
- Unless urgent action is taken, more than 8 million people will die annually from tobacco by the year 2030.
- Even if prevalence is reduced, there will be more smokers in the world for several decades to come, due to increases in population mainly in the low- and middle-income countries, and increasing longevity.
- The burden of death, disease, disability, lost productivity, and environmental costs caused by tobacco products more than outweighs any economic benefit from their manufacture and sale.
- Obstacles to tobacco control are similar around the world. These include a focus on curative not preventive medicine; tobacco tax revenue but not the debit is seen; misperceived concerns about economic losses if tobacco control measures are taken, governments preoccupied with other events or diseases that cause far fewer deaths than tobacco, inadequate funding to reduce the epidemic and the tobacco industry.
- Proven measures already exist to reduce the epidemic, such as those outlined in the WHO FCTC and MPOWER. All countries need to put much greater and immediate emphasis on price policies and smoking cessation.

References

1 Mackay J, Ritthiphakdee B, Reddy S: Tobacco Control in Asia. Lancet 2013;381:1581–1587.
2 World Health Organization: Tobacco. Fact sheet 339. http://www.who.int/mediacentre/factsheets/fs339/en/Leading cause of death, illness and impoverishment.
3 World Health Organization: Global Burden of Disease Related to Second-Hand Smoke. Executive Summary. http://www.who.int/tobacco/publications/en_tfi_gbd_executive_summary.pdf?ua=1.

4 Ng M, Freeman MK, Fleming TD, Robinson M, Dwyer-Lindgren L, Thomson B, Wollum A, Sanman E, Wulf S, Lopez AD, Murray CJL, Gakidou E: Smoking prevalence and cigarette consumption in 187 countries, 1980–2012. JAMA 2014;311:183–192.
5 Eriksen M, Mackay J, Ross H: The Tobacco Atlas, ed 4. Atlanta, American Cancer Society/New York, World Lung Foundation, 2012, http://www.tobaccoatlas.org.

6 Asma S, Mackay J, Song SY, Zhao L, Morton J, Palipudi KM, et al: The GATS Atlas. Atlanta, CDC Foundation, 2015, pp 38.
7 Asma S, Mackay J, Song SY, Zhao L, Morton J, Palipudi KM, et al: The GATS Atlas. Atlanta, CDC Foundation, 2015, pp 42–43.
8 Morales A, Ghahremani D, Kohno M, et al: Cigarette exposure, dependence, and craving are related to insula thickness in young adult smokers. Neuropsychopharmacology 2014;39:1816–1822.

9 Jha P, Ramasundarahettige C, Landsman V, Rostron B, Thun P, Anderson RN, McAfee T, Peto R: 21st-century hazards of smoking and benefits of cessation in the United States. N Engl J Med 2013; 368:341–350. http://www.nejm.org/doi/full/10.1056/NEJMsa1211128#t=articleTop.

10 Pirie K, Peto R, Reeves GK, Green J, Beral V; Million Women Study Collaborators: The 21st century hazards of smoking and benefits of stopping: a prospective study of one million women in the UK. Lancet 2013;381:133–141. http://www.thelancet.com/journals/lancet/article/PIIS0140-6736(12)61720-6/abstract.

11 Sakata R, McGale P, Grant EJ, Ozasa K, Peto R, Darby SC: Impact of smoking on mortality and life expectancy in Japanese smokers: a prospective cohort study. BMJ 2012;345:e7093. http://www.bmj.com/content/345/bmj.e7093.

12 Jha P, Jacob B, Gajalakshmi V, et al: A nationally representative case-control study of smoking and death in India. N Engl J Med 2008;358:1137–1147. http://www.nejm.org/doi/full/10.1056/NEJMsa0707719.

13 Centers for Disease Control and Prevention (CDC): Tobacco use and cessation counseling – Global Health Professionals Survey pilot study, 10 countries, 2005. MMWR Morb Mortal Wkly Rep 2005;54:505–509. http://www.cdc.gov/mmwr/preview/mmwrhtml/mm5420a2.htm?mobile=nocontent.

14 Asma S, Mackay J, Song SY, Zhao L, Morton J, Palipudi KM, et al: The GATS Atlas. Atlanta, CDC Foundation, 2015, pp 40–41.

15 Efroymson D, Ahmed S, Townsend J, Alam SM, Dey AR, Saha R, Dhar B, Sujon AI, Ahmed KU, Rahman O: Hungry for tobacco: an analysis of the economic impact of tobacco consumption on the poor in Bangladesh. Tob Control 2001;10:212–217.

16 Yang L, Sung HY, Mao Z, Hu TW, Rao K: Economic costs attributable to smoking in China: update and an 8-year comparison, 2000–2008. Tob Control 2011;20:266–272.

17 Li VC, Wang Q, Xia N, Tang S, Wang CC: Tobacco crop substitution: pilot effort in China. Am J Public Health 2012;102:1660–1663.

18 Assunta M, Fields N, Knight J, Chapman S: 'Care and feeding': the Asian environmental tobacco smoke consultants programme. Tob Control 2004; 3(suppl 2):ii4–ii12.

19 Sourcewatch: Whitecoats. http://www.sourcewatch.org/index.php?title=Whitecoats (accessed January 28, 2013).

20 Gaisch H: Philip Morris: organization of contacts with whitecoats. 1987. http://www.tobaccofreedom.org/issues/documents/landman/whitecoats/index.html (accessed January 28, 2013).

21 Campaign for Tobacco-Free Kids. Tobacco Control Laws: Litigation. http://www.tobaccocontrollaws.org/litigation.

22 World Health Organization: MPOWER in Action: Defeating the Global Tobacco Epidemic. http://www.who.int/tobacco/mpower/publications/mpower_2013.pdf?ua=1 (accessed December 23, 2013).

23 Mackay J, Bettcher D, Minhas R, Schotte K: Successes and new emerging challenges in tobacco control: addressing the vector (editorial). Tob Control 2012;21:77–79.

24 Parties to the WHO Framework Convention on Tobacco Control. http://www.who.int/fctc/signatories_parties/en/.

25 World Health Organization: Tobacco Free Initiative (TFI): WHO Report on the Global Tobacco Epidemic 2013: Enforcing Bans on Tobacco Advertising, Promotion and Sponsorship. http://apps.who.int/tobacco/global_report/2013/en/.

26 Hirayama T: Non-smoking wives of heavy smokers have a higher risk of lung cancer: a study from Japan. Br Med J (Clin Res Ed) 1981;282:183–185.

27 Kwok MK, Schooling CM, Ho LM, Leung SSL, Mak KH, McGhee SM, Lam TH, Leung GM: Early life second-hand smoke exposure and serious infectious morbidity during the first 8 years: evidence from Hong Kong's 'Children of 1997' birth cohort. Tob Control 2008;17:263–270.

28 Ding D, Fung JWH, Zhang Q, Yip GWK, Chan C-K, Yu C-M: Effect of household passive smoking exposure on the risk of ischaemic heart disease in never-smoke female patients in Hong Kong. Tob Control 2009;18:354–357.

29 Centers for Disease Control and Prevention: Smoking & Tobacco Use. Global Tobacco Control. http://www.cdc.gov/tobacco/global/index.htm (accessed January 28, 2013).

30 International Tobacco Control Policy Evaluation Project. http://www.itcproject.org/.

31 Godlee F, Malone R, Timmis A, Otto C, Bush A, Pavord I, Groves T: Journal policy on research funded by the tobacco industry. HYPERLINK "http://www.ncbi.nlm.nih.gov/pubmed/24129479" \l "comments" See comment in PubMed Commons belowBMJ 2013;347:f5193. doi: 10.1136/bmj.f5193.

32 World Health Organization: Tobacco Free Initiative. Quitting Smoking. http://www.who.int/tobacco/quitting/en/.

33 World Health Organization: Tobacco Free Initiative. Mobile Health (mHealth) for Tobacco Control. http://www.who.int/tobacco/mhealth/en/.

34 Canadian Cancer Society: Cigarette Package Health Warnings: International Status Report, ed 4. http://global.tobaccofreekids.org/files/pdfs/en/WL_status_report_en.pdf.

35 Asian Development Bank: Tobacco Taxes: A Win-Win Measure for Fiscal Space and Health. November 2012. http://www.adb.org/publications/tobacco-taxes-win-win-measure-fiscal-space-and-health.

36 Campaign for Tobacco Free Kids. Broken Promises to Our Children. The 1998 State Tobacco Settlement 14 Years Later. http://www.tobaccofreekids.org/what_we_do/state_local/tobacco_settlement/ (accessed June 6, 2014).

37 Lopez AD, Collishaw NE, Piha T: A descriptive model of the cigarette epidemic in developed countries. Tob Control 1994;3:242–247.

Dr. Judith Mackay, SBS, OBE, FRCP(Edin), FRCP(Lon)
Hong Kong Office, World Lung Foundation
Riftswood, 9th milestone, DD 229, Lot 147 Clearwater Bay Road
Kowloon, Hong Kong, SAR (China)
E-Mail jmackay@worldlungfoundation.org

Chapter 3

Loddenkemper R, Kreuter M (eds): The Tobacco Epidemic, ed 2, rev. and ext.
Prog Respir Res. Basel, Karger, 2015, vol 42, pp 27–36 (DOI: 10.1159/000369322)

The Tobacco Epidemic and the Commercial Sector: Tobacco Industry Strategies to Increase Profits and Prevent Regulation

Heide Weishaar

MRC/CSO Social and Public Health Sciences Unit, University of Glasgow, Glasgow, UK

Abstract

Being produced and promoted by large transnational corporations, tobacco provides a fascinating opportunity for investigating the detrimental impacts of commercial interests on health. This chapter critically reflects on the role of tobacco companies in the production, distribution and marketing of tobacco, their vested interests in tobacco control, and tobacco industry strategies to maintain a regulatory environment which allows them to continue running an exceptionally profitable business. First, a summary of the six major transnational tobacco companies and their efforts to exert political influence is presented. The chapter then outlines controversies about tobacco industry engagement in tobacco control before presenting three case studies of tobacco industry strategies to enhance profits and prevent regulation. The first case study describes tobacco companies' business and lobbying strategies in developing countries; the second focuses on British American Tobacco's success in building alliances to ensure political engagement at European Union level, and the final case discusses recent tobacco companies' efforts to establish themselves as legitimate stakeholders in harm reduction debates. By presenting evidence of tobacco industry success in increasing profits, building coalitions and preventing effective tobacco control policy, the chapter draws attention to the underlying political and economic factors which are crucial in understanding the tobacco epidemic.

© 2015 S. Karger AG, Basel

Epidemics, including malaria, cholera or influenza, are typically defined by a host, an environment and an agent. The host of an epidemic is often the human being who acquires the disease; the environment comprises the conditions under which the epidemic thrives, for example a swamp, poor housing or lack of hygiene; and the agent is the transmitter of the disease, for example a mosquito or parasite. This trichotomy has been equally applied to the tobacco epidemic. However, unlike communicable diseases, which are transmitted by insects, viruses or other microorganisms, the agent of the tobacco epidemic is the tobacco industry (see fig. 1 in chapter 23). Corporations which cause, promote and financially benefit from cigarette consumption have been described as a cause of tobacco-related death and disease, and a significant 'vector' of the epidemic [1]. A book about the tobacco epidemic is thus incomplete unless it considers the role of these commercial actors which rely on the consumption of tobacco for their profits and therefore put considerable efforts into fuelling, exacerbating and sustaining the epidemic. This chapter provides an overview of transnational tobacco companies and their attempts to influence tobacco control policy. In order to critically reflect on the role of the commercial sector in tobacco control, case studies outlining tobacco company strategies to increase profits, prevent regulation and maintain a conducive regulatory environment are presented, and implications for tobacco control and public health are discussed.

The Global Tobacco Market

Tobacco is an exceptionally profitable business. Worldwide, nearly 6 trillion cigarettes are produced annually, and production continues to rise [2] (see also chapter 2). In addition to tax collectors, manufacturing companies benefit from the giant share of the profits made from tobacco [2] (see also chapter 11). Figures show that in 2010 alone, the six top tobacco companies, which share more than 80% of the global tobacco market, generated total net revenues of nearly USD 346 billion and profits of USD 35 billion, equalling the combined profits of Coca-Cola, Microsoft and McDonalds [2]. The companies' wealth is reflected in their chief executive officers' annual compensations, which range from USD 2.4 million (Nicandro Durante, British American Tobacco, BAT) to USD 24 million (Michael Szymanczyck, Altria/Philip Morris USA) [2]. If Big Tobacco was a country, its gross domestic product would be similar to that of Poland, Sweden, Venezuela or Saudi Arabia [2].

Due to major privatization and mergers, six major tobacco companies currently dominate the global tobacco market: the China National Tobacco Corporation, Philip Morris International (PMI), Altria/Philip Morris USA, British American Tobacco (BAT), Japan Tobacco International (JTI) and the Imperial Tobacco Group (ITG). The China National Tobacco Corporation, the company with the biggest market share of approximately 37%, almost exclusively sells its products in the Republic of China and, as the largest state-owned tobacco company, produces more cigarettes than any of the private companies [2, 3]. PMI (17% market share), BAT (12%), JTI (10%), ITG (5%), Altria/Philip Morris USA (3%), as well as a few smaller companies share the rest of the global tobacco market [2]. PMI, a spin-off of Altria, and Altria/Philip Morris USA own the premium global brand Marlboro as well as Copenhagen, Skoal and Black & Mild [3]. BAT, a market leader in over 50 countries, sells brands like Dunhill, Kent, Lucky Strike and Pall Mall [2]. JTI, which operates in more than 120 countries around the globe, owns Winston, Camel, Mild Seven and several other brands [3]. Finally, ITG sells a portfolio of brands, including Davidoff, in over 160 countries around the world [3]. In addition to their core cigarette business, all major tobacco companies produce and sell other forms of tobacco, including cigars, roll-your-own tobacco and pipe tobacco. As outlined in detail below, international tobacco companies have also recently branched out into the market of alternative tobacco and nicotine products, including electronic cigarettes, oral tobacco and other forms of smokeless tobacco [2, 4] (see also chapters 21–23).

Tobacco Industry Attempts to Influence Policy Making

The extraordinary profits generated through tobacco manufacturing and sales explain why tobacco companies are considerably incentivised and have substantial financial re-sources at their disposal to defend their interests in the political arena. Litigation against tobacco companies in the USA has led to the public release of, and access to, formerly confidential corporate documents, including tobacco companies' correspondence, corporate presentations and strategy plans [5]. Analyses of these documents have given rise to a large body of literature focusing on tobacco companies' business strategies and their attempts to influence policy making. Such research shows that tobacco companies make immense efforts to increase profits and ensure a conductive regulatory environment by influencing political decision makers and countering effective tobacco control policy.

The literature divides tobacco industry strategies to influence policy making into two broad categories: corporate framing of public and political debates and the dissemination of arguments which are beneficial to the industry's aims [6] (see also chapters 1, 2 and 12). A substantial body of research shows that tobacco companies are successful in advancing arguments which frame their business in a positive way and can be employed to counter effective tobacco control policy [6]. Industry frames include the alleged detrimental economic consequences of tobacco control policies, the incompatibility of tobacco control legislation with international trade agreements and principles of good governance, the need for what companies define as 'flexible', 'appropriate' or voluntary, as opposed to 'extreme' regulation, and the promotion of tobacco companies as socially responsibly corporations [6]. Disregarding overwhelming evidence of the link between tobacco and a wide range of diseases, including nicotine addiction, lung cancer and cardiovascular conditions [7, 8] (see also chapters 5–10), tobacco companies contested research about the harmfulness of tobacco and second-hand smoke for several decades and continue to depict tobacco consumption as a matter of individual right, liberty and freedom of choice [6] (see also chapter 1).

Tobacco companies have subsequently employed a range of tactics to disseminate corresponding industry frames. Tactics include direct lobbying of decision makers, contributing financially to political campaigns; countering, discrediting and intimidating individuals and organisations which promote comprehensive tobacco control policy; obstructing the ratification and implementation of tobacco control policies; and legally challenging existing legislation [6]. Studies show that building alliances with a variety of actors and working through front groups are crucial industry strategies in fighting against regulation. Tobacco industry allies range from tobacco growers, trade unions, factory workers, tobacco retailers and wholesalers to scientists, journalists, lawyers, consultants and representatives of other industries, including the advertising, hospitality and ventilation sector [6]. In order to covertly promote their interests and advance more aggressive arguments, tobacco companies establish and use front groups, notably smokers' rights groups and tobacco grower associations [9, 10].

The large body of evidence outlining tobacco industry efforts to counter tobacco control policy has contributed to a risen awareness among public health advocates and decision makers about the vested interests of tobacco companies and the likely repercussions of tobacco industry interference in policy making. This awareness has led to the development of article 5.3 of the World Health Organization's (WHO) Framework Convention on Tobacco Control (FCTC), which requires parties to the treaty 'to protect their public health policies with respect to tobacco control from commercial and other vested interests of the tobacco industry in accordance with national law' [11] (see also chapter 12). The guidelines to FCTC article 5.3, which were developed to assist parties to the treaty in meeting their legal obligations under the corresponding article, highlight the need to draw attention to tobacco industry interference, limit interactions and ensure transparency of any interactions that occur, reject partnerships, avoid conflicts of interests and preferential treatment, regulate activities that portray the tobacco industry as socially responsible and demand transparency and accuracy from the tobacco industry [12]. While the FCTC uses the term 'tobacco industry' to refer to commercial actors with an obvious interest in tobacco production, import, manufacturing and sales [11], the guidelines take account of the fact that tobacco companies often work through allies, consultants, front groups and other bodies to reach their goals, and therefore highlight that measures should equally apply to 'organizations and individuals that work to further the interests of the tobacco industry' [12].

In order to illustrate and reflect on the strategies that tobacco companies employ to increase their profits and counter regulation, this chapter presents three case studies. The first critically analyses tobacco companies' strategies to expand profits in developing countries. The second case study focuses on tobacco industry interference in European Union (EU) policy making and BAT's success in building alliances to ensure political engagement at EU level. The final case study investigates tobacco companies' efforts to establish themselves as legitimate stakeholders in harm reduction debates.

Importing Death and Disease: Tobacco Companies' Strategies to Expand Profits in Developing Countries

Tobacco is grown in 124 countries worldwide, with the bulk of tobacco leaves being harvested in low- and middle-income countries [2] (see also chapter 2). In a considerable number of these countries (e.g. Malawi, Zimbabwe, Cuba, Jamaica, Bulgaria, Croatia, Bangladesh, Indonesia, Japan and Korea), tobacco is grown on more than a quarter of the agricultural land, leading to a high dependence of national economies on tobacco [13, 14]. Approximately 150 different chemicals and pesticides are used in tobacco farming, some of which, due to their toxicity, are banned in developed countries, but are still used in developing countries [15]. Moreover, the tobacco plant itself has health-damaging effects on farmers who absorb nicotine through the skin, which then enters the bloodstream and causes green tobacco sickness and a range of symptoms, including weakness, headache, vomiting, dizziness, and nicotine dependence [15]. In addition to causing health problems among adults and children who pick the crop, tobacco contributes significantly to undernourishment, exploitation, poverty, child labour, land erosion, destruction of rain forests and pollution of the ground water [2, 15]. The FCTC recognises the crucial role of alternative crops in fighting the tobacco epidemic and decreasing the detrimental consequences of the tobacco dependence of developing countries and therefore promotes economically viable alternatives for tobacco workers, growers and sellers [11].

In addition to negatively impacting on tobacco farmers and local economies, tobacco has detrimental consequences on consumers in low- and middle-income countries. Contrasting considerable drops of more than 25% in Western Europe over the last two decades, cigarette consumption has increased by almost 60% over the same time period in the Middle East and Africa [2]. Recent data show that half of all cigarettes are consumed in China, India, Indonesia and the Russian Federation [16]. While in several developing countries, including Indonesia, Malaysia, India and Thailand, people have traditionally smoked locally produced tobacco products, including kreteks, bidis, oral tobacco and shishas [17], such products are increasingly replaced by commercial cigarettes. The upsurge of commercial cigarettes in these markets is largely due to transnational companies, which aggressively promote cheap, manufactured cigarettes and specifically target population groups with the highest potential for growth. Tobacco consumption considerably reduces smokers' capacities to invest in other goods, including food, clothing, education and health, thereby increasing poverty in families which already live at or below the poverty line [16] (see also chapters 9 and 11). In Indonesia, for example, households of smokers spend approximately 11.2% on tobacco, equalling their joint expenses for fish, meat, eggs and milk [17]. In contrast, only 3.2 and 2.3% are spent on education and health, respectively [17]. As elsewhere, smokers in developing countries are suffering and dying from a multitude of tobacco-related diseases. The WHO warns that the shift in the tobacco epidemic to low- and middle income countries is resulting in an immense burden of death and disease on countries where health care services are least available [16]. Already now, the annual death toll worldwide from tobacco consumption exceeds that from HIV/AIDS, tuberculosis and malaria [16], and estimates predict that by 2030, 70% of the estimated 10 million global deaths from tobacco will occur in developing countries [18] (see chapter 2).

Due to their population growth and unlocked potential of future smokers, low- and middle-income countries have been identified by tobacco companies as crucial future markets [19]. The market entrance of transnational tobacco companies is also accompanied by a loss of foreign exchange as profits are returned to shareholders in developed countries [19]. The distinct business value of developing countries lies in the relatively low average of current smoking prevalence among women, the lack of awareness of the harmful effects of tobacco, a shortage of funding for tobacco control measures and the difficulties in implementing tobacco control legislation [19]. Trade liberalisation allows tobacco companies to enter these markets, thereby contributing to amplified competition, lower prices, higher demand for cigarettes and increases in tobacco-related burden of disease [14, 20]. Research shows that in order to exploit the potential of developing markets, tobacco companies strongly lobby the governments of corresponding countries. Kenya, for example, where BAT owns approximately two thirds of the national tobacco production [13], is an example of tobacco companies' success to secure market leadership and fight opposition of local companies [21]. Building on the national government's interests as the second largest shareholder of BAT Kenya, BAT appointed influential politicians as non-executive directors and built connections with Kenyan presidents, ministers and members of parliament, thereby securing high-level support for policies which contributed to the company's business success [21]. As a result of its close links with high-level politicians, BAT effectively lobbied the Kenyan government to support BAT's market leadership and suppress commercial opposition [21]. A key success was the 1994 adoption of a tobacco production law which BAT claimed 'was actually drafted by us but the Government is to be congratulated on its wise actions' [21]. In fact, the law was strikingly similar to earlier proposals submitted by BAT and consolidated the company's control over, and exploitation of, Kenyan tobacco farmers [21].

In addition to lobbying governments on tobacco growing and production issues, research shows that tobacco companies counter the implementation of tobacco control policies in developing countries [19, 21]. One of the most popular industry strategies in the fight against effective tobacco control are intimidation tactics and the employment of threats that tobacco control measures will lead to job losses and detrimental effects on national economies, reduce foreign earning and deepen developing countries' economic dependency on foreign aid [22]. While the dissemination of economic frames is a well-established industry strategy, which has been successfully applied in other legislative contexts [10, 23], such framing seems to meet with particular success in countries which are highly dependent on tobacco [22].

Another industry strategy which is increasingly being employed to gain market access and counter effective tobacco control policies is the use of trade agreements to reduce trade barriers and increase foreign investment [14]. Such strategies exploit the widespread assumption that low tariffs and other trade preferences improve economic productivity, expand exports and increase economic growth [14]. Research, however, contrasts these alleged positive consequences and shows that increasing trade and investment liberalisation provides opportunities for tobacco companies to prey open highly profitable markets in developing countries [20]. A recent WHO report outlines how transnational tobacco companies lobby US authorities to threaten countries with retaliatory trade sanctions unless they open up their markets to foreign tobacco products, invade local markets by launching aggressive production and promotion campaigns, and mount legal challenges in international trade courts to contest national bans on sales and promotion of foreign tobacco products [20]. It is of even greater concern that tobacco companies increasingly seem to circumvent the World Trade Organization's trade agreements as e.g. the Transatlantic Trade and Investment Partnership (TTIP) which presently is negotiated between the EU and the USA and the arbitration of legal challenges in international trade courts by using bi- and multilateral trade and investment agreements to challenge national tobacco legislation [20]. One of the most recent examples of this strategy is a legal case presented by Philip Morris under a bilateral investment treaty between Switzerland and Uruguay which challenges Uruguay's decision to increase health warning labels on tobacco packs and introduce plain packaging [24]. Philip Morris argues that such measures infringe intellectual property rights and obstruct the company's competitiveness in the local market [24]. Uruguay is sued for USD 2 billion, equalling one sixth of the country's national budget. A decision can be expected in 2015.

As outlined above, transnational tobacco companies employ a comprehensive set of strategies to exploit developing markets. Their often perfidious strategies contribute to tobacco industry control over conditions of tobacco farming, crop prices and tobacco export, and the erosion of local tobacco control policies, some of which have long been implemented in developing countries and established as international best practice [19]. Such strategies are in stark contrast to the industry's alleged societal concerns which tobacco companies promote as part of their corporate social responsibility programmes. Considering their exploitation of the world's most vulnerable populations, tobacco companies' support of local communities, sponsorship of soccer fields and tournaments and claims to help eliminate child labour seem treacherous attempts to divert attention away from their misconduct [14, 25]. Similarly, the establishment and financial support of tobacco farmers' associations, like the International Tobacco Growers' Association [26], can be seen as part of a comprehensive industry strategy aimed at portraying tobacco companies as responsible corporations which are concerned about working conditions and societal issues [14]. This case study of tobacco companies' strategies to increase profits in developing countries provides a persuasive example of the deceitfulness of the industry's corporate social responsibility agenda and its ruthlessness in increasing the burden of tobacco-related death and disease, enhancing poverty, inequality and lack of economic development in low-income countries and exploiting vulnerable populations.

Building Alliances to Secure Political Engagement at European Union Level: British American Tobacco and the European Union's 'Better Regulation' Agenda

Tobacco companies' polished corporate websites and social responsibility programmes provide evidence of the industry's concern about its public reputation and efforts to present themselves as responsible corporations. A crucial part of tobacco companies' strategies of improving their public and political profile is to heavily invest in so-called 'stakeholder marketing' and lobbying of political decision makers [27].

Given their crucial role in international trade, policy making and product regulation, European decision makers present key targets for industry lobbying, a fact that is mirrored in the industry's expenditures on EU interest representation. Official figures suggest that individual tobacco companies spend between EUR 600,000 and 1,750,000 annually on representing their interests in Brussels [28–30]. In addition to showing presence via company-specific public relation offices, tobacco manufacturers work through national and European associations and collaborate with European umbrella organisations representing other actors with commercial interests in the production, manufacture, wholesale and retail of tobacco. Organisations like the Confederation of European Community Cigarette Manufacturers, European Smoking Tobacco Association, European Cigar Manufacturers Association, European Confederation of Tobacco Retailers and European Tobacco Wholesalers Association thus support individual companies in their fight against EU regulation.

In line with the industry's financial investment in EU level lobbying, plenty of research provides evidence of tobacco industry success in preventing, stalling and derailing EU tobacco control policy. The European tobacco advertising ban constitutes presumably the most prominent example of tobacco industry opposition to EU tobacco control [31]. Research shows that industry representatives managed to counter the 1989 proposal for a comprehensive EU-wide tobacco advertising ban over more than a decade by framing debates on the alleged detrimental economic impacts, lobbying decision makers at EU and national levels, discrediting the tobacco control community, and challenging the competence of the EU to legislate on the issue [32]. Tobacco industry efforts culminated in a legal challenge in the European Court of Justice, which resulted in the annulment of the original directive in October 2000 and the adoption of a weaker directive focused on cross-border advertising in June 2001 [32]. The literature suggests that tobacco companies employed similar strategies, including direct lobbying of decision makers, mobilisation of allies, manipulation of media coverage and a legal challenge, to derail the 2001 tobacco product directive, an EU directive regulating the manufacture, presentation and sale of tobacco and related products [33]. More recently, the industry strongly opposed the revision of the tobacco product directive by mobilising allies and factory workers to submit responses to the EU consultation, using front groups to argue against product regulation, critiquing the policy process and claiming that EU institutions had insufficient competence to adopt the policy proposal [34]. As part of a comprehensive strategy, the industry submitted 2,320 responses to the European Commission's public consultation about the revision of the tobacco products directive, highlighting the sector's opposition to the initiative. Moreover, the industry mobilised tobacco retailers and other tobacco sector representatives to oppose the revised proposal, resulting in a total of 85,513 submissions to the consultation and considerable delays to the policy process [35]. Leaked industry documents show that PMI alone engaged 161 employees and consultants to combat a proposed directive, met with one third of all members of the European Parliament and spent GBP 1.25 million in the first half of 2012 alone for meetings with public officials [36]. The broad body of literature on tobacco industry interference in EU tobacco control suggests that tobacco companies have managed to secure access to, and build broad support among, EU decision makers [27]. While research suggests that tobacco company representatives sometimes face difficulties in gaining access to decision makers whose primary interest lies in public health, it shows that decision makers representing trade, agriculture, finances and taxation are often more amenable to, and willing to support, tobacco industry interests [23, 37].

In addition to studies outlining tobacco companies' strategies in preventing effective EU tobacco control, recent research by Smith et al. [38] uncovered how tobacco companies were able to influence EU policy making at a more profound level. Providing evidence that BAT worked with other representatives of the commercial sector to implement fundamental, structural changes within the EU policy process, their research points to an unprecedented level of industry interference [38]. Their analysis of tobacco documents shows that BAT and its allies were able to promote the concept of 'better regulation' (a term BAT employed to push for less regulation and the inclusion of business interests in the policy process) and establish ground rules for EU policy making, which subsequently led to the inclusion of commercial interests at early stages of policy development and increased opportunities for companies to promote concerns about the economic and administrative burden of policies to businesses and challenge potential and existing legislation [38]. In order to secure binding changes which would implement the concept of better regulation within the EU Treaty via the 1997 Treaty of Amsterdam, BAT launched a major campaign aimed at enlisting other actors in respective policy debates [38]. Allies comprised representatives of other industry sectors, including the pharmaceutical, oil, food, beverage, financial and automobile industry, business and employers' associations and key politicians [38]. Rather than fronting the campaign itself, BAT recruited and finan-

cially supported the European Policy Centre, a Brussels-based, industry-oriented think tank, to advance the issue. This strategy allowed BAT to hide its company-specific interests and maintain a low political profile, while simultaneously shaping the direction of the campaign. BAT's efforts seemed to lead to the anticipated success and resulted in considerable amendments to the EU policy process, including requirements for EU decision makers to minimise legislative burdens on businesses, conduct routine evaluation of the economic impact of legislative proposals and consult widely with stakeholders when developing policies [38]. Research suggests that tobacco companies subsequently obstructed the EU policy process by calling for increased stakeholder consultation and economic impact assessment, thereby delaying the adoption and implementation of effective tobacco control policy and promoting policies that advance tobacco industry profits rather than public health [38].

This overview of tobacco industry interference in EU policy making draws attention to the ability of tobacco companies to build opposition against regulations which threaten to undermine their profits. Previous studies provide plenty of evidence that alliances are crucial in countering tobacco control policies at national, regional and international levels [6, 39, 40]. While alliances against effective tobacco control often comprise tobacco growers, manufacturers, wholesalers, retailers, smokers' rights groups and other actors with a clear interest in tobacco consumption, the research by Smith et al. [38] illustrates BAT's success in enlisting a wide range of like-minded companies in a broader coalition opposing EU level regulation. By embedding its industry-specific interests in broader political debates and following a Trojan horse strategy, BAT was able to avoid political isolation and overcome the looming threat of increasing exclusion from the policy process deriving from its loss of credibility following litigation in the US. Moreover, the case study provides compelling evidence of BAT's use of the European Policy Centre as a front group to rally support, provide a cover for commercial interests and push for fundamental changes in the EU policy process. It thus illustrates how the tobacco industry employs its large financial resources to build strategic alliances that help in obscuring tobacco industry interests, subtly infiltrate the political sphere and influence political processes. By outlining tobacco companies' track records of shaping EU policy making and ensuring that their interests are taken into account, this case study highlights how companies use their financial resources to lobby and shape the regulatory environment, thereby safeguarding their future ability to make profits. This vicious cycle contributes to the industry's prosperity and the continuity of the tobacco epidemic.

Utilising Harm Reduction: Tobacco Companies' Strategies to Rebuild Their Corporate Image and Restore Legitimacy

Despite the massive efforts of the tobacco industry to counter tobacco control policy at all levels of governance, comprehensive tobacco control policies, including tobacco advertising bans, product regulation, smoke-free policies, health warning labels and recently, plain packaging provide evidence of the immense progress that has been made in countering the tobacco epidemic over the last decades. The implementation of comprehensive tobacco control policies has resulted in declining smoking prevalence in many European countries [41] and focused debates on how to tackle the remaining 'hard core' smokers who cannot or do not want to quit smoking. In the context of harm reduction debates, the role of alternative tobacco and nicotine products, including smokeless tobacco, nicotine inhalers and electronic cigarettes, has been discussed.

Mirroring the increasing importance of alternative tobacco and nicotine products, transnational tobacco companies increasingly venture into corresponding emerging markets [4]. The market of alternative tobacco and nicotine products is constantly and rapidly changing, evidenced by several mergers and joint ventures between transnational tobacco companies and smokeless tobacco manufacturers, and the increasing adoption of nicotine products in the portfolio of major tobacco companies [4, 42]. By acquiring previously independent smokeless tobacco companies and entering the market of non-tobacco nicotine products, transnational tobacco companies have managed to restrict competition, enhanced their pricing power and reached control over the market for most cigarette substitutes [42]. Although the revenue generate from the sales of alternative tobacco and nicotine products remains relatively low compared to the industry's total revenues [42], products which are less harmful than traditional cigarettes generate new sales without threatening existing profits [43]. By allowing tobacco companies to promote nicotine use among young people, and encourage dual use and consumption in places where smoking is prohibited, alternative tobacco and nicotine products seem to play important roles in augmenting cigarette consumption [44]. The marketing of alternative products, and particularly of products which resemble cigarettes, are further assumed to be used to re-normalise smoking, constitute a gateway to promote cigarette consumption and allow the industry to re-gain visibility through advertisement [44].

Arguably more importantly, recent developments in the market of alternative tobacco and nicotine products, and the establishment of transnational tobacco companies as providers of products which cause less harm to health and are discussed as viable alternatives to traditional cigarettes, mean that tobacco companies have emerged as important political players. Peeters and Gilmore's [43] research shows that investments into less harmful products allow tobacco companies to seek common ground and engage in dialogue with public health policy makers, experts and scientists, and signal alignment of tobacco industry and public health interests. Responding to emerging harm reduction debates, tobacco companies harness the public health rhetoric in discussions with high-level policy makers and highlight their contribution to tobacco control as suppliers of less harmful products in the context of policy debates, often citing public health experts' views on harm reduction as a crucial part of a comprehensive approach to tackle the harms caused by tobacco [45, 46].

As reflected in chapters 21–23 of this edition and evidenced by two recent letters to the WHO Director-General Margaret Chan [47, 48], the tobacco control community is divided over the issue of harm reduction and the industry's role in corresponding debates. Several tobacco control researchers and advocates see smokeless tobacco and nicotine products as a unique opportunity for advancing tobacco control and reducing tobacco-related morbidity and mortality [49]. Proponents highlight the benefits of these products as suitable alternatives to cigarettes and their potential in reducing health inequalities by reaching smokers of low socio-economic status, among which smoking prevalence is particularly high [49]. Opponents argue that focusing on less harmful products, smoking cessation and individual-level interventions will occur at the expense of population-based tobacco control measures [49]. Critical voices argue that the acquisition of smokeless tobacco and nicotine products facilitates the companies' access to, and dialogue with, political decision makers, and allows tobacco companies to publicly re-position themselves as responsible corporations and legitimate stakeholders in harm reduction debates and as partners rather than adversaries in achieving public health gains [43]. Concerns are raised that such developments form an integral part of the industry's comprehensive corporate social responsibility strategy, that their establishment as producers of potentially less harmful products presents tobacco companies with a unique opportunity to increase corporate credibility and re-build the industry's reputation, and that it allows tobacco companies to re-enter the policy arena from which they have been excluded in line with FCTC article 5.3 [42, 43].

Recent developments in the production, marketing and public presentation of alternative tobacco and nicotine products show that tobacco companies have managed to turn less harmful products into a business as well as a political opportunity [42]. Tobacco companies' acknowledgement that cigarettes are harmful and alternative products are needed provides them with a strong basis to engage in harm reduction debates. Given the history of tobacco industry deceit and previous misleading, alleged industry concerns about the harms caused by tobacco products, companies' current alleged concerns about the harms caused by cigarettes and attempts to present themselves as part of the solution to tackle the tobacco epidemic have to be treated with caution. Mirroring such doubts about the industry's commitment to harm reduction, public health and medical experts have recently argued that tobacco companies, were they to have a genuine interest in reducing the harms caused by their products, should announce target dates to stop manufacturing, marketing and selling cigarettes, and desist from aggressively opposing effective tobacco control policies [48]. The fact that tobacco companies have managed to establish a strong presence in the market of less harmful products and their apparent success to participate in contemporary tobacco control debates arguably presents the greatest contemporary challenge to the tobacco control movement. Evidenced by the divergent positions of tobacco control academics and advocates, the issue of harm reduction risks splitting the formerly largely unified community into those promoting individual-level interventions and those favouring population-based approaches. How the movement responds to the issue of harm reduction and positions itself with regard to tobacco industry efforts to engage in tobacco control debates will be a crucial determinant of the future direction of tobacco control.

Conclusion

This chapter provided a critical analysis of tobacco industry strategies to increase profits and prevent regulation. By outlining tobacco industry efforts to exploit existing and emerging markets in developing countries, shape the regulatory environment at EU level and engage in current policy debates on harm reduction, the analysis draws attention to the role of the commercial sector in fuelling, promoting and sustaining the tobacco epidemic. Tobacco has been hailed as a unique health problem and tobacco control as an unprecedented policy success with potential implications for other areas of public health policy [50, 51]. Not least, an account of tobacco industry strategies to increase profits and prevent regulation provides valuable lessons about the controversies between commercial interests and public health, and the detrimental impact which commercial players can have on health policy, thereby increasing understanding of the underlying political and economic determinants of health.

Key Points

- Corporations which cause, promote and financially benefit from cigarette consumption significantly fuel, exacerbate and sustain the tobacco epidemic.
- Following a long history of working to ensure a conducive regulatory environment by derailing tobacco control policies, tobacco companies continue to influence political debates by advancing frames and disseminating arguments to counter effective tobacco control and increase the industry's corporate image.
- Article 5.3 of the Framework Convention on Tobacco Control (FCTC), which advises decision makers to protect tobacco control policies from the vested interests of the tobacco industry, is employed by public health advocates to draw attention to the political dimension of, and the detrimental impact of economic interests on, the tobacco epidemic.
- Transnational tobacco companies employ a comprehensive set of strategies to ensure the industry's control over conditions of tobacco farming, crop prices and tobacco export, exploit developing markets and undermine local tobacco control policies.
- Research shows that tobacco companies have been successful in building alliances, using front groups and using their financial resources to counter effective tobacco control policy and shape the regulatory environment at European Union level.
- Recent developments suggest that tobacco companies increasingly employ harm reduction debates to publicly re-position themselves as responsible corporations and legitimate stakeholders in the policy process, engage in dialogue with political decision makers and re-enter the policy arena, from which they have been excluded in line with FCTC article 5.3.

References

1 LeGresley EM: A 'vector analysis' of the tobacco epidemic. Bull Medicus Mundi 1999;72. http://www.medicusmundi.ch/de/bulletin/mms-bulletin/kampf-dem-tabakkonsum/grundlagentexte-zur-tabakepidemie/a-vector-analysis-of-the-tobacco-epidemic.

2 Eriksen M, Mackay JM, Ross H: The Tobacco Atlas. Atlanta, American Cancer Society, 2012.

3 Tiessen J, Hunt P, Celia C, et al: Assessing the impacts of revising the Tobacco Products Directive. Study to support a DG SANCO impact assessment. Final report. 2010. http://ec.europa.eu/health/tobacco/docs/tobacco_ia_rand_en.pdf (accessed August 8, 2012).

4 Bialous SA, Peeters S: A brief overview of the tobacco industry in the last 20 years. Tob Control 2012;21:92–94.

5 Legacy Tobacco Documents Library. About the Library. 2012. http://legacy.library.ucsf.edu/about/about_the_library.jsp;jsessionid=634660FE3DF6FA6C5AE6039B77A23545.tobacco03 (accessed December 7, 2012).

6 Weishaar H, Collin J, Smith KE, Grüning T, Mandal S, Gilmore A: Global health governance and the commercial sector: a documentary analysis of tobacco company strategies to influence the WHO Framework Convention on Tobacco Control. PLoS Med 2012;9:e1001249.

7 Hirayama T: Non-smoking wives of heavy smokers have a higher risk of lung cancer: a study from Japan. Br Med J (Clin Res Ed) 1981;282:183–185.

8 Doll R, Peto R, Boreham J, Sutherland I: Mortality in relation to smoking: 50 years' observation on male British doctors. BMJ 2004;328:1519.

9 Smith EA, Malone R: 'We will speak as the smoker': the tobacco industry's smokers' rights groups. Eur J Public Health 2007;17:306–313.

10 Mamudu HM, Hammond R, Glantz SA: Tobacco industry attempts to counter the World Bank report 'Curbing the Epidemic' and obstruct the WHO Framework Convention on Tobacco Control. Soc Sci Med 2008;67:1690–1699.

11 World Health Organization: WHO Framework Convention on Tobacco Control. Geneva, World Health Organization, 2003.

12 World Health Organization: WHO Framework Convention on Tobacco Control. Guidelines for Implementation. Article 5.3; Article 8; Article 11; Article 13. Geneva, World Health Organization, 2009.

13 Graen L: Tabak Produktion in Afrika: Knebelverträge im Trend. 2014. http://www.unfairtobacco.org/wp-content/uploads/Tabakproduktion-in-Afrika.-Knebelvertr%C3%A4ge-im-Trend.pdf (accessed June 5, 2014).

14 Otanez MG, Mamudu HM, Glantz S: Global leaf companies control the tobacco market in Malawi. Tob Control 2007;16:261–269.

15 von Eichborn S: Big Tobacco: profits and lies. Tabakanbau im globalen Süden. 2009. http://www.unfairtobacco.org/wp-content/uploads/Big-Tobacco_Broschuere.pdf (accessed June 5, 2014).

16 World Health Organization: WHO Report on the Global Tobacco Epidemic. The MPOWER Package. Geneva, World Health Organization, 2008.

17 Weber J: Doppelte Standards. Big Tobacco in Asien. 2012. http://www.unfairtobacco.org/wp-content/uploads/Doppelte-Standards-Big-Tobacco-in-Asien.pdf (accessed June 5, 2014).

18 Gajalakshmi CK, Jha P, Ranson K, Nguyen S: Global patterns of smoking and smoking-attributable mortality; in Jha P, Chaloupka F (eds): Tobacco Control in Developing Countries. Oxford, Oxford University Press, 2000.

19 Mackay J: The tobacco problem: commercial profit versus health – the conflict of interests in developing countries. Prev Med 1994;23:535–538.

20 World Health Organization: Confronting the Tobacco Epidemic in a New Era of Trade and Investment Liberalization. Geneva, World Health Organization, 2012.

21 Patel P, Collin J, Gilmore A: 'The law was actually drafted by us but the Government is to be congratulated on its wise actions': British American Tobacco and public policy in Kenya. Tob Control 2007;16:e1.

22 Otañez MG, Mamudu HM, Glantz SA: Tobacco companies' use of developing countries' economic reliance on tobacco to lobby against global tobacco control: the case of Malawi. Am J Public Health 2009;99:1759–1771.

23 Grüning T, Weishaar H, Collin J, Gilmore A: Tobacco industry attempts to influence and use the German government to undermine the WHO Framework Convention on Tobacco Control. Tob Control 2012;21:30–38.

24 Lencucha R: Philip Morris versus Uruguay: health governance challenged. Lancet 2010;376:852–853.

25 Otañez MG, Muggli ME, Hurt RD, Glantz SA: Eliminating child labour in Malawi: a British American Tobacco corporate responsibility project to sidestep tobacco labour exploitation. Tob Control 2006;15:224–230.

26 Must E: International Tobacco Growers' Association (ITGA). ITGA uncovered: unravelling the spin – the truth behind the claims. 2001. http://www.healthbridge.ca/assets/images/pdf/Tobacco/Publications/itgabr.pdf (accessed August 11, 2010).

27 Hastings G, Angus K: The influence of the tobacco industry on European tobacco-control policy; in: Tobacco or Health in the European Union. Past, Present and Future. Luxembourg, Office for the Official Publications of the European Communities, 2004, pp 195–222.

28 European Union: Transparency Register. Profile of Philip Morris International Inc. 2011. http://ec.europa.eu/transparencyregister/public/consultation/displaylobbyist.do?id=51925911965-76 (accessed December 14, 2011).

29 European Union: Transparency Register. Profile of British American Tobacco. 2011. http://ec.europa.eu/transparencyregister/public/consultation/displaylobbyist.do?id=2427500988-58 (accessed December 14, 2011).

30 European Union: Transparency Register. Profile of Japan Tobacco International SA. 2011. http://ec.europa.eu/transparencyregister/public/consultation/displaylobbyist.do?id=71175716023-03 (accessed December 14, 2011).

31 Godfrey F: An overview of European Union tobacco control legislation. Cent Eur J Public Health 2000;8:128–131.

32 Bitton A, Neuman M, Glantz SA: Tobacco Industry Attempts to Subvert European Union Tobacco Advertising Legislation. San Francisco, University of California, Center for Tobacco Control Research and Education, 2002.

33 Mandal S: Tobacco Industry Efforts to Influence the 2001 European Union Tobacco Products Directive. London, London School of Hygiene and Tropical Medicine, 2006.

34 Tobacco Tactics: PMI's lobbying campaign to undermine the TPD. 2014. http://www.tobaccotactics.org/index.php/PMI%E2%80%99s_Lobbying_Campaign_to_Undermine_the_TPD (accessed June 25, 2014).

35 Directorate General Health and Consumers: Public consultation on the possible revision of the Tobacco Products Directive 2001/37/EC. 2012. http://ec.europa.eu/health/tobacco/consultations/tobacco_cons_01_en.htm (accessed August 8, 2012).

36 Doward J: Tobacco giant Philip Morris 'spent millions in bid to delay EU legislation'. The Guardian, September 7, 2013. http://www.theguardian.com/business/2013/sep/07/tobacco-philip-morris-millions-delay-eu-legislation (accessed July 23, 2014).

37 Princen S: Advocacy coalitions and the internationalisation of public health policies. Int Public Policy 2007;27:13–33.

38 Smith KE, Fooks G, Collin J, Weishaar H, Mandal S, Gilmore AB: 'Working the system' – British American Tobacco's influence on the European Union Treaty and its implications for policy: an analysis of internal tobacco industry documents. PLoS Medicine 2010;7:e1000202.

39 Dearlove JV, Bialous SA, Glantz SA: Tobacco industry manipulation of the hospitality industry to maintain smoking in public places. Tob Control 2002;11:94–104.

40 Mandal S, Gilmore AB, Collin J, Weishaar H, Smith KE, McKee M: Block, amend, delay: tobacco industry efforts to influence the European Union's Tobacco Products Directive (2001/37/EC). 2009. http://www.smokefreepartnership.eu/IMG/pdf/EU_TI_TPD_report_May_2012.pdf (accessed July 3, 2012).

41 Directorate General Health and Consumers: Attitudes of Europeans towards Tobacco. 2012. http://ec.europa.eu/health/tobacco/docs/eurobaro_attitudes_towards_tobacco_2012_en.pdf (accessed October 31, 2012).

42 Gilmore AB: Understanding the vector in order to plan effective tobacco control policies: an analysis of contemporary tobacco industry materials. Tob Control 2012;21:119–126.

43 Peeters S, Gilmore A: Understanding the emergence of the tobacco industry's use of the term tobacco harm reduction in order to inform public health policy. Tob Control 2014, DOI: 10.1136/tobaccocontrol-2013–051502, Epub ahead of print.

44 Gartner CE, Hall W, Chapman S, Freeman B: Should the health community promote smokeless tobacco (snus) as a harm reduction measure? PLoS Med 2007;4:e185.

45 International Smokeless Tobacco Company Inc: Submission in relation to Green Paper. Toward a Europe free from tobacco smoke: policy options at EU level. 2007. http://ec.europa.eu/health/archive/ph_determinants/life_style/tobacco/documents/r-124_en.pdf (accessed June 18, 2012).

46 European Smokeless Tobacco Council: ESTOC submission in response to the possible revision of the tobacco products directive 2001/37/EC public consultation document DG SANCO. 2010. http://www.estoc.org/uploads/Documents/documents/ESTOC%20response%20TPDR%20public%20consultation%20-%20leave%20behind.pdf (accessed June 25, 2014).

47 Statement from specialists in nicotine science and public health policy to Dr Margaret Chan. Reducing the toll of death and disease from tobacco – tobacco harm reduction and the Framework Convention on Tobacco Control (FCTC). 2014. http://nicotinepolicy.net/documents/letters/MargaretChan.pdf (accessed June 4, 2014).

48 129 public health and medical authorities from 31 countries write WHO DG Chan urging evidence-based approach to ecigs (letter). 2014. http://tobacco.ucsf.edu/129-public-health-and-medical-authorities-31-countries-write-who-dg-chan-urging-evidence-based-appro (accessed June 24, 2014).

49 Fox BJ, Cohen JE: Tobacco harm reduction: a call to address the ethical dilemmas. Nicotine Tob Res 2002;4(suppl 2):S81–S87.

50 Brand H: From 'public health in Europe' to 'European public health'. Eur J Public Health 2010;20:127–129.

51 A framework convention on alcohol control. Lancet 2007;370:1102.

Heide Weishaar
Research Fellow
MRC/CSO Social and Public Health Sciences Unit University of Glasgow
200 Renfield Street
Glasgow G2 3QB (UK)
E-Mail Heide.Weishaar@glasgow.ac.uk

Chapter 4

Loddenkemper R, Kreuter M (eds): The Tobacco Epidemic, ed 2, rev. and ext.
Prog Respir Res. Basel, Karger, 2015, vol 42, pp 37–46 (DOI: 10.1159/000369323)

Chemistry and Primary Toxicity of Tobacco and Tobacco Smoke

Friedrich J. Wiebel

Institute of Toxicology, Helmholtz Zentrum München, German Research Center for Environmental Health, Neuherberg, Germany

Abstract

Tobacco smoke contains thousands of organic and inorganic chemicals. Two thirds of these originate from pyrolysis and pyrosynthesis in the burning or smoldering of tobacco products. The rest is transferred unchanged from the tobacco into the smoke. The components in tobacco leaves and processed tobacco differ widely with the type of tobacco plant, and method of cultivation, harvesting and curing. Major toxic constituents of tobacco smoke are volatile organic chemicals, free radicals, nonvolatile polycyclic aromatic hydrocarbons, aromatic amines, heterocyclic amines and metals. N-nitrosamines, in particular tobacco-specific N-nitrosamines, in processed tobacco are of major health concern. They are distilled into the smoke but are also present in 'smokeless' tobacco products. The distribution of tobacco smoke constituents between the particulate and gaseous phase largely determines their site of deposition and, hence, action. Reactive compounds in tobacco smoke interact with cellular macromolecules to cause lipid peroxidation, protein modification and DNA damage. In addition, free radicals, foremost reactive oxygen and nitrogen species, disturb the equilibrium of physiological messenger substances. Together, this leads to malfunctioning of signaling pathways, cytotoxicity, cell necrosis and apoptosis, impaired growth control and gene mutation, initial steps in the development of cardiovascular disease, lung disorders and cancer.   © 2015 S. Karger AG, Basel

This chapter reviews the state of knowledge about the chemistry and primary toxicity of tobacco and tobacco smoke. It focuses on manufactured cigarettes and deals to a lesser extent with other nicotine-containing products, such as hand-rolled cigarettes, cigars, cigarillos, waterpipe tobacco or smokeless tobacco products (see also chapters 21 and 22). The newly marketed so-called electronic cigarettes (e-cigarettes) are covered in chapter 23. A survey of other 'less' harmful cigarette products such as nonburning cigarettes or electrically heated cigarettes has been given by Kleinstreuer and Feng [1].

There exists a wealth of information on the presence of toxic, mutagenic or carcinogenic agents in tobacco leaves, processed tobacco and tobacco smoke [2]. The individual agents are, with few exemptions, most notably the tobacco-specific nitrosamines (TSNAs), not unique to tobacco. Their chemical features and adverse effects fill textbooks of chemistry and toxicology. Tobacco smoke shares the major features of other air pollutants, such as smog, effluents of waste incinerators or smoke of wood stoves. However, tobacco smoke is unusual in that it is inhaled at very high concentrations over long time periods and is exceptional in that it contains an alkaloid that drives the consumers to inhale the conglomerate of toxic agents again and again: nicotine (see chapter 5).

Chemistry

Tobacco smoke contains thousands of inorganic and organic chemicals [2]. Their highest estimated number surpasses 9,500 [3]. Two thirds of the compounds in tobacco smoke are estimated to be products of pyrolysis and pyrosynthesis formed during burning or smoldering of the tobacco. The rest is already present in the tobacco leaf or processed tobacco and is transferred unchanged into the tobacco smoke.

Components in the Tobacco Leaf

The components of toxicological concern differ considerably between tobacco plants and the methods with which these are cultivated and harvested [2]. For example, fertilization with sewage sludge and irrigation with polluted water increases the uptake of metals into the tobacco plant. Fertilization with nitrates boosts the nitrate content in tobacco plants leading to an increase in the formation of carcinogenic amino-, nitroso- and nitro-products. Another source of concern is pesticides, which are applied during cultivation of tobacco plants and during tobacco storage.

Methods of tobacco plant cultivation and harvesting are also essential determinants of the nicotine content in leaves and stems used to manufacture the various tobacco products [2]. The metabolism and biological effects of nicotine are described in chapter 5.

Components in Processed Tobacco

The procedure for the processing of tobacco, 'curing', depends to a large degree on the type of the tobacco used. Three types of tobacco predominate in cigarettes: Virginia, Oriental and Burley tobacco. Virginia tobaccos are primarily 'flue cured', Oriental tobacco 'sun cured' and Burley tobacco 'air cured' [4]. At high temperatures and short heating times, as applied during flue curing, enzymatic activities come to a quick halt and the components in the tobacco leaf are largely preserved. In contrast, during air drying of Burley tobacco, many components are metabolically degraded, leading for example to the desired formation of tasty metabolic products but also to the loss of beneficial components. The latter is the case for the degradation of sugars [5], which are important for adjusting the pH in tobacco smoke.

Aside from the fact that the composition of the tobacco differs considerably between products, the design of tobacco products and the way the products are used greatly modifies the level of the components taken up by the consumer. Clearly, there is no such thing as a 'standard cigarette'.

Table 1. Tobacco additives: examples of the diverse substances permitted for use in tobacco products [44]

Ammonium	3-Hexyl-2-acrolein	Pigment red 184
Bicarbonate		Piperonal
Hydroxide	Iron oxides	Propionic acid
Sulfide		Propylene glycol
Trans-anethole	Lecithin	Pyridine
	Levulinic acid	
1,3-Butylene glycol	D-Limonene	Rum
	Liquid paraffin BP	
Chlorophyll		Saccharin
	Magnesium salts	Salicylaldehyde
Dextrin	Menthol	Shellac
Dimethyl pyrazine	*p*-Methyl anisole	Sugars
	Methyl cellulose	
Farnesol	Methyl pyrazine	Tartrazine yellow
D-Fructose	Methyl salicylate	Thiabendazole
		Titanium dioxide
D-Glucose	1-Octanol	
L-Glutamic acid		Urea
Glycerol	*o*-Phosphoric acid	
Glycyrrhizin	Pectin	Vanillin
Hexanal		

Tobacco Additives[1]

Depending on the jurisdiction, manufacturers of tobacco products can add any of about 600 chemicals to their products [6]. The added materials may comprise 10–20% of the total weight of a cigarette. Tobacco additives are members of virtually all classes of organic molecules, aliphatic or aromatic compounds of various size and charge, saturated and unsaturated, nonsubstituted and substituted, or of natural or synthetic origin (table 1). Tobacco additives may also consist of mixtures of substances such as liquorice, honey, syrups, molasses and extracts or oils of basically all fruits and spice plants. The additives were initially authorized for use in food stuff. Later, they were simply adopted to be used in tobacco products[2] without taking into consideration that their toxic potential may be greater when they are inhaled [7].

---

[1] The terms 'additives' and 'ingredients' are used interchangeably in EU Directive 2001/37/EC and its recently revised version EU Directive 2014/40/EU [10]. However, in some cases, the term 'ingredients' also denotes tobacco-derived components in smoke such as tar, nicotine and carbon monoxide. The term 'additive' will be used throughout this chapter.
[2] In Europe, the status of the current lists of compounds that are authorized as tobacco additives/ingredients ('positive lists') is uncertain. The new EU Directive 2014/40/EU [10] requires the establishment of 'negative lists', i.e. a list of compounds that are prohibited as tobacco additives/ingredients.

Tobacco additives serve many purposes. They are added to improve the taste of tobacco products, to mitigate the harsh tobacco flavor and to act as humectants or antioxidants. Tobacco additives also serve to adjust the pH level in tobacco products. Prominent representatives of pH modulators are ammonium compounds and other alkaline substances, such as the amino acid lysine, which release ammonia. By raising the pH, they convert nicotine from its ionized (protonated) form into a nonionized (unprotonated) form, which is thought to be faster absorbed by the smoker than the ionized substance providing him with a nicotine boost soon after inhalation of the tobacco smoke [8]. Other frequently used substances are sugars, which are added to supplant the sugars lost, e.g. during the air curing process of Burley tobacco [5].

Generally, the toxic potential of the authorized tobacco additives, even when inhaled, is rather low. However, when burned during smoking, they share the fate of the constitutive compounds in tobacco, i.e. they are subjected to combustion to form toxic, mutagenic and carcinogenic products [7, 9]. Beyond that, many of the additives make tobacco products more attractive and palatable, which increases tobacco consumption and consequently health hazards. A prime example is menthol. The substance has been targeted by regulators [10] not because of its potential toxicity but because of its physiological and sensory effects, i.e. 'taste', which may incite people, in particular youths, to start smoking.

Tobacco Smoke

Smoke from combustible tobacco products, cigarettes, cigars, cigarillos and cut tobacco for pipes contains the same toxic substances. However, their relative amounts differ to some extent depending on the type of tobacco used and the design features of the product. For example, the extended fermentation of tobacco used in cigars causes the formation of higher concentrations of the carcinogenic TSNAs. Also, cigar wrappers are less porous than cigarette wrappers making the combustion of cigars less complete. As a result, cigar smoke has higher concentrations of certain toxic substances than cigarette smoke. Although such differences might have an effect on the type and severity of health outcomes of smokers, it is the way combustible tobacco products are consumed, e.g. depth of inhalation and frequency of use, that primarily determines the extent of exposure to the smoke and the resulting health risks [11].

Formation of Tobacco Smoke

Smoke is formed when a tobacco product is lit and puffs are taken (mainstream smoke) and when the cigarette smolders between puffs (sidestream smoke). During smoking, chemical compounds in tobacco can be distilled into smoke or can be subjected to pyrolysis and/or pyrosynthesis to yield products that, in turn, are distilled into smoke [2]. Conventionally, the newly formed compounds are referred to as pyrolysis products. As pointed out above, very few compounds are specific for the tobacco plant. This pertains also to the pyrolysis products in tobacco smoke. For example, polycyclic aromatic hydrocarbons (PAHs) are formed by incomplete combustion of natural organic matter such as wood or petroleum. Heterocyclic aromatic amines occur in heated food stuff, such as grilled meats, poultry or fish [2].

Phases of Tobacco Smoke

Smoke from a burning cigarette can be regarded as an aerosol of liquid particles suspended in an atmosphere of gaseous compounds. Particulate and gaseous matters are divided into two phases by operational definition. The particulate phase is defined as material that is trapped, when smoke generated in a smoking machine passes through a Cambridge glass fiber filter that retains 99% of all particulate matter with a size >0.1 μm [2]. Accordingly, the gaseous phase consists of the smoke that passes through the filter. The term 'tar' refers to the particulate matter minus the fraction of nicotine.

The distribution of tobacco smoke constituents in the particulate and gaseous phase constitutes an important element for risk assessment, since they differ in their deposition pattern and hence their sites of toxic action.

Particulate Phase. The number of particles, more appropriately termed 'droplets', is about 10^{10}/ml. They have a mean aerodynamic diameter of about 0.3–0.4 μm with a range of about 0.05–1.0 μm. The diameter of the particles is not constant. It grows as the particles coalesce after their formation or shrink as the smoke dilutes and particles lose semivolatile components.

Tobacco smoke particles/droplets are composed of porous carbonaceous material on which non- or semivolatile compounds are absorbed, such as PAHs, TSNAs, aromatic amines, carboxylic acids, phenols, heavy metals, water and nicotine. The compounds contained in the particles comprise more than 80% of the total tobacco smoke components [1].

Gaseous Phase. The gaseous phase of cigarette smoke consists largely of the inorganic compounds nitrogen (N_2), oxygen (O_2), carbon monoxide (CO), carbon dioxide (CO_2), hydrogen cyanide (HCN), nitric acid, hydrogen sulfide (H_2S) and a large number of volatile organic compounds such as acetaldehyde, acrolein, ammonia, methanol, certain nitrosamines and carbonyls. The total mass of compounds in the gaseous phase amounts to 0.4–0.5 g/cigarette.

Some individual chemical constituents may almost exclusively occur in the particulate phase (e.g. PAHs) or gaseous phase (e.g. CO). However, many others, e.g. formaldehyde and cyanide, pass between the phases as the smoke dissipates.

Mainstream and Sidestream Smoke
Mainstream smoke and sidestream smoke differ quantitatively but not qualitatively in their composition (see also chapters 9 and 10). The differences are largely attributable to the burning conditions, when the two types of smoke are formed. Mainstream smoke is generated at a temperature reaching 900°C during puffing. Sidestream smoke is formed between puffs, when the temperature falls to about 400°C. This is not the only difference. Sidestream smoke evolves under conditions where less oxygen is available and where the alkalinity and water content is relatively high [12]. Overall, this causes the formation of higher levels of PAHs, nitrosamines, aza-arenes, aromatic amines, CO, ammonia, pyridine, 1,3-butadiene, acrolein, isoprene, benzene or toluene in sidestream smoke [2]. At the same time, sidestream smoke contains less cyanide, catechol and hydroquinone than mainstream smoke [2]. The relative amounts of tobacco smoke compounds in mainstream and sidestream smoke differ with the design of the cigarettes, filter and paper porosity, and the intensity in which the product is consumed.

Deposition and Removal
The deposition of particles/droplets of tobacco smoke has been extensively reviewed [1]. In general, the deposition of inhaled particles depends on their size. Particles smaller in diameter than 2.5 μm pass through the extrathoracic and upper airways and deposit in lower bronchial and alveolar regions by sedimentation and diffusion.

Modeling the spatial distribution of particles in the lung is highly complicated by the fact that they are subject to coagulation, hygroscopic growth, condensation and evaporation, vapor formation and changes in composition. In addition, differences in puffing behaviors, smoke inlet conditions and moving along lung airway walls during breathing influence airflow characteristics and deposition patterns.

Overall, the distribution models predict that the particles deposit largely in the terminal bronchi and the alveolar region [13]. However, this is debatable. Studies including human volunteers using radiolabeled inhaled cigarette smoke indicated that the particles are deposited as if their aerodynamic diameters were 6.5 μm [14]. This has been confirmed by analyzing the deposition pattern in hollow airway replica casts [15]. The exceptionally large particles have been attributed to the formation of 'clouds' in highly concentrated smoke [16] that consist of a very larger number of particles surrounded by clear fluid. Hot spots for the deposition of these clouds are the bifurcations of bronchi and along posterior sections of tubular airways [17].

Once the particles/droplets are incorporated into the liquid that lines the epithelial layer (epithelial lining fluid, ELF), they unload their freight of water-soluble, and non- and semivolatile compounds. The fate of the residual particle 'core' is uncertain. Extrapolating from what is known about the removal of uniform particles from the lung, particles deposited in the ELF are transported outwards by the mucociliary escalator. Particles reaching the alveoli are taken up by regional macrophages and, thus, compartmentalized. The macrophages can migrate to bronchioli and bronchi to be removed by the mucociliary apparatus or can find their way to the lymph system. However, if the macrophages are overloaded with smoke particles, they may perish and release the particles into the ELF. Set free, the particles can damage the alveolar septum, induce fibrous tissue and remain there [18]. Clearly, substantial amounts of the particular matter remain in the lung [19], giving it a dark tinge after years of smoking [2].

Particles of nanometer size (<0.1 μm) can penetrate through the alveolar epithelial layer and interstitium, enter the pulmonary blood vessels and are transported to other organs. Inhaled gases are absorbed into the ELF depending on their solubility. Highly soluble gases (e.g. NH_3 or SO_2) are removed high in the respiratory tract. Poorly soluble gases (e.g. CO or NO) may reach the alveoli and diffuse across the alveolar-capillary membranes to find their way into the blood system [2].

Constituents of Tobacco Smoke

The following presents a brief overview over the major classes of organic compounds in tobacco smoke (table 2) and of their metabolism [reviewed in ref. 2]. Separate sections will be devoted to metals and free radicals.

Wiebel

Table 2. Major classes of tobacco smoke constituents

N-nitrosamines
  N-nitrosodimethylamine[1]
  N-nitrosodiethylamine[1,3]
  N-nitrosopyrrolidine[1]
  N-nitrosopiperidine[1]
  N-nitrosodi-N-butylamine
  N-nitrososarcosine[1]
  N-nitrosodiethanolamine[1]
  TSNAs
    NNN[1,2]
    NNK[1-3]
PAHs
  Anthracene[1]
  Benzene[1,2]
  Benz(a)anthracene[1]
  Benzo(a)pyrene[1-3]
  Benzo(b)fluoranthene[3]
  Benzo(j)fluoranthene[1]
  Benzo(k)fluoranthene[1,3]
  Dibenz(a,h)anthracene[3]
  Dibenzo(a,i)pyrene[1]
  Dibenzo(a,e)pyrene[1]
  Indeno(1,2,3-cd)pyrene[1,3]
  5-Methylchrysene[1,3]
Aromatic amines
  Aniline
  2-Toluidine[1-3]
  Dimethylaniline[1]
  2-Naphthylamine[1-3]
  4-Aminobiphenyl[1-3]
  2-Methyl-1-naphthylamine
Heterocyclic amines
  3-Amino-1,4-dimethyl-5H-pyrido(4,3-b)indole (Trp-P-1)[1]
  3-Amino-1-methyl-5H-pyrido(4,3-b)indole (Trp-P-2)[1]
  2-Amino-6-methyldipyrido(1,2-a:3',2'-d)imidazole (Glu-P-1)[1]
  2-Amino-1-methyl-6-phenylimidazo(4,5-b)pyridine (PhIP)[1]
Aliphatic hydrocarbons
  Methane
  Ethane
  Ethylene oxide[1,2]
  Isoprene[1]
  1,3-Butadiene[1,2]
  Vinylchloride[1,2]
Carbonyl compounds
  Acetone
  Butanone
  Acetaldehyde[1]
  Acrolein[4]
  Dimethylhydrazine[1]
  Ethyl carbamate[1]
  Formaldehyde[1]
Nitriles
  Acetonitrile
  Acrylonitrile[1]
Metals
  Arsenic[1-3]
  Cadmium[1-3]
  Chromium[1,2]
  Lead[1]
  Polonium-210[1,3]
  Selenium

Alkaloids
  Anabasine
  Anatabine
  Cotinine
  Nicotine
Gases/inorganic compounds
  Nitrogen (N_2)
  Oxygen (O_2)
  Nitric oxides (NO, NO_2)
  Carbon oxides (CO, CO_2)
  Hydrogen cyanide (HCN)
  Hydrogen sulfide (H_2S)
  Hydrazine[1,3]

The number of carcinogens (in parentheses) in the various classes of chemicals are N-nitrosamines (8), PAHs (10), aza-arenes (3), aromatic amines (4), heterocyclic amines (8), aldehydes (2), volatile hydrocarbons (4), nitro compounds (3), miscellaneous organic compounds (12), metals and other inorganic compounds (9): total (63) [20].
[1] Tumorigenic in experimental animals [reviewed in ref. 2].
[2] Tumorigenic in humans (limited and sufficient evidence) [reviewed in ref. 2].
[3] Tumorigenic in the lung of at least one animal species [21].
[4] Tumorigenicity to humans evaluated 'as not classifiable' by IARC 1995 (to be reevaluated [45]).

Organic Compounds

Polycyclic Aromatic Hydrocarbons. More than 500 PAHs have been identified in tobacco smoke [3]. In the burning cone at the tip of the tobacco rod, CH radicals are formed, which are precursors to the pyrosynthesis of PAHs. At least ten PAHs have been classified as carcinogens in experimental animals [20]. Some of them have been found to be tumorigenic in the lung [21], and a few are also known carcinogens in humans (table 2) [2]. Total PAH levels in mainstream smoke from commercial cigarettes are about 1–2 μg per cigarette. Individual PAHs range from 10 to 20 ng benzo(a)pyrene to approximately 500 ng naphthalene per cigarette [2].

Aromatic Amines. Aromatic amines are present in unburned tobacco and are also formed during tobacco combustion. They reside primarily in the particulate phase of smoke, except for the more volatile species such as *o*-toluidine. The levels of aromatic amines in mainstream smoke were reported to be 200–1,300 ng per cigarette [22].

Heterocyclic Amines. Heterocyclic amines arise by pyrolysis of amino acids and proteins through radical reactions or by heating mixtures of creatinine, sugars and amino acids. Heterocyclic amine levels in tobacco smoke amount to 0.3–260 ng per cigarette [20].

Aromatic and Aliphatic N-Nitrosamines. N-nitrosamines are formed by the reaction of secondary and tertiary amines in tobacco with nitrosating agents [23]. The most prominent members are the TNSAs (table 1), foremost NNN (N′-nitrosonornicotine) and NNK [4-(methylnitrosamino)-1-(3-pyridyl)-1-butanone], which are predominantly generated from nicotine and nornicotine in tobacco leaves and processed tobacco [2]. Their levels range from 2 to 12 ng of NNN and from 55 to 10,000 ng of NNK per cigarette [23]. Only minor amounts of TSNAs are transferred to the tobacco smoke. Consequently, they can be at an order of magnitude lower in mainstream smoke than in tobacco. TSNAs are almost exclusively found in the particulate phase of tobacco smoke; in contrast, aliphatic volatile nitrosamines, such as N-nitrosodimethylamine or N-nitrosodiethyamine, are primarily contained in the gaseous phase [2]. About one half of the (non-TSNAs) nitrosamines in tobacco smoke originate from processed tobacco. The remainder is formed from pyrosynthesis during smoking.

Aliphatic Compounds. The mass of the organic chemicals in tobacco smoke consists of aliphatic saturated and unsaturated hydrocarbons, including their aldehydes and ketones [24]. The most abundant hydrocarbons in cigarette smoke are methane, ethane and propane. Prominent representatives of unsaturated hydrocarbons are isoprene (70–480 μg) and 1,3-butadiene (6–55 μg). The most prevalent aldehydes are acetaldehyde (30–650 μg), acrolein (2.5–60 μg) and formaldehyde (2–50 μg); the most prevalent ketones are acetone (50–550 μg) and 2-butanone (10–130 μg) [24]. Tobacco smoke contains also appreciable amounts of nitriles such as HCN (3–200 μg) and acetonitrile (~100 μg) [24].

Metabolic Activation of Tobacco Smoke Components. Most of the organic compounds in tobacco smoke are not reactive by themselves but require metabolic activation to intermediates, generally electrophiles, which can react with nucleophilic sites in macromolecules. The metabolism of organic compounds in cigarette smoke that are of health concern is well established [2, 21].

Enzymes mediating the formation of reactive intermediates are largely members of the cytochrome P450 family. For example, PAHs are oxidized by P450 forms 1A1 and 1B1 to their reactive metabolites, aromatic amines by P450 1A2, nitrosamines by P450 forms 2A6, 2E1 and 2A13, and 1,3-butadiene by P450 2E1. Location and activity of the various P450s determine to a large extent the vulnerability of cells and tissues to the cytotoxic and carcinogenic effects of organic chemicals.

The reactive intermediates are usually inactivated by binding to endogenous molecules to form water-soluble metabolites that can be excreted. The inactivation reactions are catalyzed by a variety of enzyme families, including glutathione S-transferases, glucuronosyltransferases, N-acetyltransferases, sulfotransferases and epoxide hydrolases. Occasionally, conjugation reactions do not result in inactivation, but mediate an activation process. For example, acetyltransferases can O-acetylate the N-hydroxy metabolites of aromatic and heterocyclic amines forming the ultimate carcinogenic products of the amines [25].

A number of the 'xenobiotic metabolizing enzymes' involved in the metabolism of tobacco smoke constituents exhibit genetic polymorphisms, e.g. P450 CYP1A1, CYPD6 and CYP22C19, glutathione S-transferase GSTM1 or N-acetyltransferase NAT2 [2]. Evidence accumulates that such genetic polymorphisms play a role in the risk of lung and bladder cancer in smokers [2].

Metals

The toxicity of metals in tobacco smoke is mainly attributable to their propensity to accumulate in the body (Cd, Cr, Pb and Po). For the majority of metals, there are no clear indications that they are toxic at the amounts taken up by smokers. The lack of clarity is mainly due to the fact that these metals are usually to a greater extent derived from other sources, primarily food or ambient air, than from tobacco smoke [26].

Cadmium. Smokers absorb about 1–3 µg of Cd per day which doubles the average daily Cd intake by food [27]. In the burning cigarette, Cd is transformed to cadmium oxide which is taken up by the smoker and readily absorbed into the systemic blood circulation. In the blood of smokers, Cd levels are 4–5 times higher and in the kidney 2–3 times higher than in nonsmokers. Cd is known to be nephrotoxic, to interfere with blood pressure regulation and to increase the cancer risk [27]. It is likely that Cd in tobacco smoke contributes to these adverse effects.

Chromium. Of the various Cr species, only Cr(III) and Cr(VI) are common in the natural environment. Cr levels in mainstream smoke range from 0.2 to 500 ng per cigarette [28]. Cr(VI) is recognized by the International Agency for Cancer Research as a group I carcinogen [29]. The metal may exert its genotoxic effects by directly inducing DNA single-strand breaks [30] or may act indirectly by potentiating the DNA-damaging effects of other agents. Thus, Cr(VI) has been shown to greatly enhance benzo(a)pyrene diol epoxide-DNA binding at mutational hot spots of the p53 gene [31].

Lead. Pb is of public health concern because of its high neurotoxic potential. Children are at a particularly high risk, because Pb interferes with the development of the brain and nervous system. Blood Pb levels as low as 2 µg/dl have been associated with hyperactivity symptoms, and decreased IQ and cognition in 1- to 5-year-old children [reviewed in ref. 32]. Such low Pb levels have been found in children exposed to environmental tobacco smoke (ETS). In highly ETS-exposed children, blood Pb levels can exceed 10 µg/dl (see also chapter 9).

Selenium. Although Se is contained in tobacco smoke, its blood levels are reduced in smokers [26]. The reasons for this phenomenon have not been clarified. Low Se levels may be detrimental, since it is a cofactor of enzymes that are involved in antioxidant activity against radicals and in the repair of oxidative DNA damage.

Copper. Tobacco contains 10–15 µg Cu/g dry weight, of which very little, 0.2%, pass to the smoke [33]. Nevertheless, plasma Cu levels and erythrocyte Cu-Zn superoxide dismutase activity were observed to be higher in tobacco smokers than in nonsmokers [34]. This increase may be of importance, since Cu plasma levels correlate with the degree of lipid peroxidation in smokers [26]. The correlation is plausible in view of the fact that Cu^{2+} is an effective catalyst in the so-called Fenton reaction, which results in the production of reactive oxygen species (ROS) and concomitant lipid peroxidation.

Radioactive Compounds. ^{210}Po and its precursor ^{210}Pb are contained in the tobacco plant and are transferred at appreciable amounts from processed tobacco to tobacco smoke [reviewed in ref. 35]. The radioactive ^{210}Po has a relatively short half-life of about 138 days, but is continually replaced through the decay of ^{210}Pb, which has a half-life of 22 years. Mean tissue concentrations of ^{210}Po in smokers have been found to be more than twice those of nonsmokers [36]. The effective whole body radiation dose of ^{210}Po to the average cigarette smoker is estimated to be 0.3 mSv, i.e. 30 mrem/year [35], suggesting a low level of exposure. However, since ^{210}Pb and ^{210}Po are contained in tobacco smoke particles and deposit at rather closely circumscribed areas of the lung [36], the local radiation exposure to ^{210}Pb and ^{210}Po will be much higher. Aside from that, ^{210}Po emits α-particles, which have a range of only 40 µm in the body. Thus, cells at the site of ^{210}Po deposition are likely to receive a high radiation dose. Even then, the radionuclide has been estimated to be responsible for not more than 1% of all lung cancers in the USA [37].

Radicals

Tobacco smoke carries a high load of radicals [reviewed in ref. 38]. The particulate phase contains $>10^{17}$ radicals/puff and the gaseous phase $>10^{15}$ radicals/puff [39]. The prevalent species are derived from oxygen, nitrogen, sulfur or organic alkoxyls and peroxyls.

ROS are generated by sequential reduction of oxygen to form superoxide anions ($O_2^{.-}$) and hydroxyl radicals ($^{.}OH$). Hydroxyl radicals have a half-life of milliseconds and, thus, react immediately with organic molecules at their site of production. $O_2^{.-}$ radicals are somewhat more stable than $^{.}OH$ radicals and able to cover a distance in the range of 1 µm [40]. Reactive nitrogen species are oxidation products of NO, which is generated from nitrogen-containing compounds in tobacco during combustion. NO itself is not toxic at concentrations found in tobacco smoke. Its adverse effects are mainly caused by autoxidation to the more reactive $NO_2^{.}$ Of greater importance is the interaction of NO with $O_2^{.-}$ to form the potent oxidant peroxynitrite ($ONOO^{-}$), which can be protonated to yield peroxynitrous acid (HNO_3). The latter is highly reactive, unstable and capable of both oxidizing and nitrating aromatic molecules. HNO_3 may also isomerize, giving rise to hydroxyl and nitrogen dioxide radicals. Radicals and oxidants in cigarette smoke do not only emerge from the combustion process. They are also continuously formed and inactivated by secondary reactions in the tobacco smoke increasing in concentration as the smoke ages [38].

Radicals in the particulate phase have a much longer half-life than those in the gaseous phase [38]. They may persist for hours, weeks and even months. The principal generator of these radicals is thought to be a quinone/semiquinone/hydroquinone system that undergoes redox cycling, thereby reducing oxygen and generating ROS [38]. In consequence, the site of deposition and retention time of the particles are key determinants for the toxicity of radicals in vivo.

Concluding Comments

In view of the high number of toxic compounds in tobacco smoke and their potential interactions, it is virtually impossible to attribute an adverse effect to a single compound. An attempt has been made to assess the relative health risk of individual tobacco smoke components by taking their yields and toxic potential into consideration [41]. Based on this approach, 1,3-butadiene poses the highest cancer risk, acrolein and acetaldehyde are the strongest respiratory irritants, and cyanide, arsenic and cresols are the primary sources of cardiovascular risks. More recently, another similar assessment has been carried out to establish the potential health risks of smoke components for cancer, cardiovascular and respiratory diseases [42]. Although the two assessments differ widely in their risk estimates of individual smoke components, they agree on the overall finding that volatile small organic molecules, e.g. 1,3-butadiene, acetaldehyde, acronitrile, benzene, formaldehyde and acetamide, rate highest on the list of hazardous tobacco smoke components. N-nitrosamines and PAH, which have frequently been in the focus of attention, take only a low position on this list. Notably, radicals in tobacco smoke were not considered in the two risk assessments, even though they might be prime contributors to the toxicity of tobacco smoke. This is most likely attributable to the fact that not enough is known about their composition and their effective dose at the site of action.

Primary Toxic Effects

As shown above, there is an abundance of organic and inorganic molecules in tobacco smoke which are reactive and potentially toxic. Accordingly, the primary effects of these agents are multifaceted ranging from reversible disturbance of cell functions, impairments in the immune system to irreversible changes in growth control, which can ultimately lead to lung disease, cardiovascular failure and cancer (see also chapters 7 and 8) [2]. Tobacco smoke poses a particularly high threat to the lung, because it contains to considerable amounts of oxidants and radicals, which can directly attack the epithelial cells once they have overcome or eluded the protective shield of the ELF.

The reactive agents damage cells and tissues in various ways. They may interact with sensors and receptors at cellular membranes which signal the external threat to the cellular interior and evoke a defensive response [2]. Depending on the type of agent and affected cells, this may involve the induction of enzymes, stimulation of phagocytosis, initiation of cell replication or triggering of programmed cell death (apoptosis), for example. The reactive agents in tobacco smoke may also elicit a systemic response activating the innate immune system and, with that, inducing inflammation [2].

An essential element of the inflammatory process is the recruitment of neutrophilic leukocytes by pulmonary macrophages to the site of action. The accumulation of leukocytes in peripheral lung can be deleterious in various respects. First, leukocytes are principal producers of ROS and add substantially to the burden of reactive species derived from tobacco smoke eventually leading to oxidative stress. Second, neutrophilic leukocytes and macrophages are main sources of elastases, which degrade the elastic fibers of lung. If unchecked by their physiological counterparts, α_1-antiproteinase and tissue inhibitor metalloproteinase, elastases irrevocably reduce the elasticity of the lung causing the development of emphysema and chronic obstructive pulmonary disease (see chapter 7). Third, ROS inactivate α_1-antiproteinases by oxidizing methionine 351 and 358 in the catalytic center of the enzyme [43], tilting the elastase/anti-elastase balance further in the direction of the elastase.

Aside from their interaction with specific signal-transducing components in the cellular membrane, reactive tobacco smoke ingredients may attack cells at random. They can cause extensive lipid peroxidation and inactivation of proteins in membranes disrupting their integrity and function to the point where the cells are no longer able to maintain their regulatory control function and may, eventually, die. In the case of peripheral lung disease, tobacco smoke injures and destroys first alveolar type I cells, which line the alveolar surface. This leaves the underlying interstitial tissue and endothelial cell layer more accessible to the toxic agents, and the impact of the tobacco smoke components is amplified. Repair of the damage to alveolar type I cells may in-

Table 1. DSM-V symptom groups and criteria for tobacco use disorder

Symptom group	Criteria
Impaired control	More tobacco use or for a longer period than intended (1)
	Unsuccessful efforts to stop or cut down use (2)
	Spending a great deal of time obtaining, using or recovering from use (3)
	Craving for substance (4)
Social impairment	Failure to fulfill major obligations due to use (5)
	Continued use despite problems caused or exacerbated by use (6)
	Important activities given up or reduced because of substance use (7)
Risky use	Recurrent use in hazardous situations (8)
	Continued use despite physical or psychological problems that are caused or exacerbated by substance use (9)
Pharmacological dependence	Tolerance to effects of the substance (10)
	Withdrawal symptoms when not using or using less (11)

DSM-V defines a substance use disorder as the presence of at least 2 of the 11 criteria listed above, which are clustered in four groups. DSM-V suggests using the number of criteria met as a general measure of severity: from mild (2–3 criteria) to moderate (4–5 criteria) and severe (6 or more criteria) [13].

ational activities are reduced because of tobacco use, and (7) use of the substance continues despite recurrent physical or psychological problems caused or exacerbated by tobacco. As defined by the DSM-IV, nicotine withdrawal is a condition in which a person, after using nicotine daily for at least several weeks, exhibits at least four of the following symptoms within 24 h after reduction or cessation of tobacco use: (1) dysphoric or depressed mood; (2) insomnia; (3) irritability, frustration or anger; (4) anxiety; (5) difficulty concentrating; (6) restlessness, and (7) decreased heart rate [12].

DSM-V was published in 2013 with a threshold for tobacco use disorder set as two or more criteria across the four symptom groups listed in table 1. The criteria for tobacco use disorder are the same as those for other substance use disorders. DSM-IV did not have a category for tobacco abuse. Consequently, the criteria in DSM-V that are from DSM-IV are new for tobacco [13].

Several authors have questioned the utility of the DSM-IV classification (present/not present) and suggest that the weight of evidence indicates the criteria are ambiguous, are not used in human clinical research and are lacking the ability to predict important clinical outcomes such as relapse likelihood. They recommend including new items (smoking pattern, smoking heaviness and the severity of craving) from the instruments described below and deletion of several of the original DSM indicators of nicotine dependence, in order to simplify and strengthen future versions of the classification algorithm (e.g. DSM-V) [14, 15].

In research on nicotine dependence, the most widely used instrument to assess physical dependence is the Fagerström Test of Nicotine Dependence [16], a questionnaire consisting of 6 items to assess physical dependence (see table 2 for items, response options and scoring). The total scale score can range from 0 to 10 with a high level of nicotine dependence indicated by a score of 6 or greater. The scale score correlates highly with the total number of cigarettes smoked daily. One of the items on the Fagerström Test of Nicotine Dependence assesses the time interval from waking to smoking the first cigarette of the day. A shorter interval is thought to be a strong indicator of nicotine dependence [15].

Because modern conceptualizations view nicotine dependence as consisting of multiple constructs, two multidimensional scales, the Nicotine Dependence Syndrome Scale (NDSS) and the Wisconsin Inventory of Smoking Dependence Motives (WISDM-68), have been recently developed and are described briefly below.

NDSS [17] is a 19-item questionnaire based on Edwards's syndromal conceptualization of dependence [18]. The original NDSS consisted of five factors named *drive* (craving and withdrawal, and subjective compulsion to smoke), *priority* (preference for smoking over other reinforcers), *tolerance* (reduced sensitivity to the effects of smoking), *continuity* (regulation of smoking rate) and *stereotypy* (invariance of smoking). The other assessment tool, the WISDM-68 [19], was developed based on theoretically grounded motives for

Table 2. Items, response options and scoring for the Fagerström test for nicotine dependence [16]

Item	Response options (points)
(1) How soon after waking do you smoke your first cigarette?	Within 5 min (3) 6–30 min (2) 31–60 min (1) After 60 min (0)
(2) Do you find it difficult to refrain from smoking in places where it is forbidden?	Yes (1) No (0)
(3) Which cigarette would you hate to give up?	The first one in the morning (1) All the others (0)
(4) How many cigarettes do you smoke?	10 or less (0) 11–20 (1) 21–30 (2) 31 or more (3)
(5) Do you smoke more frequently during the first hours after waking than during the rest of the day?	Yes (1) No (0)
(6) Do you smoke if you are so ill you are in bed most of the day?	Yes (1) No (0)

drug use. The scale consists of 68 items comprising 13 subscales with adequate psychometric properties [19, 20]. This factor structure has recently been refined to include four primary dependence motives (*automaticity, craving, loss of control* and *tolerance*) and nine secondary dependence motives (*affiliative attachment, behavioral choice/melioration, cognitive enhancement, cue exposure/associated processes, negative reinforcement, positive reinforcement, social/environmental goads, taste/sensory processes* and *weight control*) [21].

Vulnerability to Nicotine Dependence

Genetics

Meta-analyses of many twin studies from Australia, the United States, Finland and Sweden, as well as analyses of other cohorts, support the conclusion that smoking initiation and persistence have a significant genetic component [22–24]. Additive genetic factors account for 35 and 52% of the total variation in smoking initiation and 60 and 45% of smoking persistence in male and female adults, respectively (see also chapter 6).

Variants in the nicotinic receptor gene cluster on chromosome 15q24–25.1 (*CHRNA5-CHRNA3-CHRNB4)* were first reported to be associated with nicotine dependence by Saccone et al. [25] from a genome-wide association study in a sample of European Americans. A subsequent series of papers (also relying on genome-wide association methodology) confirmed this association for smoking quantity [26–28]. Because nAChR subunits in this gene cluster reduce the aversive effects of nicotine and promote its consumption [29, 30], some have speculated that people with one or more single nucleotide polymorphisms (SNPs) in the gene cluster smoke more and become addicted at a younger age because they lack sufficient functional α5 nAChRs [31].

Macroenvironmental Factors

In the USA, smoking rates among women increased from 18% in 1935 to >50% in 1960 [32]. Since that time, smoking rates have declined among both men and women, but remain slightly higher among men (22.3 vs. 17.4% in 2007) [33]. A number of social, cultural and demographic factors are also associated with tobacco use and dependence. These include education, race/ethnicity, socioeconomic status and sexual orientation. Smoking rates are disproportionately high among people with lower education levels [34] (see chapter 16).

Similarly, smoking rates vary significantly among different racial and ethnic populations [33]. They are also disproportionately higher in the lesbian, gay and bisexual communities [35]. Rates of tobacco use and dependence are also higher among people with psychiatric disorders [36, 37] (see chapter 17). For a more complete discussion of macroenvironmental influences, the reader is referred to a recent review [38].

Pharmacokinetics of Nicotine

Smoking is an optimal nicotine delivery system to the brain that is under complete control by the smoker, who can regulate nicotine concentrations in the brain by the number of cigarettes smoked and the frequency of puffs and inhalations. During smoking, a large portion of the nicotine in the tobacco is burnt, but part is vaporized and inhaled into the lungs from where it is readily absorbed and distributed throughout the body via the bloodstream. Details of the pharmacokinetics and metabolism of nicotine have been reviewed by Benowitz et al. [39]. Briefly, nicotine rapidly reaches high brain concentrations, which increase sharply with each puff to a maximum level after each cigarette. The usual range of nicotine concentrations in arterial blood is 20–60 ng/ml (120–350 nM), which declines rapidly when not smoking anymore. The half-life of nicotine in human plasma is about 2 h and it is extensively metabolized in the liver by CYP2A6 and CYP2B6, with cotinine as the main metabolite. Cotinine has a half-life of 16–20 h, remains in the blood for a long time and is detectable for up to a week after the use of tobacco. Because cotinine blood concentrations (250–300 ng/ml) are much higher and more stable than those of nicotine, cotinine is used as a biomarker for nicotine exposure in cigarette smokers and passive smokers. Since nicotine is eliminated with a half-life of about 2 h, it will accumulate during a day of smoking and still be present in significant amounts after the last cigarette in the evening and during the night. The metabolism and excretion of nicotine and its metabolites are determined by genetic factors and strongly influenced among others by age, gender, race, kidney disease, smoking and the presence of drugs that can inhibit or induce the activity of CYP2A6.

Mechanisms of Nicotine Dependence

The pharmacological actions of nicotine that lead to nicotine dependence are almost exclusively mediated via nAChRs, for which the endogenous neurotransmitter is ACh. This section summarizes the structure and functioning of nAChRs, the pharmacological actions of nicotine and other nAChR ligands, and the role of nAChR subtypes that are also potential targets for new smoking cessation aids (for more details, see recent reviews [1, 5, 40] and chapter 20).

Nicotinic Acetylcholine Receptors

nAChRs belong to the family of ligand-gated ion channels and consist of 5 protein subunits arranged in a doughnut-like manner, forming a pore in their center that functions as the ion channel. There are 10 α subunits and 4 β subunits known, which are assembled into at least 14 different subtypes of nAChRs, which can be either heteromeric (made up of α and β subunits) or homomeric (containing only α subunits). Each pentameric nAChR contains two binding sites for ACh or nicotinic ligands, which are located between adjacent subunits (fig. 2a).

Functional Effects of Nicotine at Nicotinic Acetylcholine Receptors

When nAChRs are activated by brief exposure to an agonist, the ion channel opens, resulting in depolarization and excitatory postsynaptic potentials until the agonist dissociates from the binding site, in a matter of milliseconds, and the ion channel closes again. The deactivated nAChR can be activated again by another short pulse of the agonist. However, upon prolonged exposure to an agonist, the nAChR transitions into a desensitized state and can no longer be activated for an extended time. Only after the agonist concentration decreases and it starts to dissociate from the binding site, does the nAChR transition back to a deactivated, closed state and is ready to be activated again by an agonist (fig. 2b). Agonists are usually much more potent in desensitizing than in activating nAChRs (fig. 3a). This is relevant for the pharmacological effects of nicotine and smoking cessation agents, since these compounds are present much longer at nAChRs than endogenous ACh. For instance, at clinical doses, the main effect of the α4β2 agonists nicotine, varenicline, cytisine and dianicline is the desensitization of the α4β2 nAChRs [41], while efficacious concentrations of the α3β4 partial agonist AT-1001 have been shown to potently desensitize human α3β4 nAChRs [42].

The efficacy, or intrinsic activity, of an nAChR ligand indicates if it is a full agonist, a partial agonist or an antagonist (fig. 3b). Compounds that cause the same maximal activation of nAChRs as the maximal response evoked by the endogenous ligand ACh are full agonists (100% efficacy). Compounds that induce a smaller maximal effect than ACh are partial agonists (>0 and <100% efficacy), while compounds that bind to, but do not activate the nAChR and prevent full activation by ACh, are antagonists (0% efficacy). The endogenous neurotransmitter ACh is a full agonist at all nAChR subtypes, but exogenous compounds can be partial agonists at certain nAChRs and full agonists or antagonists at other subtypes. The functional activity of nAChRs can also be modulated by ligands that have no affinity for the orthosteric ligand binding sites, but interact with a different (allosteric) site on the ion channel. Such

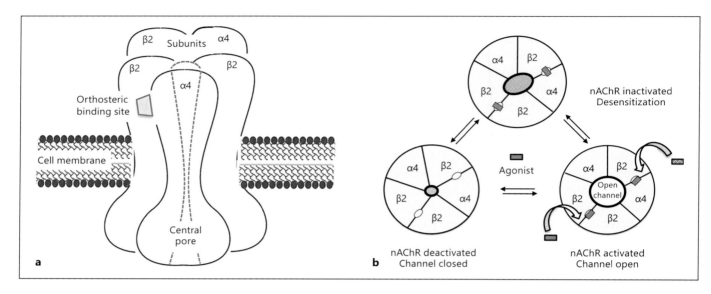

Fig. 2. Schematic representation of the structure and functional states of the α4β2 nAChR. **a** An α4β2 nAChR in the cell membrane showing 5 subunits (2 α4 and 3 β2 subunits) that form a central pore (ion channel). One of the two orthosteric binding sites between adjacent α4 and β2 subunits is also shown. **b** Binding of an agonist (e.g. ACh or nicotine) to the two binding sites of nAChR induces subtle changes in the conformation of the subunits that cause the ion channel to open (activation). Upon dissociation of the agonist, the ion channel closes again (deactivation), while prolonged exposure to an agonist causes desensitization (inactivation) of the nAChR, until the agonist dissociates again from the binding sites (reactivation).

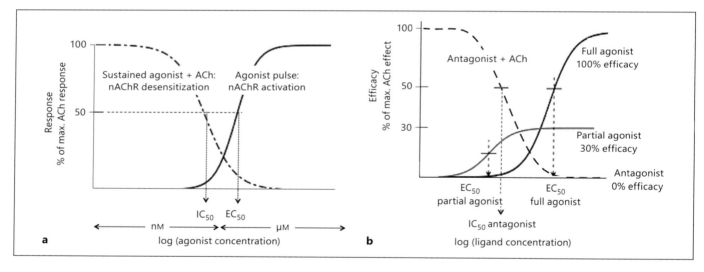

Fig. 3. Functional effects of nAChR ligands. **a** Concentration-dependent activation and desensitization of nAChRs. Short exposure to an agonist activates the nAChR. The EC_{50} indicates the activation potency of the agonist and 'agonist efficacy' is the maximal effect relative to ACh (i.e. 100% agonist efficacy denotes a full agonist). Prolonged exposure to an agonist can cause nAChR desensitization, which reduces the ACh-induced activation of nAChRs. The IC_{50} indicates the inhibitory or desensitization potency of the agonist. Agonists are usually more potent in inactivating (IC_{50} in the nM range) than activating (EC_{50} in the μM range) nAChRs. **b** nAChR ligands are full agonists, partial agonists or antagonists. Full agonists have the same maximal effect as ACh (100% efficacy), partial agonists have a lower maximal effect than ACh (<100% efficacy). In this example, the partial agonist has less efficacy (30%) than the full agonist, but is more potent (lower EC_{50} value). Antagonists bind to, but do not activate, nAChRs and will thus inhibit activation by ACh or by exogenous agonists (dotted curve; IC_{50} is the antagonist potency).

compounds can either increase the activity of nAChRs (positive allosteric modulators) or decrease nAChR activity (negative allosteric modulators).

Pharmacological Effects of Nicotine

The pharmacological responses that contribute to both the reinforcing effects of nicotine during smoking and the craving symptoms upon smoking cessation are mediated through various nAChRs subtypes located in different brain areas [1, 5]. The interaction with nicotine modulates the release of a variety of neurotransmitters, including monoamines, GABA, glutamate, corticotropin-releasing factor, neuropeptide Y, substance P and hypocretins [43].

The nicotine-induced release of dopamine in the mesolimbic reward pathway initiates a physiological response that contributes to the reinforcing effects of nicotine. Between cigarettes, brain nicotine levels gradually decrease, triggering several processes that contribute to the cycle of craving and urge to smoke that maintains nicotine dependence. It is believed that the rapidly recurring and transitory increases in mesolimbic dopamine levels following repeated exposure to, and withdrawal from, nicotine transmit salient reward and aversive signals to higher cortical centers, facilitating the learning and associations that lead to physical dependence, characterized by both somatic and psychoactive symptoms. Besides the direct effect of nicotine on mesolimbic dopamine release through the α4β2* and α4β2α6* nAChRs on dopaminergic neurons, nicotine can also modulate mesolimbic dopamine release through various nAChR subtypes that are located on glutamatergic, GABAergic and cholinergic neurons. The dopaminergic system is connected with other circuits that are involved in the regulation of various aspects of nicotine dependence, not necessarily through mesolimbic dopamine.

An important aspect of the pharmacology of nicotine is that chronic exposure can induce persistent molecular and cellular adaptations that are thought to underlie withdrawal symptoms, even after long periods of abstinence, which lead to relapse. It has been well established that chronic nicotine causes an increase in the density of nAChRs, which was observed in smokers and laboratory animals, and in cell cultures expressing nAChRs. The agonist-induced upregulation of nAChRs was a surprising finding, given that repeated exposure of agonists of other cell surface receptors causes a downregulation to compensate for the continuous activation by agonists. The nicotine-induced upregulation of nAChRs is likely a response to receptor desensitization, and several molecular mechanisms have been postulated that could mediate this type of neuroadaptation [44]. Most

nAChR upregulation studies have been performed with nicotine, but nAChR upregulation is also reported for other α4β2 nAChR agonists, as well as for α7 agonists and α4β2 antagonists [45, 46]. Interestingly, agonists are more potent at upregulating (EC_{50} in nM range) than at activating nAChRs (EC_{50} in μM range), whereas antagonists are 2–3 orders of magnitude less potent at upregulating than at antagonizing ACh-induced receptor activation. Since both agonists and antagonists can increase the density of different nAChR subtypes, receptor upregulation may have therapeutic relevance, especially if it occurs at such low concentrations that the net result of upregulation and nAChR desensitization is a gain of function.

Finally, neuroadaptive changes are thought to underlie the effect of chronic nicotine on lowering the threshold for the use of other drugs of abuse. Recent insights from molecular biology studies on the effects of nicotine show that long-term exposure to nicotine may induce changes in the acetylation state of the striatum, a brain region involved in addiction, which would create an environment conducive to activation by other drugs of abuse, particularly cocaine, marijuana and alcohol. These data have been proposed as a molecular basis for the hypothesis that nicotine acts as a 'gateway drug', i.e. that nicotine is a starting point of a sequence of drug use that can proceed to the use of other drugs (for a review, see Kandel and Kandel [47]).

Given the complexity of the effects of nicotine, it is difficult to predict the net outcome of nicotine-induced activation, desensitization and/or upregulation of nAChR subtypes located on neurons that can respond with an increase or decrease in the release of either stimulatory or inhibitory transmitters. Though this represents a challenge for the discovery of novel selective smoking cessation aids, the search for compounds that are selective for certain nAChR subtypes has led to exciting findings.

Nicotinic Acetylcholine Receptor Subtypes: Role in Nicotine Dependence and as Targets for New Medications

α4β2* Nicotinic Acetylcholine Receptors

The most prevalent nAChR in the CNS is the α4β2 nAChR, which is a major subtype involved in nicotine addiction. Nicotine has higher affinity for the α4β2 nAChR than for other subtypes and will thus preferentially bind to this subtype. Preclinical studies in genetically modified mice have provided evidence that α4β2* nAChRs located in the mesolimbic system, with cell bodies in the ventral tegmental area and terminals in the nucleus accumbens, regulate the release of mesolimbic dopamine that mediates reward and reinforcement. The important role of α4β2 nAChRs is also supported by the clinical efficacy of the selective α4β2 nAChR partial agonist varenicline as a smoking cessation aid (see chapter 20).

α6* Nicotinic Acetylcholine Receptors

Studies using neurotoxic peptides from the cone snail (conotoxins) that are selective α6β2* antagonists, have demonstrated that α6β2* nAChRs (e.g. α4α6β2β3* and α6β2β3*) in the nucleus accumbens and striatum are the main regulators of mesolimbic dopamine release. Given the key role of α6* nAChRs in nicotine-induced reinforcement, partial or full agonists at α6* nAChR might be expected to aid smoking cessation, possibly with better efficacy than α4β2 nAChR partial agonists. Interestingly, recent studies revealed that the α4β2* nAChR partial agonist varenicline is also a high-affinity, potent α6β2* partial agonist and stimulates [³H]-dopamine release in rat and monkey striatal synaptosomes both via α4β2* and α6β2* nAChRs, an effect that may contribute to the efficacy of varenicline for nicotine dependence [48].

α3β4* Nicotinic Acetylcholine Receptors

As mentioned earlier, several human genetic association studies found that single nucleotide polymorphisms in the gene cluster CHRNA5-CHRNA3-CHRNB4, encoding for α3, α5 and β4 subunits, are closely associated with the risk for heavy smoking, inability to quit and increased sensitivity to nicotine [49–53]. Unlike the wide distribution of α4β2 nAChRs in the brain, α3 and β4 subunits are expressed in a restricted number of brain areas, mainly the medial habenula (MHb) and interpeduncular nucleus (IPN), which are major cholinergic tracts in the brain recently associated with various aspects of nicotine dependence [29, 30, 54–56]. Studies in transgenic mouse and rat models have shown that the β4 subunit is necessary for nicotine withdrawal [57] and that α3β4 nAChRs in the MHb-IPN tract are highly activated upon nicotine exposure during nicotine withdrawal [55]. Consistent with genetic studies, overexpression of the α5, α3 and β4 nAChR subunit genes in mice increased nicotine self-administration [58].

Given the prominence of the α3β4* and α3β4α5* subtypes in nicotine dependence and their high expression in the MHb-IPN tract, the α3β4 nAChR has become a promising target in the search for novel smoking cessation agents. Recently, it was shown that a selective, high-affinity α3β4 nAChR ligand, AT-1001, potently blocks nicotine self-administration in rats at doses that do not affect nonspecific food responding [59]. Subsequent studies found that AT-1001 blocks nicotine prime and stress-induced reinstatement of extinguished nicotine seeking in rats. Interestingly, it was recently shown that AT-1001 causes desensitization of human α3β4 nAChRs at concentrations at which it functions as a partial agonist [42]. These mechanisms may underlie its behavioral effects in inhibiting nicotine seeking, suggesting that α3β4* ligands such as AT-1001 could represent new smoking cessation agents with a novel mechanism of action.

α5* Nicotinic Acetylcholine Receptors

The human CHRNA5 gene that encodes for the α5 subunit, which is part of the gene cluster CHRNA5-CHRNA3-CHRNB4, is closely associated with aspects of smoking behavior, including increased sensitivity to nicotine. Studies in transgenic animals confirmed that the presence of an α5 subunit in nAChRs in the MHb and IPN plays an important role in nicotine dependence, as it can significantly impact the functional response to nicotine and the regulation of nicotine intake. For instance, deletion of the α5 subunit causes an increase in nicotine self-administration, whereas reexpression of the α5 subunit in the MHb of α5 knockout mice restored nicotine intake to control levels [29]. These results show that α5* nAChRs mediate the aversive response to nicotine and participate in reward control mechanisms, implying that greater activation of α5* nAChRs than that caused by nicotine will increase aversion to nicotine and may be a potential novel mechanism for treating nicotine dependence. At this time, there are no compounds in development that specifically target α5* nAChRs.

α7 Nicotinic Acetylcholine Receptors

The α7 subtype may also play a role in nicotine dependence, based on the association of CHRNA7 genes with smoking behavior and on the finding that the expression of α7 nAChRs is reduced in the brain of schizophrenic patients. This suggests that these patients could be heavy smokers because of the reduced activation of α7 nAChRs. Preclinical studies with α7 nAChR ligands have mixed results, in that α7 nAChR antagonists were found either not to affect or to decrease nicotine intake. Other behavioral and neurochemical studies reported that inactivation or deletion of α7 nAChRs stimulates nicotine intake and potentiates nicotine-evoked dopamine release, while activation of α7 nAChRs reduced nicotine self-administration. Opposing the effect of nicotine by activating α7 nAChRs could therefore be a promising smoking cessation strategy [60].

Conclusions

Significant progress made in the past decade has increased our understanding of the genetics and mechanisms of nicotine dependence. These efforts are beginning to unravel several new approaches to curb the impact of the tobacco epidemic on public health and mortality. The elucidation of genetic factors influencing nicotine dependence is already shaping the clinical assessments of smoking cessation trials and factors underlying successful abstinence. The ongoing effort to elucidate the neurobiological mechanisms of nicotine dependence is uncovering several new targets, such as other nAChR subtypes and various neurotransmitter systems, for pharmacotherapeutic interventions that will likely result in new treatments to assist smoking cessation. Continued momentum on all these fronts will be required to further reduce the serious health consequences of nicotine dependence.

Key Points

- New approaches to assess nicotine dependence have become available besides the Fagerström Test, i.e. the DSM-V measure of the severity of tobacco use disorder, the Nicotine Dependence Syndrome Scale and the Wisconsin Inventory of Smoking Dependence Motives.
- The well-established association between variants in the nicotinic gene cluster on chromosome 15q24–25.1 (*CHRNA5-CHRNA3-CHRNB4*) and nicotine dependence led to the identification of novel therapeutic targets.
- Elucidation of genetic factors influencing nicotine dependence is shaping the clinical assessment of smoking cessation trials and factors underlying successful abstinence.
- Chronic exposure to nicotine can induce persistent molecular and cellular adaptations that underlie withdrawal symptoms and can lead to relapse, even after long periods of abstinence.
- The addictive effects of nicotine are almost exclusively mediated via its interactions with nAChRs, which modulate the release of several neurotransmitters.
- Elucidation of the neurobiological mechanisms is uncovering new promising targets for pharmacotherapeutic interventions to assist smoking cessation, such as $\alpha3\beta4^*$ nAChRs. AT-1001 is the first example of a selective, high-affinity $\alpha3\beta4$ nAChR ligand that blocks nicotine self-administration in rats.

Acknowledgements

The authors wish to acknowledge the following sources of grant support from the National Institute on Drug Abuse: R43DA033744 and R44DA033744 (N.Z.), and U01DA20830 (G.E.S.).

References

1 D'Souza MS, Markou A: Neuronal mechanisms underlying development of nicotine dependence: implications for novel smoking-cessation treatments. Addict Sci Clin Pract 2011;6:4–16.

2 Henningfield JE, Miyasato K, Jasinski DR: Abuse liability and pharmacodynamic characteristics of intravenous and inhaled nicotine. J Pharmacol Exp Ther 1985;234:1–12.

3 Shiffman SM, Jarvik ME: Smoking withdrawal symptoms in two weeks of abstinence. Psychopharmacology (Berl) 1976;50:35–39.

4 Hughes JR: Effects of abstinence from tobacco: etiology, animal models, epidemiology, and significance: a subjective review. Nicotine Tob Res 2007;9:329–339.

5 Benowitz NL: Neurobiology of nicotine addiction: implications for smoking cessation treatment. Am J Med 2008;121:S3–S10.

6 Schnoll RA, Leone FT: Biomarkers to optimize the treatment of nicotine dependence. Biomark Med 2011;5:745–761.

7 Hughes JR, Keely J, Naud S: Shape of the relapse curve and long-term abstinence among untreated smokers. Addiction 2004;99:29–38.

8 Javitz HS, Swan GE, Lerman C: The dynamics of the urge-to-smoke following smoking cessation via pharmacotherapy. Addiction 2011;106:1835–1845.

9 Javitz HS, Lerman C, Swan GE: Comparative dynamics of four smoking withdrawal symptom scales. Addiction 2012;107:1501–1511.

10 Brody AL, Mandelkern MA, London ED, Olmstead RE, Farahi J, Scheibal D, Jou J, Allen V, Tiongson E, Chefer SI, Koren AO, Mukhin AG: Cigarette smoking saturates brain alpha 4 beta 2 nicotinic acetylcholine receptors. Arch Gen Psychiatry 2006;63:907–915.

11 Dani JA, Heinemann S: Molecular and cellular aspects of nicotine abuse. Neuron 1996;16:905–908.

12 Diagnostic and Statistical Manual of Mental Disorders, ed 4. Washington, American Psychiatric Association, 2000.

13 Diagnostic and Statistical Manual of Mental Disorders, ed 5. Washington, American Psychiatric Association, 2013.

14 O'Brien C: Addiction and dependence in DSM-V. Addiction 2011;106:866–867.

15 Baker TB, Breslau N, Covey L, Shiffman S: DSM criteria for tobacco use disorder and tobacco withdrawal: a critique and proposed revisions for DSM-5. Addiction 2012;107:263–275.

16 Heatherton TF, Kozlowski LT, Frecker RC, Fagerström KO: The Fagerström Test for Nicotine Dependence: a revision of the Fagerström Tolerance Questionnaire. Br J Addict 1991;86:1119–1127.

17 Shiffman S, Waters A, Hickcox M: The nicotine dependence syndrome scale: a multidimensional measure of nicotine dependence. Nicotine Tob Res 2004;6:327–348.

18 Edwards G: The alcohol dependence syndrome: a concept as stimulus to enquiry. Br J Addict 1986; 81:171–183.

19 Piper ME, Piasecki TM, Federman EB, Bolt DM, Smith SS, Fiore MC, Baker TB: A multiple motives approach to tobacco dependence: the Wisconsin Inventory of Smoking Dependence Motives (WISDM-68). J Consult Clin Psychol 2004;72: 139–154.

20 Piper ME, McCarthy DE, Bolt DM, Smith SS, Lerman C, Benowitz N, Fiore MC, Baker TB: Assessing dimensions of nicotine dependence: an evaluation of the Nicotine Dependence Syndrome Scale (NDSS) and the Wisconsin Inventory of Smoking Dependence Motives (WISDM). Nicotine Tob Res 2008;10:1009–1020.

21 Piasecki TM, Piper ME, Baker TB, Hunt-Carter EE: WISDM primary and secondary dependence motives: associations with self-monitored motives for smoking in two college samples. Drug Alcohol Depend 2011;114:207–216.

22 Lessov-Schlaggar CN, Pergadia ML, Khroyan TV, Swan GE: Genetics of nicotine dependence and pharmacotherapy. Biochem Pharmacol 2008;75:178–195.

23 Li MD, Cheng R, Ma JZ, Swan GE: A meta-analysis of estimated genetic and environmental effects on smoking behavior in male and female adult twins. Addiction 2003;98:23–31.

24 Swan GE, Lessov-Schlaggar CN: Tobacco addiction and pharmacogenetics of nicotine metabolism. J Neurogenet 2009;23:262–271.

25 Saccone SF, Hinrichs AL, Saccone NL, Chase GA, Konvicka K, Madden PA, Breslau N, Johnson EO, Hatsukami D, Pomerleau O, Swan GE, Goate AM, Rutter J, Bertelsen S, Fox L, Fugman D, Martin NG, Montgomery GW, Wang JC, Ballinger DG, Rice JP, Bierut LJ: Cholinergic nicotinic receptor genes implicated in a nicotine dependence association study targeting 348 candidate genes with 3713 SNPs. Hum Mol Genet 2007;16:36–49.

26 Amos CI, Wu X, Broderick P, Gorlov IP, Gu J, Eisen T, Dong Q, Zhang Q, Gu X, Vijayakrishnan J, Sullivan K, Matakidou A, Wang Y, Mills G, Doheny K, Tsai YY, Chen WV, Shete S, Spitz MR, Houlston RS: Genome-wide association scan of tag SNPs identifies a susceptibility locus for lung cancer at 15q25.1. Nat Genet 2008;40:616–622.

27 Hung RJ, McKay JD, Gaborieau V, Boffetta P, Hashibe M, Zaridze D, Mukeria A, Szeszenia-Dabrowska N, Lissowska J, Rudnai P, Fabianova E, Mates D, Bencko V, Foretova L, Janout V, Chen C, Goodman G, Field JK, Liloglou T, Xinarianos G, Cassidy A, McLaughlin J, Liu G, Narod S, Krokan HE, Skorpen F, Elvestad MB, Hveem K, Vatten L, Linseisen J, Clavel-Chapelon F, Vineis P, Bueno-de-Mesquita HB, Lund E, Martinez C, Bingham S, Rasmuson T, Hainaut P, Riboli E, Ahrens W, Benhamou S, Lagiou P, Trichopoulos D, Holcatova I, Merletti F, Kjaerheim K, Agudo A, Macfarlane G, Talamini R, Simonato L, Lowry R, Conway DI, Znaor A, Healy C, Zelenika D, Boland A, Delepine M, Foglio M, Lechner D, Matsuda F, Blanche H, Gut I, Heath S, Lathrop M, Brennan P: A susceptibility locus for lung cancer maps to nicotinic acetylcholine receptor subunit genes on 15q25. Nature 2008;452:633–637.

28 Thorgeirsson TE, Geller F, Sulem P, Rafnar T, Wiste A, Magnusson KP, Manolescu A, Thorleifsson G, Stefansson H, Ingason A, Stacey SN, Bergthorsson JT, Thorlacius S, Gudmundsson J, Jonsson T, Jakobsdottir M, Saemundsdottir J, Olafsdottir O, Gudmundsson LJ, Bjornsdottir G, Kristjansson K, Skuladottir H, Isaksson HJ, Gudbjartsson T, Jones GT, Mueller T, Gottsater A, Flex A, Aben KK, de Vegt F, Mulders PF, Isla D, Vidal MJ, Asin L, Saez B, Murillo L, Blondal T, Kolbeinsson H, Stefansson JG, Hansdottir I, Runarsdottir V, Pola R, Lindblad B, van Rij AM, Dieplinger B, Haltmayer M, Mayordomo JI, Kiemeney LA, Matthiasson SE, Oskarsson H, Tyrfingsson T, Gudbjartsson DF, Gulcher JR, Jonsson S, Thorsteinsdottir U, Kong A, Stefansson K: A variant associated with nicotine dependence, lung cancer and peripheral arterial disease. Nature 2008;452:638–642.

29 Fowler CD, Lu Q, Johnson PM, Marks MJ, Kenny PJ: Habenular α5 nicotinic receptor subunit signalling controls nicotine intake. Nature 2011;471:597–601.

30 Frahm S, Slimak MA, Ferrarese L, Santos-Torres J, Antolin-Fontes B, Auer S, Filkin S, Pons S, Fontaine JF, Tsetlin V, Maskos U, Ibanez-Tallon I: Aversion to nicotine is regulated by the balanced activity of β4 and α5 nicotinic receptor subunits in the medial habenula. Neuron 2011;70:522–535.

31 De Biasi M, Dani JA: Reward, addiction, withdrawal to nicotine. Annu Rev Neurosci 2011;34:105–130.

32 US Department of Health and Human Services: Women and Smoking: A Report of the Surgeon General. Atlanta, Centers for Disease Control and Prevention, National Center for Chronic Disease Prevention and Health Promotion, Office on Smoking and Health, 2001.

33 Centers for Disease Control and Prevention (CDC): Cigarette smoking among adults – United States, 2007. MMWR Morb Mortal Wkly Rep 2008;57:1221–1226.

34 Centers for Disease Control and Prevention (CDC): Cigarette smoking among adults and trends in smoking cessation – United States, 2008. MMWR Morb Mortal Wkly Rep 2009;58:1227–1232.

35 Lee JG, Griffin GK, Melvin CL: Tobacco use among sexual minorities in the USA, 1987 to May 2007: a systematic review. Tob Control 2009;18:275–282.

36 Diaz FJ, James D, Botts S, Maw L, Susce MT, de Leon J: Tobacco smoking behaviors in bipolar disorder: a comparison of the general population, schizophrenia, and major depression. Bipolar Disord 2009;11:154–165.

37 George TP, Ziedonis DM: Addressing tobacco dependence in psychiatric practice: promises and pitfalls. Can J Psychiatry 2009;54:353–355.

38 David SP, McClure JB, Swan GE: Nicotine dependence; in Weiner I (ed): Handbook of Psychology, ed 2. Hoboken, Wiley, 2013, vol 9: Health Psychology, Nezu A, Nezu CM, Geller PA (vol eds), pp 149–181.

39 Benowitz NL, Hukkanen J, Jacob P 3rd: Nicotine chemistry, metabolism, kinetics and biomarkers. Handb Exp Pharmacol 2009;192:29–60.

40 Hurst R, Rollema H, Bertrand D: Nicotinic acetylcholine receptors: from basic science to therapeutics. Pharmacol Ther 2013;137:22–54.

41 Rollema H, Shrikhande A, Ward KM, Tingley FD 3rd, Coe JW, O'Neill BT, Tseng E, Wang EQ, Mather RJ, Hurst RS, Williams KE, de Vries M, Cremers T, Bertrand S, Bertrand D: Pre-clinical properties of the alpha4beta2 nicotinic acetylcholine receptor partial agonists varenicline, cytisine and dianicline translate to clinical efficacy for nicotine dependence. Br J Pharmacol 2010;160:334–345.

42 Zaveri NT, Bertrand S, Yasuda D, Bertrand D: Functional characterization of AT-1001, an α3β4 nicotinic acetylcholine receptor (nAChR) ligand, at human α3β4 and α4β2 nAChR. Nicotine Tob Res 2014;pii:ntu170. Epub ahead of print.

43 Harmey D, Griffin PR, Kenny PJ: Development of novel pharmacotherapeutics for tobacco dependence: progress and future directions. Nicotine Tob Res 2012;14:1300–1318.

44 Govind AP, Walsh H, Green WN: Nicotine-induced upregulation of native neuronal nicotinic receptors is caused by multiple mechanisms. J Neurosci 2012;32:2227–2238.

45 Christensen DZ, Mikkelsen JD, Hansen HH, Thomsen MS: Repeated administration of alpha7 nicotinic acetylcholine receptor (nAChR) agonists, but not positive allosteric modulators, increases alpha7 nAChR levels in the brain. J Neurochem 2010;114:1205–1216.

46 Buisson B, Bertrand D: Chronic exposure to nicotine upregulates the human (alpha)4(beta)2 nicotinic acetylcholine receptor function. J Neurosci 2001;21:1819–1829.

47 Kandel ER, Kandel DB: Shattuck Lecture. A molecular basis for nicotine as a gateway drug. N Engl J Med 2014;371:932–943.

48 Bordia T, Hrachova M, Chin M, McIntosh JM, Quik M: Varenicline is a potent partial agonist at α6β2* nicotinic acetylcholine receptors in rat and monkey striatum. J Pharmacol Exp Ther 2012;342:327–334.

49 Weiss RB, Baker TB, Cannon DS, von Niederhausern A, Dunn DM, Matsunami N, Singh NA, Baird L, Coon H, McMahon WM, Piper ME, Fiore MC, Scholand MB, Connett JE, Kanner RE, Gahring LC, Rogers SW, Hoidal JR, Leppert MF: A candidate gene approach identifies the CHRNA5-A3-B4 region as a risk factor for age-dependent nicotine addiction. PLoS Genet 2008;4:e1000125.

50 Berrettini W, Yuan X, Tozzi F, Song K, Francks C, Chilcoat H, Waterworth D, Muglia P, Mooser V: Alpha-5/alpha-3 nicotinic receptor subunit alleles increase risk for heavy smoking. Mol Psychiatry 2008;13:368–373.

51 Saccone NL, Wang JC, Breslau N, Johnson EO, Hatsukami D, Saccone SF, Grucza RA, Sun L, Duan W, Budde J, Culverhouse RC, Fox L, Hinrichs AL, Steinbach JH, Wu M, Rice JP, Goate AM, Bierut LJ: The CHRNA5-CHRNA3-CHRNB4 nicotinic receptor subunit gene cluster affects risk for nicotine dependence in African-Americans and in European-Americans. Cancer Res 2009;69:6848–6856.

52 Caporaso N, Gu F, Chatterjee N, Sheng-Chih J, Yu K, Yeager M, Chen C, Jacobs K, Wheeler W, Landi MT, Ziegler RG, Hunter DJ, Chanock S, Hankinson S, Kraft P, Bergen AW: Genome-wide and candidate gene association study of cigarette smoking behaviors. PLoS One 2009;4:e4653.

53 Schlaepfer IR, Hoft NR, Collins AC, Corley RP, Hewitt JK, Hopfer CJ, Lessem JM, McQueen MB, Rhee SH, Ehringer MA: The CHRNA5/A3/B4 gene cluster variability as an important determinant of early alcohol and tobacco initiation in young adults. Biol Psychiatry 2008;63:1039–1046.

54 Grady SR, Moretti M, Zoli M, Marks MJ, Zanardi A, Pucci L, Clementi F, Gotti C: Rodent habenulo-interpeduncular pathway expresses a large variety of uncommon nAChR subtypes, but only the alpha3beta4* and alpha3beta3beta4* subtypes mediate acetylcholine release. J Neurosci 2009;29: 2272–2282.

55 Gorlich A, Antolin-Fontes B, Ables JL, Frahm S, Slimak MA, Dougherty JD, Ibanez-Tallon I: Reexposure to nicotine during withdrawal increases the pacemaking activity of cholinergic habenular neurons. Proc Natl Acad Sci U S A 2013;110: 17077–17082.

56 Dani JA, De Biasi M: Mesolimbic dopamine and habenulo-interpeduncular pathways in nicotine withdrawal. Cold Spring Harb Perspect Med 2013; 3:a012138.

57 Salas R, Pieri F, De Biasi M: Decreased signs of nicotine withdrawal in mice null for the beta4 nicotinic acetylcholine receptor subunit. J Neurosci 2004;24:10035–10039.

58 Gallego X, Molas S, Amador-Arjona A, Marks MJ, Robles N, Murtra P, Armengol L, Fernandez-Montes RD, Gratacos M, Pumarola M, Cabrera R, Maldonado R, Sabria J, Estivill X, Dierssen M: Overexpression of the CHRNA5/A3/B4 genomic cluster in mice increases the sensitivity to nicotine and modifies its reinforcing effects. Amino Acids 2012;43:897–909.

59 Toll L, Zaveri NT, Polgar W, Jiang F, Khroyan TV, Zhou W, Xie X, Stauber GB, Costello MR, Leslie FM: AT-1001: a high affinity and selective α3β4 nicotinic acetylcholine receptor antagonist blocks nicotine self-administration in rats. Neuropsychopharmacology 2012;37:1367–1376.

60 Brunzell DH, McIntosh JM, Papke RL: Diverse strategies targeting α7 homomeric and α6β2* heteromeric nicotinic acetylcholine receptors for smoking cessation. Ann NY Acad Sci 2014;1327: 27–45.

Gary E. Swan, PhD
Department of Medicine, Stanford Prevention Research Center, Stanford University School of Medicine
Medical School Office Building
1265 Welch Road
Stanford, CA 94305-5411 (USA)
E-Mail gswan@stanford.edu

Loddenkemper R, Kreuter M (eds): The Tobacco Epidemic, ed 2, rev. and ext.
Prog Respir Res. Basel, Karger, 2015, vol 42, pp 58–71 (DOI: 10.1159/000369325)

The Psychology of the Smoker

David G. Gilbert[a] · Michele L. Pergadia[b, c]

[a]Southern Illinois University, Carbondale, Ill., [b]Charles E. Schmidt College of Medicine, Florida Atlantic University, Boca Raton, Fla.,
and [c]Washington University School of Medicine, St. Louis, Mo., USA

Abstract

Vulnerability to becoming a smoker, the likelihood of smoking in a given situation and individual differences in smoking patterns are influenced by complex interactions of nicotine with genetically influenced differences in brain functioning, psychological traits, learning and responses to contextual states. This review addresses these interactions using the recently developed Research Domain Criteria (RDoC) of the National Institute of Mental Health (NIMH) that provide new ways of classifying neuropsychiatric disorders based on basic dimensions across multiple units of analysis, from genes to neural circuits to behavior, that cut across disorders as traditionally defined. NIMH expects that the RDoC approach will lead to new and better-focused treatments. The RDoC research domains/constructs are: (1) negative valence systems (fear, anxiety and loss); (2) positive valence systems (reward learning and reward valuation); (3) cognitive systems (attention, perception, working memory and cognitive control); (4) systems for social processes (attachment formation, social communication, perception of self and perception of others), and (5) arousal/modulatory systems (arousal, circadian rhythm and sleep wakefulness). The smoker status and the acute effects of smoking/nicotine and smoking abstinence have well-established and significant effects on all of these systems, though the nuances of the subcategories articulated in the RDoC have only recently received attention in studies of smokers.   © 2015 S. Karger AG, Basel

The psychology of smoking and the smoker is based on the complex interplay of nicotine, genetic, learning, emotional, reward and punishment sensitivity, and environmental factors (e.g. family and peers) that characterize the individual smoker [1, 2]. Substantial evidence indicates that there are many differences between smokers and the factors that drive their smoking and influence their quitting smoking [1, 2]. A number of these differences result from genetically influenced cognitive and affective functioning, including temperamental differences in dispositions to experience high versus low degrees of positive and negative emotionality, cognitive efficiency and general vulnerabilities to experience clinical and subclinical forms of psychopathology [3]. While there are large differences between smokers, as a group, smokers tend to exhibit suboptimal and frequently dysfunctional cognitive and affective traits with regard to the risk of smoking. These suboptimal traits can be characterized by the Research Domain Criteria (RDoC) developed by the US National Institute of Mental Health (NIMH) [4]. The RDoC provide new ways of classifying neuropsychiatric disorders based on dimensions of observable behavior and neurobiological measures. The NIMH goal is to 'define basic dimensions of functioning to be studied across multiple units of analysis, from genes to neural circuits to behaviors, cutting across disorders as traditionally defined' [4]. NIMH expects that the RDoC approach will lead to new and better-focused treatments when combined with well-characterized interactions with the current contextual factors, including social factors and stressors. The major RDoC research domains/constructs are: (1) negative valence systems (NVS; fear, anxiety and loss); (2) positive valence systems (PVS; reward learning and reward valuation); (3) cognitive systems (CoS; attention, perception, working memory (WM), and cognitive control); (4) systems for social processes (SSoP; attachment formation, social communication, perception of self and perception of others), and (5) arousal/modulatory systems (ARMS; arousal, circadian rhythm, sleep and wakefulness).

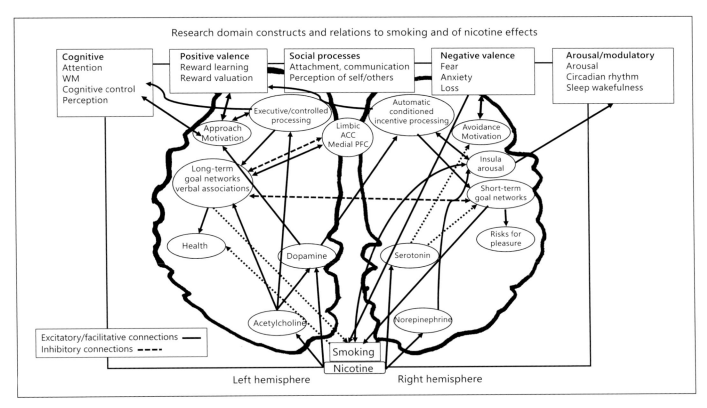

Fig. 1. The effects of acute smoking/nicotine and smoking abstinence on the five RDoC constructs and their subcomponents are indicated by excitatory and inhibitory neural network connections. Activation of one node spreads or inhibits activation in other nodes in the network. Changes in activation of any one network component result in direct or indirect changes in other components. Components in one hemisphere are generally more tightly associated with each other than with components in the other hemisphere. Note that this figure is simply meant to depict hypothesized, sometimes relatively lateralized, processes and activations. Thus, the specific location of a specified node within a hemisphere is not meant to suggest that the specified process takes place only in that hemisphere or at the location within the hemisphere. Neural networks associated with even simple psychological processing and associated RDoC constructs typically involve widely distributed, parallel processes in both hemispheres [48]. For example, acetylcholine and dopamine are widely distributed within both hemispheres, though evidence suggests that they may be relatively denser in the left hemisphere, while serotonin and norepinephrine are relatively denser in the right hemisphere [3]. Based on nicotine binding at and modulation of nicotinic cholinergic receptors, acute smoking/nicotine leads to the release and modulation of dopamine, serotonin and other neurotransmission-related transmitters and modulators that in concert with nicotine itself modulate the activities of brain systems underlying the RDoC systems and subsystems. The effects of nicotine on the RDoC systems varies across individuals and across situations within an individual as a function of genetically influenced factors such as neurotransmission-related receptor polymorphisms that promote differences in receptor number and sensitivity to nicotine and other neurotransmitters, as well as structural factors. ACC = Anterior cingulate cortex; PFC = prefrontal cortex.

Figures 1 and 2 provide a visual summary and overview of the relations of the RDoC systems, their components, and hypothesized relationships to contextual, genetic and neurobiological factors related to nicotine effects, and state and trait vulnerabilities to smoke. Nicotine-induced and other changes in neural activation of any one RDoC system component result in direct or indirect excitatory and inhibitory changes in other components (fig. 1). Figure 2 provides an overview of the activation of the five RDoC constructs as a function context/situation, smoking/nicotine and individual differences in the trait tuning/neurocircuitry of RDoC con-

structs. The RDoC tuning/neurocircuitry results in large part from complex interactions of genetic sources with each other and with early environment [1, 3], and is modified by subsequent nicotine exposure, and chronic and acute environmental factors, including smoking and smoking abstinence. Additional information related to these figures is reviewed in subsequent chapter sections. A more detailed account of the relationships of the environment with the temperamental tuning is provided by the situation by trait adaptive response model of smoking and the effects of nicotine [3] and its lateralized neural network model of situation by trait interac-

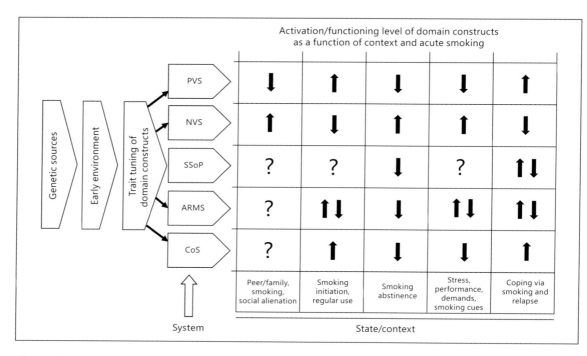

Fig. 2. The activation of the five RDoC constructs as a function context/situation, smoking/nicotine and individual differences in the trait tuning/neurocircuitry of RDoC constructs. The RDoC tuning/neurocircuitry results in large part from complex interactions of genetic sources with each other and with early environment [1, 3] and is modified by subsequent nicotine exposure, and chronic and acute environmental factors, including smoking and smoking abstinence.

tions. The lateralized neural network model is based on evidence that acetylcholine and dopamine receptors and neurocircuitry are relatively denser in the left hemisphere, while serotonin and norepinephrine, which are also modulated by nicotine, are relatively denser in the right hemisphere [reviewed in ref. 3]. Given that nicotine is a cholinergic agonist that also promotes dopaminergic functioning [2, 3], the situation by trait adaptive response model proposes that nicotine is especially effective in promoting left-hemisphere frontal functioning, including active coping, reward sensitivity and activation of verbal generation (inferior frontal) and executive functioning (dorsal lateral prefrontal) that inhibit the influences of limbic (NVS-related) areas of the brain, such as the subgenual anterior cingulate [3]. The model also suggests that the ability of nicotine to reduce some forms of NVS activity and to enhance sustained attention may in part reflect its enhancement of somewhat right-lateralized serotonergic and noradrenergic functions, respectively.

Many of the acute effects of smoking/nicotine and of smoking abstinence have been well established [3] and include significant effects on one or more components of at least four of the five RDoC systems [3], though the understanding of the smoker status and the effects of nicotine on

RDoC component subsystems is minimal to nonexistent for several of the RDoC. Generally, the nuances of the component subcategories have only recently begun to receive attention in studies of smokers. A major goal of this review is to provide a brief systematic review of these oft-ignored but potentially clinically and theoretically important differences in subcomponents of each of the RDoC (e.g. anxiety versus fear facets of the NVS). RDoC reflect both states and traits of individuals. An individual may be in a suboptimal cognitive state due a temporary state, such as sleep deprivation, or due to more permanent trait factors, including genetically and environmentally induced deviations in brain structure and function. RDoC is not a complete diagnostic system, but at this time is meant to provide a framework for organizing research on the large range of factors relating to mental health problems, both clinical and subclinical, using a dimensional, rather than categorical perspective [4].

The NIMH RDoC constructs are designed to provide an organizing framework for understanding mental health and behavioral problems at a deeper level than in current symptom-based disorder analyses. The expectation is that this new framework will allow greater precision to understanding these problems based on detailed scientific research from molecular to social and learning determinants and associated mechanisms. The framework encourages assessment and integration of each of these five systems at seven levels of an overall matrix that consists of: (1) genes, (2) molecules, (3) cells, (4) circuits, (5) physiology, (6) behavior and (7) self-reports. The matrix also includes a column listing well-validated paradigms for the study of each construct. This chapter focuses primarily on the genetic, behavioral and self-report level, but also touches briefly on the neurocircuitry of smoking, something that along with molecular and cellular levels will be needed to more completely understand the situation state-trait vulnerability interactions that influence who becomes a smoker, when the smoker smokes and the effects of smoking versus abstaining.

Below, we review evidence indicating that smoker status, nicotine abstinence responses and the acute effects of smoking abstinence may be viewed as being moderated by state and trait functioning of multiple interacting RDoC. Figure 1 outlines hypothesized interactions among the RDoC constructs and their relationships to brain systems, and the effects of nicotine and smoking.

A better understanding of individual differences between smokers in RDoC-related traits can provide new and more precise insights into differences among smokers concerning when and why they are motivated to smoke. Differences in RDoC vulnerability profiles interacting with social and cultural factors may account for the growing proportion of smokers who are light smokers – individuals who never progressed to heavy smoking or once heavy smokers who now are light and nondaily smokers [5]. Light smokers, including nondaily users, comprise a growing group of about 25% of all US smokers and are significantly more likely than other smokers to be less than 30 years of age [5]. About 12% of smokers in the US smoke fewer than 5 cigarettes per day and 8% of current smokers smoke less than 1 cigarette per day [5]. Across 2 years, approximately 21–35% of young light smokers (<5 cigarettes per day) increase to >5 per day, while about 27–32% quit smoking, and the rest maintain their baseline smoking rates [6]. The growing population of light smokers in the US poses a significant challenge for some of the major existing models of smoking reinforcement, maintenance and trajectories [6]. For example, compared to heavier smokers, they report smoking in highly specific situational contexts and in response to particular affective, cognitive and social situations, and desired outcomes such as to reduce negative affect when stressed, enhance cognitive functioning when fatigued or when studying, and to enhance enjoyment in social situations [1, 3, 6]. There is also reason to believe that, relative to nonsmokers, individuals in the shrinking group of heavy

smokers in the US generally have more problematic functions on one or more of the RDoC (e.g. negative affect, depression, low positive affect, cognitive impairment and impulsive traits) [3], and these changing characteristics of smokers challenge traditional notions of smoking being driven by simple models of nicotine dependence or addiction [6]. Figure 2 depicts some of the complex multifactorial interplays among RDoC constructs and the environment that appear to influence smoking motivation, reinforcement and relapse.

Some of the factors that differentiate smokers from nonsmokers are well established. However, in recent years, the very question of who is or is not a smoker has changed with the advent of electronic cigarettes and with light and occasional smokers, and smokeless tobacco products. These changes in smoking patterns are likely a result of public health interventions and societal changes that have led to reduced social acceptability of and greater restrictions on smoking. These societal changes have led to a greatly reduced percentage of Americans who smoke (from 45% in 1965 down to 18.1% in 2012, Centers for Disease Control) [7] (see chapter 16). This downward trend is consistent with the hypothesis that smoking is progressively becoming more prevalent in individuals with psychological characteristics that may make it difficult for them to cope with the demands of modern life (see chapter 17). This chapter concludes with a discussion of potential new and more efficacious prevention and intervention strategies.

Below, we first briefly review how traditional dimensions of personality, psychopathology and cognitive functioning, and associated RDoC are related to smoking status, motivation, progression and relapse. New directions for future research, methodological issues, situation (context) by RDoC interactions and clinical implications are addressed. It is important to note that the RDoC approach to understanding is based on continuous, as opposed to categorical (all or none), measures of smoking, smoking motivation, and clinical and subclinical psychopathology. The tentatively suggested RDoC indices of the basic construct include self-report questionnaires, task performance indices and neurobiological measures [4].

Predictors of Smoking Status, Progression and Relapse – The Broad Scope

Smoking and the effects of nicotine and nicotine replacement therapy are relatively strongly related to basic dimensions of personality/temperament, cognitive and educational status, and psychiatric disorders [3, 8] (see also chapters 16 and 17). Latent genetic influences have been estimated to explain approximately 30–50% of the variance in each of the major personality dimensions [9], smoking behavior [10, 11] and smoking-related psychiatric disorders [3, 12]. There is also evidence to suggest the possibility of shared familial influences, at least for some measures of depression and smoking [11]. In terms of measured genetic effects, tobacco-related phenotypes, relative to other substances, have thus far evidenced relatively greater success with genome-wide association studies, and genome-wide significant results ($p < 5 \times 10^{-8}$) have emerged for logical biological variants in α_5/α_3 cholinergic nicotinic receptors genes *(CHRNA5/CHRNA3)*, namely rs16969968, a nonsynonymous single nucleotide polymorphism in *CHRNA5* (or its proxy rs1051730 in *CHRNA3*) [13] (see also chapter 5). The risk allele in rs16969968(A) results in an amino acid change (aspartic acid to asparagine) that decreases the function of the subunit, and *CHRNA5* knockout mice evidence increased nicotine administration [13]. However, the most compelling results from smoking-related genome-wide association studies have not converged with those for personality dimensions [14] or psychiatric disorders [15]. This lack of convergence may, in part, be attributable to the self-report assessment utilized in these genome-wide association studies to date. Endophenotypes may be viewed as lying in the space between genes and global vulnerability factors, and they may allow for a greater understanding of the biology across these associated behaviors. Each of the RDoC subcomponent factors may be viewed within an endophenotype framework that has the potential to enlighten mechanistic and related clinical intervention studies.

Smoking is associated with higher neuroticism/negative affectivity (N, RDoC-NVS), extraversion/positive affectivity (E, RDoC-PVS) and psychoticism/impulsive-unsocialized sensation seeking (P-IUSS, likely a combination of suboptimal RDoC SSoP combined with suboptimal cognitive and negative systems). P-IUSS consists of impulsivity, cynicism, coldness, alienation, antisocial attitudes, novelty/sensation seeking, and low agreeableness, conscientiousness and constraint [3, 8]. E-PVS is composed of facets including gregariousness, dominance, assertiveness, positive affect, warmth and activity level. Low positive affectivity [anhedonia] is associated with a significantly elevated prevalence of smoking, likely through an association with clinical and subclinical depressive affect [8], while the gregarious and outgoing component of E-PVS has also been associated with a greater prevalence of smoking, especially in contexts and times when smoking is approved by the social context [3]. N-NVS is composed of a number of facets of lower-order dimensions, including anxiety, depression, psychological vulnerability and anger/hostility. N-NVS is predictive of and genetically associated with depressive and anxiety disorders [3, 8]. To the degree that nicotine reduces emotionality or negative affect, smoking would be expected to be more reinforcing in high N-NVS than low N-NVS individuals. Not surprisingly, N-NVS correlates with reported smoking for stress/negative affect relief and nicotine dependence [3, 16]. While little is known about reported reasons for smoking in those high in psychoticism (P-IUSS) and the unsocialized disinhibitory disorders, it may be that high P-IUSS and individuals with cognitive deficits related to impulsivity smoke in part to reduce their impulsivity and enhance their attentional efficacy [3, 17].

Self-Reported Smoking Motivation and Effects of Smoking Abstinence

Numerous investigations have shown smokers to report that they smoke in part because smoking helps them reduce negative affect (RDoC-NVS) and weight/appetite, provides pleasurable relaxation (RDoC-PVS) and enhances their concentration (RDoC-CoS) [3, 16]. Abstaining from smoking in dependent smokers is associated with self-reported and objectively assessed sleep disturbances (RDoC-ARMS) [18]. While there is a great deal of variability in the reported intensity of the effects of smoking and smoking abstinence [19], heavy, occasional and very light smokers report emotional calming effects (RDoC-NVS) from smoking [20]. These smoking motives and effects of smoking are to some extent specific to individuals and situations [3, 21]. On one occasion, an individual may feel drowsy and smoke to become more stimulated and/or to focus his/her attention in order to complete an important task. On another occasion, the same individual may experience a dysphoric mood (NVS) and smoke to reduce subjective distress. When smoking is used as a conscious psychological resource/coping mechanism, individuals with poor coping skills and those with high chronic stress would be expected to consciously choose to smoke more frequently and thus have a greater chance of eventually smoking in a habitual manner. More generally, individuals genetically or otherwise predisposed towards various forms of affective, attentional, cognitive and behavioral dysfunction would likely become smokers and eventually smoke habitually because they find the cognitive-enhancing and negative-affect-reducing effects of smoking rewarding (i.e. positively and negatively reinforcing). Fully conscious, controlled choices to smoke would be expected to occur prior to habitual smoking and would be expected to constitute a higher proportion of light smokers than heavy smokers' behavior. Consistent with such psychological resource/self-medication conceptions of smoking motivation, smokers tend to smoke more during stressful situations [20] and those attempting to quit smoking tend to relapse during stressful situations, even years after quitting [16]. A recent study [21] found that nicotine reduced anxiety most when unpleasant pictures were presented in combination with neutral pictures, but it had no effect on anxiety when unpleasant pictures were presented in combination with pleasant pictures or when unpleasant pictures were not presented. In contrast, nicotine only reduced depressive affect when the participant had attentional choice between pleasant and unpleasant pictures. Nicotine also enhanced overall positive affect and reduced overall negative affect as measured by the positive and negative affect schedule, but these generalized effects were not moderated by task manipulations. Overall, the findings support the view that the ability of nicotine to reduce specific negative affects is moderated by emotional context and the precision of the RDoC-NVS measures used (global NVS versus NVS components such as anxiety and loss/depression).

While self-report indices are a critical part of understanding the effects of smoking and smoking abstinence, there are numerous well-documented limitations of self-report measures. These limitations include individual differences in presentation bias, demand effects, measurement drift associated with repeated questionnaire administration [19], and insensitivity to rapidly changing and nonconscious processes. Thus, the following discussions of mechanisms associated with each of the RDoC are largely focused on carefully conducted laboratory experimental studies that focus on objective brain and behavioral mechanisms and measures that are supplemented in some cases with self-report indices.

Negative Valence Systems

As noted in the preceding sections, traits related to negative affect are associated with a higher prevalence of smoking [3, 8]. The five constructs included in the RDoC NVS domain are: (1) responses to acute threat (fear); (2) responses to potential harm (anxiety); (3) responses to sustained threat; (4) frustrative nonreward and (5) loss. The RDoC working group acknowledged that 'these NVS constructs and definitions are not intended to be definitive or all-inclusive and that it is expected that modifications will

be made and additional constructs will be added to the framework as science progresses. Constructs such as guilt, shame and disgust, which were not included because the working group was constrained to focus on constructs that had the best fit with the stated criteria for construct definition and the proposed units of measurement' [4]. In the case of smoking and theory development, this group of largely social constructs has been studied only rarely in relationship to smoking and nicotine. Individuals who experience frequently high levels of a given NVS component, activation can be said to be high in that NVS trait. However, given the intensely provoking circumstance, almost any individual can experience acute (state) activation of one or more NVS domain constructs whether or not they are high in a general or specific component NVS trait. Both state and trait NVS baseline-dependent effects of nicotine and smoking have been observed. For example, Korhonen et al. [22] found that prequit baseline depressive symptoms (loss NVS) predicted the impact of nicotine replacement therapy on the mood profile after cessation. Similarly, angry and depressive traits, as well as generalized NVS/neuroticism/negative affectivity have been found to predict NVS mood responses/withdrawal symptoms and EEG patterns during smoking abstinence, as well as responses to nicotine [3, 16, 19].

Anxiety versus Fear Constructs Related to Smoking and the Effects of Nicotine
The differentiation of responses to acute threat (fear) from potential harm (anxiety) and sustained threat is well based in the scientific literature on emotion in humans and lower animals [23]. In a 1989 review, Gilbert and Welser [24] interpreted findings as suggesting that nicotine reduces distal potential threat (anxiety) but not acute proximal threat (fear). The hypothesized reason for this was that nicotine promotes attention to salient proximal stimuli and also tends to promote attention to emotionally positively valent stimuli, relative to negatively valent stimuli. Subsequent findings have supported this model [25, 26] and more generally support the view that dopamine release by the actions of nicotine in the brain tends to promote attention to salient emotional stimuli [21, 27].

Sustained Threat/Stress Effects Related to Smoking, the Smoker and the Effects of Nicotine
The relationship of chronic stress to the effects of nicotine on NVS is important given that evidence suggests that chronic stress interacts with brain networks supporting both negative and positive reinforcement [28]. Also, nico-

tine has many of the hormonal effects of a low-level stressor, including increases in blood cortisol concentration and generalized arousal [3]. However, smokers report that they subjectively feel less stress and NVS affects when they smoke, as compared to when they abstain from smoking, and acute administration studies tend to support this view [3].

Frustrative Nonreward Response Relationships to Smoking and the Effects of Nicotine
Reactions elicited in response to withdrawal/prevention of reward (the inability to obtain positive rewards following repeated or sustained efforts) is the definition of both frustrative nonreward and a characteristic that differentiates many smokers from nonsmokers. Self-report measures suggested by the NIMH RDoC working committee included measures of proactive and reactive aggression. On average, smokers are higher in self-report measures of trait anger and hostility [3]. Trait anger/hostility is also one of the most reliable and strongest predictors of relapse, and increases in state anger during smoking abstinence are greater in individuals highest in trait anger/hostility [1, 3, 29]. The measures of trait and state anger/hostility used in these studies appear to be more reactive anger/irritability/hostility than proactive measures of aggression. The role of state and trait frustrative nonreward to smoking status, withdrawal symptoms and responses to nicotine is an active area of investigation [1, 29].

Loss Construct Relationships to Smoking and the Effects of Nicotine
The RDoC loss constructs are essentially those typically associated in severe degrees with clinical depression and nicotine withdrawal, and in less severe forms and combinations to measures of N-NVS traits. RDoC self-report indices include changes in attributional style and hopelessness, while listed behavioral indices are: rumination, withdrawal, worry, crying, sadness, loss-relevant recall bias, attentional bias to negative-valenced information, guilt, morbid thoughts, psychomotor retardation, anhedonia, increased self-focus, deficits in executive function (e.g. impaired sustained attention), loss of drive (sleep/appetite), decreased libido, shame, amotivation, memory impairments and intrusive thoughts. Prequit baseline depressive symptoms (loss NVS) have been found to predict the impact of nicotine replacement therapy on the mood profile after cessation [19, 22]. Those with greater baseline loss-construct activation levels exhibit larger increases in loss-construct levels after cessation (e.g. anhedonia and other

depressive NVS symptoms) than those low in baseline loss NVS levels. More generally, high levels of trait loss NVS activity (especially anhedonia and depressed affect) have been found to predict larger increases in loss NVS levels during smoking abstinence and higher levels of relapse [19, 26].

Prevention and Intervention Strategies Based on Negative Valence Constructs
The above-reviewed evidence shows that NVS and associated psychiatric diagnoses are common among treatment-seeking smokers and are related to increased motivation to smoke, relatively more severe withdrawal symptoms, lack of response to treatment and impaired ability to quit smoking. These findings could guide treatment assignment algorithms and treatment development for smokers high in trait NVS functioning and those with NVS-related diagnoses [26]. Consistent with this hypothesis, a recent meta-analysis found that smokers with current or past clinical depression benefitted significantly from psychosocial mood management training combined with standard smoking cessation interventions compared with a standard treatment alone [30]. In general, it seems reasonable to suggest that treatments should be individualized and focused on the RDoC situational and trait vulnerabilities of the given smoker [3]. Research findings and theory suggest that nicotine may bias attention away from negative stimuli when equally salient positive or benign stimuli are present, especially when the affective cues are conditioned or reflect distal threat (anxiety) [3, 31]. Attentional modification procedures could prove to be effective for individuals high in NVS traits, though there is little evidence to support this view at this time.

Positive Valence Systems

Five constructs are included in the PVS and are all related to approach behavior: (1) approach motivation consisting of four components [(a) reward valuation; (b) effort valuation/willingness to work; (c) expectancy/reward prediction error, and (d) action selection/preference-based decision making]; (2) initial responsiveness to reward attainment; (3) sustained/longer-term responsiveness to reward attainment; (4) reward learning, and (5) habit. The RDoC committee noted that 'approach behavior can be directed toward innate or acquired cues (including those resulting from Pavlovian conditioning), and implicit or explicit goals. Expectancy/reward prediction error, and action selection/decision making are also part of the PVS' [4]. Sophisticated subhuman animal work and an associated large knowledge base exist for these PVS constructs. Less is known about how these PVS constructs are related to smoker status and the effects of nicotine. However, recent evidence supports the view that PVS constructs play a critical role in the reinforcing effects of nicotine and the adverse subjective cognitive effects of nicotine abstinence [2].

Approach Motivation – Reward Valuation
'Processes by which the probability and benefits of a prospective outcome are computed and calibrated by reference to external information, social context (e.g., group input, counterfactual comparisons), and/or prior experience. This calibration is influenced by pre-existing biases, learning, memory, stimulus characteristics, and deprivation states. Reward valuation may involve the assignment of incentive salience to stimuli' [4]. Consistent with the importance of prospective outcomes and social context, peer and family smoking and socioeconomic status are highly predictive of smoking status and failure to successfully maintain smoking cessation efforts [1, 3]. Nicotine has been found to enhance reward valuation in both human and subhuman species [2, 3, 27, 32].

Approach Motivation – Effort Valuation/Willingness to Work
'Processes by which the cost(s) of obtaining an outcome is computed; tendency to overcome response costs to obtain a reinforcer' [4]. Nicotine can promote the highjacking of attention to smoking cues via its ability to promote the release of dopamine in the nucleus accumbens and frontal lobes [27]. Dopamine also has a motivation-enhancing effect for salient environmental stimuli that may tend to enhance hedonic tone and reward sensitivity [2, 3, 32, 33]. In rodent models, nicotine enhances the willingness to work as assessed by the breakpoint at which animals will no longer work for reinforcers (see also chapter 5) [1].

Approach Motivation – Expectancy/Reward Prediction Error
'A state triggered by exposure to internal or external stimuli, experiences or contexts that predict the possibility of reward. Reward expectation can alter the experience of an outcome and can influence the use of resources (e.g. cognitive resources)' [4]. Nicotine enhances dopamine release in reinforcement/reward circuits in the brain and thereby may be associated with increased attention to and effort for reward-related stimuli (see also chapter 5, fig. 1) [1, 2, 27].

Approach Motivation – Action Selection/Preference-Based Decision Making
'Processes involving an evaluation of costs/benefits and occurring in the context of multiple potential choices being available for decision-making' [4]. The delay discounting literature indicates that smokers, compared to non-smokers and light smokers, tend to prefer immediate but smaller rewards compared to delayed but larger rewards in non- and light smokers [1]. It is not clear whether or not acute doses of nicotine or chronic smoking influence delay discounting [1]. Longitudinal studies suggest that impulsive traits are reliable predictors of the development of nicotine dependence and delay discounting is considered to be a behavioral index of impulsivity [1, 3]. The willingness to delay gratification for greater rewards is an excellent example of what smokers do not do with their tobacco habit. They seek the immediate rewards of smoking over the long-term costs and the rewards of a most likely longer life.

Initial Responsiveness to Reward Attainment
'Mechanisms/processes associated with hedonic responses – as reflected in subjective experiences, behavioral responses, and/or engagement of the neural systems to a positive reinforcer – and culmination of reward seeking' [4]. Nicotine has been found by a number of investigators to enhance attentional bias toward motivation-related (affect-inducing stimuli) [27], and some studies and theory suggest that nicotine may reduce attention and associative processes to unpleasant stimuli when the alternative pleasant stimuli are present. The overall findings provide mixed evidence in support of the view that nicotine biases attention towards pleasant and away from unpleasant stimuli when equally salient pleasant and unpleasant stimuli are present [3, 21, 31]. Nicotine has also been found to enhance hedonic tone and reward sensitivity [2, 3, 32], something that individuals with temperamentally or environmentally induced low hedonic tone may find highly reinforcing [2, 3] (see also chapter 5; fig. 1).

Sustained/Longer-Term Responsiveness to Reward Attainment
'Mechanisms/processes associated with the termination of reward seeking, e.g. satisfaction, satiation, regulation of consummatory behavior' [4]. While tolerance to the effects of nicotine across time might be viewed as a means to terminate smoking behavior, individuals typically increase the amount used to derive the same level of satisfaction initially experienced. In addition, after overnight ab-

stinence (while sleeping), a majority of smokers find the first cigarette of the day to be particularly satisfying, promoting a sustained cycle of cigarette use [11, 20] (see also chapter 5).

Reward Learning
'A process by which organisms acquire information about stimuli, actions, and contexts that predict positive outcomes, and by which behavior is modified when a novel reward occurs or outcomes are better than expected. Reward learning is a type of reinforcement learning, and similar processes may be involved in learning related to negative reinforcement' [4]. Consistent with putative reinforcement-enhancing properties of acute nicotine exposure, Barr et al. [32] found that a nicotine patch, relative to placebo, enhanced reward responding on a probabilistic reinforcement task in nonsmokers. Likewise, during withdrawal from nicotine, in both heavy smoking humans and rats chronically administered nicotine, Pergadia et al. [2] found significant reductions in reward responsiveness following 24-hour abstinence from nicotine using the same probabilistic reward task.

Habit
'Sequential, repetitive, motor, or cognitive behaviors elicited by external or internal triggers that, once initiated, can go to completion without constant conscious oversight. Habits can be adaptive by virtue of freeing up cognitive resources. Habit formation is a frequent consequence of reward learning, but its expression can become resistant to changes in outcome value. Related behaviors could be pathological expression of a process that under normal circumstances subserves adaptive goals' [4]. Cigarette smoking for heavy smokers is a classic habitual process and a model system to inform this RDoC construct. However, factors other than habit contribute to the smoking in many individuals, especially in light and occasional smokers [6]. According to Shiffman [6], a majority of smokers in nondeveloped countries are not daily smokers, a fact that indicates that factors other than simple habit influences smoking in many smokers. It has been argued with significant empirical support that in addition to habit systems, executive-system-chosen self-medication of state- or trait-high NVS activity, low PVS functioning (e.g. anhedonia in depression) and suboptimal cognitive system functioning exert a powerful influence on smoking reinforcement and smoking in specific situations, as well as the development of nicotine dependence [2, 3].

Prevention and Intervention Strategies Based on Positive Valence System Constructs
Prevention and cessation strategies that offer effective healthy rewarding alternatives to smoking may help to offset blunting of PVS functioning that may be typical of smokers as a trait and is frequently experienced during smoking cessation [2]. Evidence suggests that alternatives may be particularly helpful for smokers with a vulnerability to depression [2] (see also chapter 17).

Cognitive Systems

CoS constructs are: (1) attention – processes that regulate access to capacity-limited systems, including awareness, higher perceptual processes and motor action; (2) perception – processes that alter sensory data to construct and transform representations of the environment; (3) declarative memory – the encoding, storage and consolidation, and retrieval of representations of facts and events; (4) language – the system of shared symbolic representations of the world, self and thoughts; (5) cognitive control – the system that modulates other cognitive and emotional systems, in the service of goal-directed behavior, and (6) WM – the combination of short-term memory with information processing. Baseline-dependent individual differences in the effects of nicotine have been observed for many CoS construct indices, such as suboptimal cognitive performance as assessed with objective, computer-based cognitive tasks including memory, WM and sustained attention [34, 35], which are listed as RDoc CoS indices [4]. Individuals with poor cognitive performance when nicotine deprived benefit more from the effects of nicotine than do individuals with higher baseline performance. This baseline-dependent effect of nicotine on cognitive enhancement has also been found in nonsmokers [35].

It has been argued that some clinical and subclinical populations with cognitive deficits (e.g. patients with schizophrenia or attention deficit disorder) may smoke or initiate smoking as an effort to self-medicate preexisting clinical or subclinical psychopathology [36, 37]. In a 25-year longitudinal study of a birth cohort of 1,265 children, Fergusson et al. [38] found a highly significant correlation between the intelligence quotient (IQ) during childhood and nicotine dependence later in life. Higher IQ predicted a lower likelihood of progressing to nicotine dependence. This association remained significant after adjustment for childhood conduct problems. This relationship between IQ and smoking prevalence may reflect several factors, including the level of awareness of the health risks associated with smoking, higher stress levels associated with lower socioeconomic status, self-medication for cognitive dysfunction, and prevalence of smoking and deviant behavior in social networks. IQ-related cognitive capacity and integrity may result in enhanced emotional control, coping and cognitive efficiency that reduces the benefits of smoking and nicotine.

In their systematic review, Heishman et al. [39] found significant beneficial effects of nicotine in both habitual smokers and nonsmokers on six components of cognitive functioning: fine motor, alerting attention accuracy and response time, orienting attention response time, short-term episodic memory accuracy, and WM response time with effect sizes from 0.30 to 0.86. Thus, nicotine and smoking have clear objectively assessed acutely beneficial effects on cognition that may promote nicotine use and dependence. These six cognitive components are subsumed by four of the six CoS constructs: (1) CoS attention, (2) CoS declarative memory, (3) CoS cognitive control and (4) CoS WM. The two remaining CoS constructs, perception and language, were not addressed in the their review. However, nicotine has been found to increase accuracy of perception/identification of briefly presented visual stimuli. Consistent with lateralized neural-network models of NVS traits and states, and the effects of nicotine on affective information processing [3], nicotine has been found to enhance the perception of briefly presented visual stimuli in a manner that is moderated by NVS traits, the visual field of the target stimulus and the affective valence of the stimulus [40, 41].

Prevention and Intervention Strategies Based on Cognitive System Constructs
There is reason to believe that CoS WM capacity, both as a trait and as a state, is an important mediator and moderator of smoker-nonsmoker differences and of risk situations given that WM is defined as the active maintenance and flexible updating of goal/task-relevant information (e.g. items, goals and strategies) in a form that has limited capacity and resists interference [4]. However, cognitive control processes associated with smoker-nonsmoker differences and the beneficial effects of nicotine [35] appear to be distinguishable from WM by virtue of the fact that they involve processes that are not present in WM, including motivation, goal selection, motor inhibition and error conflict monitoring [4]. Differentiation of and interactions among all RDoC research domains and their subconstructs in differing social and affective contexts are likely to be important in understanding factors that promote smoking and the development of new efficacious smoking interventions.

Systems for Social Processes

The SSoP include: (1) affiliation and attachment formation; (2) social communication; (3) perception of self, and (4) perception of others [4]. There is currently minimal knowledge of the effects of acute/chronic nicotine exposure and smoking on SSoP or the effects of individual differences in SSoP on smoking progression and the effects of nicotine. New research in these areas could conceivably provide important information that might in turn lead to new interventions (e.g. social training). The limited work on learning refusal skills in adolescents may be relevant to early prevention efforts. Procedures to enhance affiliation and social communication may indirectly increase PVS activation in those with deficits in this area by increasing alternatives to smoking for those low in sources for PVS activation.

Affiliation and Attachment
'Affiliation is the engagement in positive social interactions with other individuals' [4]. Given the high association of an individual's smoking with peer smoking behavior, as well as evidence supporting the view that nicotine may modulate brain processes associated with social bonding [3], it is surprising that there are virtually no experimental data on the effects of nicotine on such processes. Given that many smokers smoke outside with others who are smoking, the possibility that nicotine or other components of tobacco smoke promote social bonding among smokers is an interesting one because such groups of smokers may support each other's choice to continue smoking [1]. For example, giving up the bonding time of smoking may also mean the loss of time together with one's attachment to smoking friends. Ongoing clinical trials and other studies are currently assessing the effects of oxytocin, the social bonding hormone, on responses to smoking cues and stress. Such studies are designed to assess the potential of oxytocin as an aide for smoking abstinence.

Social Communication: Four Subsets
'(a) Reception of Facial Communication: The capacity to perceive someone's emotional state non-verbally based on facial expressions. (b) Production of Facial Communication: The capacity to convey one's emotional state non-verbally via facial expression. (c) Reception of Non-Facial Communication: The capacity to perceive social and emotional information based on modalities other than facial expression, including non-verbal gestures, affective prosody, distress calling, cooing, etc. (d) Production of Non-Facial Communication: The capacity to express social and emotional infor-

mation based on modalities other than facial expression, including non-verbal gestures, affective prosody, distress calling, cooing, etc.' [4]. Findings [41] suggest that other smokers are a potent stimulus for smoking. It seems reasonable to hypothesize that numerous other forms of social communication, both cognitive and affective, are critical factors in influencing smoking and the effects of nicotine.

Perception and Understanding of Self

'The processes and/or representations involved in being aware of, accessing knowledge about, and/or making judgments about the self' [4]. It is reasonable to hypothesize that identifying oneself as a smoker or as a person in need of smoking or medication to cope with temperamental disposition (one or more suboptimal RDoC traits) may play an important role in the likelihood of progressing to nicotine dependence and the likelihood of initiating or maintaining abstinence. Consistent with this view, some smokers with dispositions to depressive affect and clinical depression experience clinical or subclinical depression or depressive affect during quit attempts [2, 8]. Unpublished findings of the first author indicate that some light and occasional smokers do not label themselves as smokers, something that may reflect a dedication to and protection from escalating to greater levels of tobacco consumption.

Perception and Understanding of Others

'The processes and/or representations involved in being aware of, accessing knowledge about, reasoning about, and/or making judgments about other animate entities' [4]. To the degree that acute doses of nicotine enhance general cognitive information processing efficiency [39], one might expect smoking to enhance the perception and understanding of others. However, there appears to be no specific evidence to support this hypothesis. However, evidence that acute doses of nicotine enhance a number of cognitive processes in individuals with poor understanding of others (e.g. schizophrenia and attention-deficit/hyperactivity disorder) [39] is consistent with the hypothesis that nicotine may enhance the perception and understanding of others, especially those who have deficits in these areas.

Prevention and Intervention Strategies Based on Constructs of Systems for Social Processes

New knowledge concerning the effects of nicotine and smoking status on the SSoP constructs could potentially lead to more efficacious prevention and treatment approaches for smoking, especially in those with deficits in these areas [34, 39]. New knowledge could also suggest new

brain and behavioral mechanisms that differentiate smokers from nonsmokers and the effects of nicotine. Better understanding of these brain-related correlates of smoking and nicotine-related effects on SSoP constructs could potentially lead to novel pharmacological and behavioral intervention and prevention strategies for smoking. Current findings indicate that other smokers are cues for smoking, and recent and ongoing studies are systematically assessing these effects and their relationships to brain activity and to subtle stimulus manipulations [42].

Arousal/Modulatory Systems

The ARMS include arousal, sleep and wakefulness, and circadian rhythm constructs that modulate and are modulated by the other four RDoC systems, as well as by nicotine and smoking abstinence. 'Arousal is a continuing sensitivity of the organism to stimuli, both external and internal. Distinct arousal-related neural circuitry can be activated under appetitive and aversive conditions. Other arousal systems may be activated under either appetitive or aversive conditions, controlling specific, affectively-neutral behaviors that are associated with the elevated arousal levels' [4]. Eysenck [37] provided the earliest detailed model of the influence of nicotine and smoking on ARMS. He was also the first to describe how individual differences in genetically influenced personality traits (e.g. extraversion) and the arousal potential of the environment interact to influence when introverts versus extraverts experience nicotine/smoking benefits. Eysenck's model assumes that in situations with moderate arousal potentials introverts are ideally aroused or overaroused while extraverts in the same situation are underaroused. Given that nicotine was hypothesized to have an inverted-U relationship to arousal (cortical activation), nicotine was hypothesized to reduce cortical activation in introverts in environments while increasing arousal in extraverts. There is some support for the view that the effects of and motivations for nicotine vary as a function of extraversion [3, 37]. However, there is strong evidence to support Eysenck's [37] hypothesis that nicotine increases brain activation and cognitive performance to a greater degree in situations and individuals with low arousal potential and in those who have low baseline arousal and performance [4, 34]. Given that extraversion is correlated with positive affect and RDoC PVS [3], it would be interesting for the field to better characterize the contributions of PVS and NVS, as well as context-specific state arousal/brain activation on the effects of nicotine and nicotine abstinence [3] given that several studies have observed traits related to PVS and NVS to modulate electrocortical and other brain indices of activation/arousal [43].

Sleep and wakefulness are reliably altered by nicotine and nicotine abstinence in nicotine-dependent individuals [18, 43, 44]. Increased sleep disturbances (delay in falling asleep and in awakenings) occur during the first weeks of smoking abstinence [43]. In addition, bupropion SR (a pharmacotherapy to facilitate smoking abstinence) increases sleep disturbance during withdrawal, as well as during nonwithdrawal EEG-verified sleep studies (see also chapter 20) [18]. Deprived smokers report increased drowsiness relative to nondeprived conditions and exhibit EEG slowing (deactivation/low arousal) [44]. However, it is not known whether the effects of nicotine and smoking/nicotine deprivation on sleep are moderated by E-PVS or other RDoC systems.

Studies of the effects of smoking/nicotine on circadian rhythms are limited in number and size, but studies of the effects of nicotine and nicotine withdrawal in rodents and humans suggest that nicotine may alter circadian rhythm sleep and eating patterns [43]. The potentially moderating effects of RDoC on nicotine-associated ARMS have not be assessed.

Finally, though the current version of RDoC systems does not include brain default mode networks (DMN) as a subcomponent of ARMS or other RDoC, there is a great deal of interest in DMN systems in neuroscience, and these systems are highly related to the effects of smoking and nicotine. Nicotine has been found to influence the task-negative component of the DMN (TN-DMN), a set of brain regions, including the medial prefrontal cortex, medial temporal lobes and posterior cingulate cortex/retrosplenial cortex, implicated in episodic memory processing and associated with an internal, rather than an external, focus of attention [45]. The DMN is defined by the functional connectivity of brain regions through low-frequency neuronal oscillations typically using functional magnetic resonance imaging, though EEG can also index DMN activity. TN-DMN abnormalities have been found in a variety of disorders, including interference by network activity during task performance, altered patterns of antagonism between task-specific and nonspecific elements, altered connectively and integrity of the TN-DMN and altered psychological functions served by the TN-DMN. TN-DMN abnormalities have been found in individuals with a variety of disorders, including dementia, schizophrenia, epilepsy, anxiety, depression, autism and attention deficit/hyperactivity disorder. A recent review concluded that nicotine and smoking appear to have acute effects on DMN activity [46]. Evidence suggests that DMN activity is related to attentional and other cognitive and valence RDoC constructs, as well as to alterations in DMN functioning in a large range of disorders, including schizophrenia, attention-deficit/hyperactivity disorder and clinical depression [45]. Alterations in the interplay between task positive (TP) and TN elements of the DMN have been proposed as a risk factor for clinical depression [45]. There is also reason to believe that the DMN construct may prove to be useful in characterizing the beneficial cognitive and affective effects of nicotine in reducing TN and enhancing TP neural network activity. Researchers have proposed and provided evidence that nicotine withdrawal is associated with a dysfunctional internally focused cognitive state as well as a failure to attenuate TN activity in the transition from rest to task [3, 24, 46]. Similarly, Marchetti et al. [45] proposed that the TN-TP imbalance as the overarching neural mechanism involved in crucial cognitive risk factors for recurrent depression, namely rumination, impaired attentional control and cognitive reactivity. Given that nicotine and tobacco smoking abstinence modulate the DMN, reducing TN-DMN activity [3, 45], and given the above-noted associations of DMN activation to clinical depression, attention-deficit/hyperactivity disorder and other psychiatric disorders that are associated with a high prevalence of nicotine dependence, future work in this area seems important and promising.

Prevention and Intervention Strategies Based on Constructs of Arousal/Modulatory Systems
Given the adverse effects on sleep produced by smoking abstinence, pharmacological aids for smoking cessation (nicotine replacement therapy and bupropion SR) [18, 43], stress and psychopathology [32], as well as the effects of nicotine and smoking abstinence on objective measures of brain arousal/activation, it is crucial that smoking interventions address issues related to ARMS constructs. There is a clear need for future randomized clinical trials to assess the effects of different cessation treatments as a function of individual differences in ARMS constructs, including sleep patterns and general cognitive functions related to arousal. Given the adverse effects of smoking abstinence and pharmacotherapies to promote smoking abstinence, the authors encourage systematic assessments and interventions focused on sleep disturbances and other ARMS constructs.

Conclusion

Smoking status, smoking abstinence and nicotine influence many of the components of each of the higher-order RDoC constructs – NVS, PVS, CoS, SSoP and ARMS. There is reason to believe that many of these smoking-related effects combine in differing degrees across different smokers to reinforce smoking and constitute important endophenotypes with multiple, genetic, state- and trait-dependent effects on the development of smoking and cessation processes. Clinical and preventative interventions to promote smoking abstinence would likely benefit from the routine and systematic assessment of these constructs in combination with information about specific situations that promote smoking initiation and maintenance, and those that make it difficult for a given individual or groups of individuals with specific RDoC dysfunctions to refrain from smoking.

Key Points

- The psychology of the smoker and the likelihood to become a smoker varies between individuals, depending on trait factors related to individual differences in genetics, nicotine exposure, temperament, and chronic environmental and social factors.

High chronic (trait) NVS activation (e.g. anxious and depressive traits), suboptimal positive affect-related PVS functioning and suboptimal cognitive system functioning are predictive of both increased prevalence of smoking and failed attempts to quit smoking.

- The current state activations of the various research domain criteria (RDoC) constructs vary across time as a function of changes in situations across time. Changes in the state activation of these constructs influence the likelihood of smoking at a given moment by a given smoker.
- The likelihood of smoking by an individual varies as a function of both inhibitory and facilitative internal (e.g. negative moods) and external contexts (e.g. smokers in the environment) combined with the relative balance of neural control systems and motivations associated with the cognitive control constructs.
- RDoC of the National Institute of Mental Health provide new ways of assessing and classifying smoking based on basic dimensions across multiple units of analyses, from genes to neural circuits to behavior. There is good reason to expect that the RDoC approach will lead to new and better-focused smoking intervention treatments.

References

1 Audrain-McGovern J, Nigg JT, Perkins K: Endophenotypes for nicotine dependence risk at or before initial nicotine exposure; in NCI Tobacco Control Monograph Series, No 20: Phenotypes and Endophenotypes: Foundations for Genetic Studies of Nicotine Use and Dependence. Bethesda, National Cancer Institute, 2009, chapt 8.
2 Pergadia ML, Der-Avakian A, D'Souza MS, Madden PAF, Heath AC, Shiffman S, Markou A, Pizzagalli DA: Association between nicotine withdrawal and reward responsiveness in humans and rats. JAMA Psychiatry 2014;71:1238–1245.
3 Gilbert DG: Smoking: Individual Differences, Psychopathology, and Emotion. Washington, Taylor & Francis, 1995.
4 National Institute of Mental Health: Research Domain Criteria (2011). http://www.nimh.nih.gov/research-priorities/rdoc/nimh-research-domain-criteria-rdoc.shtml.
5 Centers for Disease Control and Prevention (CDC): Cigarette smoking among adults – United States, 2006. MMWR Morb Mortal Wkly Rep 2007;56:1157–1161.
6 Shiffman S: Light and intermittent smokers: background and perspective. Nicotine Tob Res 2009; 11:122–125.
7 Agaku IT, King BA, Dube SR; Centers for Disease Control and Prevention(CDC): Current cigarette smoking among adults – United States, 2005–2012. MMWR Morb Mortal Wkly Rep 2014;63: 29–34.

8 Kahler CW, Daughters SB, Leventhal AM, Rogers ML, Clark MA, Colby SM, Boergers J, Ramsey SE, Abrams DB, Niaura R, Buka SL: Personality, psychiatric disorders, and smoking in middle-aged adults. Nicotine Tob Res 2009;7:833–841.
9 Pergadia ML, Madden PAF, Lessov CN, et al: Genetic and environmental influences on extreme personality dispositions in adolescent female twins. J Child Psychol Psychiatry 2006;47:902–909.
10 Pergadia ML, Heath AC, Martin NG, Madden PAF: Genetic analyses of DSM-IV nicotine withdrawal in adult twins. Psychol Med 2006;36:963–972.
11 Lessov-Schlaggar CN, Pergadia ML, Khroyan TV, Swan GE: Genetics of nicotine dependence and pharmacotherapy. Biochem Pharmacol 2008;75: 178–195.
12 Burmeister M, McInnis MG, Zöllner S: Psychiatric genetics: progress amid controversy. Nat Rev Genet 2008;9:527–540.
13 Bierut LJ, Johnson EO, Saccone NL: A glimpse into the future – personalized medicine for smoking cessation. Neuropharmacology 2014;76:592–599.
14 de Moor MH, Costa PT, Terracciano A, Krueger RF, de Geus EJC, Toshiko T, et al: Meta-analysis of genome-wide association studies for personality. Mol Psychiatry 2012;17:337–349.
15 Cross-Disorder Group of the Psychiatric Genomics Consortium: Identification of risk loci with shared effects on five major psychiatric disorders: a genome-wide analysis. Lancet 2013;381:1371–1379.

16 Zuo Y, Gilbert DG, Rabinovich NE, Riise H, Needham R, Huggenvik JI: DRD2-related TaqIA polymorphism modulates motivation to smoke. Nicotine Tob Res 2009;11:1321–1329.
17 Pritchard WS: The link between smoking and P: a serotonergic hypothesis. Pers Individ Differ 1991; 12:1187–1204.
18 Colrain IM, Trinder J, Swan GE: The impact of smoking cessation on objective and subjective markers of sleep: review, synthesis, and recommendations. Nicotine Tob Res 2004;6;913–925.
19 Gilbert DG, McClernon FJ, Rabinovich NE, Plath LC, Masson CL, Anderson AE, Sly KF: Mood disturbance fails to resolve across 31 days of cigarette abstinence in women. J Consult Clin Psychol 2002;70:142–152.
20 Shiffman S, Paty J: Smoking patterns and dependence: contrasting chippers and heavy smokers. J Abnorm Psychol 2006;115:509–523.
21 Gilbert DG, Riise H, Dillon A, Huber J, Rabinovich NE, Sugai C: Emotional stimuli and context moderate effects of nicotine on specific but not global affects. Exp Clin Psychopharmacol 2008; 16:33–42.
22 Korhonen T, Kinnunen TH, Garvey AJ: Impact of nicotine replacement therapy on post-cessation mood profile by pre-cessation depressive symptoms. Tob Induc Dis 2006;3:17–33.
23 Gray JA, McNaughton N: The Neuropsychology of Anxiety. New York, Oxford University Press, 2000.
24 Gilbert DG, Welser R: Emotion, anxiety, and smoking; in Ney T, Gale A (eds): Smoking and Human Behavior. Chichester, Wiley, 1989, pp 171–196.

25 Kassel JD, Stroud LR, Paronis CA: Smoking, stress, and negative affect: correlation, causation, and context across stages of smoking. Psychol Bull 2003;129:270–304.

26 Hogle JM, Kaye JT, Curtin JJ: Nicotine withdrawal increases threat-induced anxiety but not fear: neuroadaptation in human addiction. Biol Psychiatry 2010;68:719–725.

27 Robinson TE, Berridge KC: The psychology and neurobiology of addiction: an incentive-sensitization view. Addiction 2000;95(suppl 2):91–117.

28 Al'Absi M: Current and future directions of research on stress and addictive behaviors; in Al'Absi M (ed): Stress and Addiction: Biological and Psychological Mechanisms. Burlington, Elsevier, 2007, pp 349–371.

29 Gilbert DG, Zuo Y, Rabinovich NE, Riise H, Needham R, Huggenvik JI: Neurotransmission-related genetic polymorphisms, negative affectivity traits, and gender predict tobacco abstinence symptoms across 44 days with and without nicotine patch. J Abnorm Psychol 2009;118:322–334.

30 van der Meer RM, Willemsen MC, Smit F, Cuijpers P: Smoking cessation interventions for smokers with current or past depression. Cochrane Database Syst Rev 2013;8:CD006102.

31 Asgaard GL, Gilbert DG, Malpass D, Sugai C, Dillon A: Nicotine primes attention to competing affective stimuli in the context of salient alternatives. Exp Clin Psychopharmacol 2010;18:51–60.

32 Barr RS, Pizzagalli DA, Culhane MA, Goff DC, Evins AE: A single dose of nicotine enhances reward responsiveness in nonsmokers: implications for development of dependence. Biol Psychiatry 2008;63:1061–1065.

33 Pizzagalli DA, Bogdan R, Ratner KG, Jahn AL: Increased perceived stress is associated with blunted hedonic capacity: potential implications for depression research. Behav Res Ther 2007;45:2742–2753.

34 Perkins KA: Baseline-dependency of nicotine effects: a review. Behav Pharmacol 1999;10:597–615.

35 Wachter NJ, Gilbert DG: Nicotine differentially modulates antisaccade eye-gaze away from emotional stimuli in nonsmokers stratified by pre-task baseline performance. Psychopharmacology (Berl) 2013;225:561–568.

36 Kollins SH, McClernon FJ, Fuemmeler BF: Association between smoking and ADHD symptoms in a population-based sample of young adults. Arch Gen Psychiatry 2005;62:1142–1147.

37 Eysenck HJ: Personality and the maintenance of the smoking habit; in Dunn WL (ed): Smoking Behavior: Motives and Incentives. Washington, Winston, 1973, pp 113–146.

38 Fergusson DM, Horwood LJ, Ridder EM: Show me the child at seven II: childhood intelligence and later outcomes in adolescence and young adulthood. J Child Psychol Psychiatry 2005;46:850–858.

39 Heishman SJ, Kleykamp BA, Singleton EG: Meta-analysis of the acute effects of nicotine and smoking on human performance. Psychopharmacology (Berl) 2010;210:453–469.

40 Carlson JM, Gilbert DG, Riise H, Rabinovich NE, Froeliger B, Sugai C: Serotonin transporter genotype and depressive symptoms moderate effects of nicotine on spatial working memory. Exp Clin Psychopharmacol 2009;17:173–180.

41 McClernon FJ, Gilbert DG, Radtke R: Effects of transdermal nicotine on lateralized identification and memory interference. Hum Psychopharmacol 2003;18:339–343.

42 Conklin CA, Salkeld RP, Perkins KA, Robin N: Do people serve as cues to smoke? Nicotine Tob Res 2013;15:2081–2087.

43 Van Veen MM, Kooij JJ, Boonstra AM, Gordijn M: Delayed circadian rhythm in adults with attention-deficit/hyperactivity disorder and chronic sleep-onset insomnia. Biol Psychiatry 2010;67:1091–1096.

44 Gilbert DG, McClernon FJ, Rabinovich NE, Sugai C, Plath LC, Asgaard G, Zuo Y, Huggenvik JI, Botros N: Effects of quitting smoking on EEG activation and attention last for more than 31 days and are more severe with stress, dependence, DRD2 A1 allele, and depressive traits. Nicotine Tob Res 2004;6:249–267.

45 Marchetti I, Koster EHW, Sonuga-Barke EJ, De Raedt R: The default mode network and recurrent depression: a neurobiological model of cognitive risk factors. Neuropsychol Rev 2012;22:229–251.

46 Lerman C, Louhed J, Ruparel K, Yang Y, Stein EA: Large-scale brain network coupling predicts acute nicotine abstinence effects on craving and cognitive function. JAMA Psychiatry 2014;71:523–530.

47 Taylor DJ, Lichstein KL, Durrence HH, Reidel BW, Bush AJ: Epidemiology of insomnia, depression, and anxiety. Sleep 2005;28:1457–1464.

48 Pulvermüller F: Hebb's concept of cell assemblies and the psychophysiology of word processing. Psychophysiology 1996;33:317–333.

David G. Gilbert, PhD
Department of Psychology, LSII, Room 281, Mail Code: 6502, Southern Illinois University
1125 Lincoln Drive
Carbondale, IL 62901-6502 (USA)
E-Mail dgilbert@siu.edu

Loddenkemper R, Kreuter M (eds): The Tobacco Epidemic, ed 2, rev. and ext.
Prog Respir Res. Basel, Karger, 2015, vol 42, pp 72–84 (DOI: 10.1159/000369327)

Respiratory Disorders Related to Smoking Tobacco

John F. Murray[a] · A. Sonia Buist[b]

[a]University of California San Francisco, San Francisco, Calif., and [b]Oregon Health and Science University, Portland, Oreg., USA

Abstract

Respiratory disorders are among the most frequent causes of death and severe disability from the steadily worsening global pandemic of smoking tobacco. Two disorders stand out: lung cancer and chronic obstructive pulmonary disease (COPD). First, lung cancer caused 1.59 million deaths worldwide in 2012, more than the next two top cancer causes combined (liver and stomach). Tobacco smoke induces pathologic changes in the bronchial epithelium that often progress to fatal invasive lung cancer. For the first time, the recent US National Lung Screening Trial reported a significant (20%) reduction in lung cancer mortality in current or previous heavy smokers detected by low-dose, spiral computed tomography. Second, dramatic advances in understanding COPD include the recognition that it is a complex, multisystem disease that involves many organs – not just the lungs. COPD results from an inflammatory process leading to narrowing and scarring of small airways and destruction of lung parenchyma causing emphysema. Tobacco smoke remains the most important risk factor for COPD globally, but occupational and environmental exposures play increasing roles. Tobacco smoke is also the principal cause of certain interstitial lung diseases and worsens others. Both prenatal and postnatal tobacco exposure contribute to impairment in lung growth and development, and increase the risk of acquiring infectious pneumonias and tuberculosis.   © 2015 S. Karger AG, Basel

Virtually all steady smokers eventually suffer from nagging, chronic respiratory symptoms, chiefly cough, sputum production and intermittent breathlessness, which impair the quality of life and shorten its duration by a decade. Smoking has adverse health effects on the structure and function of the lungs and reduces lung defenses against infection.

Smokers also suffer from many other chronic health conditions so the effects of smoking are not confined to the lungs (see table 1 in chapter 8). Exposure to cigarette smoke impairs lung growth and functional development, starting in utero and extending into infancy and childhood (see also chapter 9). Smoking is by far the number one cause of preventable mortality and disability throughout the world, and respiratory diseases have long topped the list of smoking-determined origins of death and illness (see fig. 1 in chapter 2). Furthermore, the cost of respiratory diseases is gigantic; according to the European Lung White Book, 'The cost of respiratory disease in the 28 countries of the EU alone amounts to more than EUR 380 billion annually. Approximately half of the economic burden of respiratory disease is attributable to smoking' [1].

This chapter mainly discusses the two principal smoking-related respiratory diseases, first, lung cancer, by far the biggest killer among malignancies, and, second, not far behind, chronic obstructive pulmonary disease (COPD) [2–4].

Emphasis in these chapters is placed on epidemiology, pathogenesis, diagnosis, management and prevention. Briefly considered are interstitial lung diseases (ILDs), asthma, pre- and postnatal development and pulmonary infections – which are all greatly worsened by tobacco smoking. The benefits of smoking cessation and reducing smoking worldwide is an important priority to improve global health.

Lung Cancer

Epidemiology

The World Health Organization (WHO) has just launched its latest (2014) report from the International Agency for Research on Cancer that warns both health professionals and the general public about the alarming increase in new cases of cancer and related deaths: a veritable 'tidal wave' of malignancies, which includes a global burden of cancer estimated to have increased to 14 million cases [5]. Moreover, cancer is 'a leading' cause of death worldwide; WHO data in 2012 indicated there were 1.59 million deaths from lung cancer alone, more than the total number of deaths from the next two top causes of cancer deaths – liver (745,000) and stomach (723,000) – combined [6].

History

The growth of new cases and deaths from lung cancer during the last century has been truly amazing. In all the years leading up to 1912, a total of only 374 cases had been reported in the entire world's medical literature [7]; by contrast, in 2012, exactly 100 years later, 1.8 million new lung cancer cases were diagnosed that *single year alone*, including (as mentioned) 1.59 million deaths [6]. In addition, as everyone knows, the cause of this astronomic explosion of disease and deaths is tobacco, chiefly from smoking cigarettes [8].

Tobacco has a long history of use by Native Americans dating back to thousands or more years. The rest of the world learned about tobacco after Christopher Columbus brought some back from the New World to Spain, from which it quickly spread to other regions. Not long afterward, tobacco was smoked in pipes and cigars, inhaled as snuff, and had a variety of supposed therapeutic properties. Cultivation of tobacco during the 17th and 18th centuries in the southern states of America greatly increased its availability and popularity. Hand-rolled cigarettes became increasingly smoked during the Civil War, but usage soared in 1891 after James Bonsack invented the cigarette-making machine (for more details, see chapter 1).

The seminal event in the evolving epidemiologic history of the use of tobacco occurred with the publication in 1964 of the first US Surgeon General's Report that conclusively established that cigarette smoking caused lung cancer in men, and that the linkage between the two conditions outweighed the importance of all other causative factors [9]. The evidence in women pointed in the same direction – that cigarette-smoking caused lung cancer – but was not yet definitive.

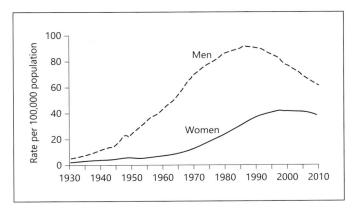

Fig. 1. Graph showing age-adjusted lung and bronchus cancer death rates in men (dotted line) and women (solid line) from 1930 to 2010 (source: US Mortality Volumes 1930 to 1959 and US Mortality Volumes 1960 to 2010. National Center for Health Statistics, Centers for Disease Control and Prevention. ©2014 American Cancer Society, Inc., with permission).

The 1964 Surgeon General's Report had considerable public impact and led to an immediate reduction in cigarette smoking by Americans. Looking back now, it is of interest to reflect on the magnitude of smoking in adults at the time: 52.9% of men and 31.5% of women. Astonishingly, in 1964 also, two thirds of all men aged 21–24 years (67.0%!) and well over 40% of women in the same age range (41.9%) smoked cigarettes [7]. Most young people today do not remember that not long ago nearly everyone smoked in restaurants, movie theaters, airplanes, offices and even hospitals. In the 50 years since that first blockbuster publication – which definitively linked lung cancer in men with smoking cigarettes – the US Surgeon General has issued 30 additional reports that have examined the tobacco versus health connection from every conceivable angle. Naturally, last year's stupendous and comprehensive 50th-anniversary report celebrated The Health Consequences of Smoking – 50 Years of Progress: A Report of the Surgeon General, 2014 [10].

Mortality

As shown by the data in figure 1, the age-adjusted mortality rates from lung cancer in the US, both in males and females, changed dramatically from 1930 to 2010 [11]. Mortality rates in men peaked in the early 1990s and then began to decline substantially; by contrast, those in women rose more slowly, then plateaued for over a decade before declining slightly about 2002. These patterns reflect differences in prevailing smoking habits between men and women over time, which have narrowed the mortality difference between the two sexes.

Roughly similar patterns have evolved in Canada and the United Kingdom, but there are marked regional variations in age-standardized mortality rates from lung cancer in various countries and regions. Mortality remains high in most of Europe, which has a notable preponderance of men over women [12]. Lung cancer mortality rates in many poor countries, though low, are increasing as incomes and prosperity have improved.

Fifteen to 20% of American victims of lung cancer have never smoked cigarettes or used tobacco in any form, and the number appears to be growing. Exposure to radon, diagnostic radiation, occupational hazards, air pollution and some infections, all increase the risk of developing lung cancer [13]. Among the most frequent of these exposures is secondhand smoke from two different sources: first and more important, the smoke from the end of a burning cigarette or other tobacco product, and second, the smoke that has been exhaled from a smoker's lungs (see chapter 10).

Secondhand smoke causes a variety of dangerous respiratory disorders in infants and children (see chapter 9), and an enhanced risk of cardiovascular disease, especially in adults already afflicted with heart disease. Secondhand smoke exposure at home or work by Americans increases the risk of acquiring lung cancer by 20–30% and is estimated to cause over 7,300 lung cancer deaths every year in nonsmokers [14].

Pathogenesis

Tobacco smoke is a mixture of gases and fine particles that contains more than 5,000 toxic chemicals, including about 70 that are carcinogenic (see chapter 4). But the mechanisms that lead from exposure of carcinogen-laden tobacco smoke to the onset of lung cancer are incompletely understood. The beginnings of this multistep process fit in with the concept of what is called 'field cancerization': the induction of pathologic abnormalities by a carcinogenic agent – such as tobacco smoke – that lead to histologically defined premalignant precursor lesions. The next step insofar as the lungs are concerned is characterized by the formation of one or more zones of genetic and epigenetic alterations of bronchial epithelium having malignant potential, especially dysplasia and carcinoma in situ. The final step in the evolution of lung cancer is for lesions to become invasive and fatal carcinomas (see chapter 8, fig. 2).

'Only' 10–15% of all current and former cigarette smokers develop progressive pulmonary malignancies, which suggests that risk factors besides tobacco, such as other exposures and/or genetic predisposition, may play an additive role [15].

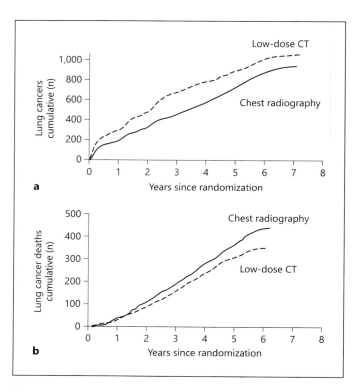

Fig. 2. a Cumulative number of lung cancers that were diagnosed from the date of randomization through December 31, 2009. **b** Cumulative number of deaths from lung cancer that occurred from the date of randomization through January 15, 2009 (reproduced with permission from Aberle et al. [17]).

Eighty-five percent of lung cancers are classed as nonsmall-cell lung carcinomas, of which there are three principal histologic types – adenocarcinoma, squamous cell carcinoma and large cell carcinoma – plus a few atypical cellular variants; the remaining 15% of lung cancers are small-cell lung carcinomas, which are aggressively malignant, virtually incurable, and respond transiently to radiation and chemotherapy.

Since the early 1990s, adenocarcinoma has replaced squamous cell carcinoma as the predominant cell type, perhaps owing to the use of different types of cigarettes and/or smoking habits [12]; an increased prevalence of adenocarcinoma in nonsmokers, especially women, is also playing a role. Of note, considerable progress has been made in staging non-small-cell lung carcinomas and in using immunohistochemical techniques to identify biological markers (e.g. epidermal growth factor receptor and Alk-gene rearrangement) that identify specific targeted antineoplastic regimens, which, in turn, have improved prognosis in individuals bearing the responsible marker [16].

Screening

Considerable interest and excitement greeted the long-awaited report published in the *New England Journal of Medicine* in June 2011 announcing the outcome of the US National Lung Screening Trial, a collaborative effort between the National Cancer Institute and the American College of Radiology Imaging Network [17]. This epic study resulted in the largest (53,454 subjects) and longest (enrollment started in 2002) randomized comparison ever performed to determine the benefits of screening for lung cancer with low-dose spiral computed tomography (CT) versus ordinary chest X-ray examinations. The trial was stopped in October 2010 – earlier than expected – by the Data Safety and Monitoring Board, which regularly evaluates the growing amount of information; the cutoff was mandated because interim analysis at the time showed a statistically significant 20.0% reduction in lung cancer mortality in the CT arm of the study compared with the chest X-ray arm; in addition, there was also a significant reduction (6.7%) in overall mortality in the subjects tested by CT, largely owing to fewer lung cancer deaths (fig. 2).

The outcome of the National Lung Screening Trial represents a tremendous scientific and organizational achievement. Starting in the 1970s, several chest X-ray screening studies of heavy smokers, sometimes supplemented by cytological (Papanicolaou smears) examinations, mostly failed to lower death rates from lung cancer. Low-dose CT, however, is much more sensitive and accurate than an ordinary chest X-ray in detecting various kinds of small lesions. In fact, 24% of the CT studies showed one or more abnormalities, a surprisingly high yield [17]. But the downside of the more sensitive technique is that a remarkable 96% of the lesions proved to be benign.

Treatment

Surgical resection of potentially malignant tumors demands appropriate caution and a high level of judgment; removal of lung nodules represents a major diagnostic undertaking with considerable cost and inevitable side effects, including occasional deaths. Semisolid or solid lesions that were undetectable on previous radiographic examinations are highly suspect, as are spiculated nodules and those with notches and other discernable morphologic characteristics of malignancy. Another decisive reason for surgical removal is obvious growth documented by serial CTs. But because the growth rates of lung nodules authenticated by repeat examinations vary, different study intervals may be required [18]. Another serious concern over lung cancer

screening is the undeniable and unavoidable hazard of radiation itself as the proximate cause of lung cancer and other malignancies.

To further define the presence or absence of malignancy in radiologically detectable nodules, Patz et al. [19] have developed a serum assay combining three markers, carcinoembryonic antigen, α_1-antitrypsin and squamous cell carcinoma antigen, which documented 80% sensitivity and 89% specificity in a logistic regression model. Additional such tests may help differentiate true-positive from false-positive outcomes of lung nodule detection.

Finally, the joy inherent in finding a curable lung cancer by screening is often overshadowed by the expense of the undertaking, which is colossal and dependent on the criteria for selecting who gets screened. The bottom line of the Lung Cancer Screening Trial indicates that screening lowers the stage at which lung cancer is detectable and therefore curable for some but by no means all surveyed subjects [8]. Widespread screening will cost a lot of money. Guidelines are already in place that rely heavily on age, the pack-years of cigarette smoking, how long ago someone quit (smoking cessation should be part of lung cancer screening programs) and how often examinations should be repeated [20]. Preliminary US estimates concerning the 5-year cost of lung cancer screening are enormous, upwards of USD 10 billion. So far, the prevailing gospel from America has been that saving lives is paramount and that costs are secondary. Debate is underway about the cost-effectiveness of lung cancer screening in prosperous European and Asian countries.

Other Malignancies

According to the American Cancer Society [11], besides the huge number of lung cancer deaths, cigarette smoking is a major cause of death from cancers arising in other anatomic sites, such as upper air passages [mouth, lips, nose, sinuses pharynx (throat) and larynx (voice box)], esophagus (swallowing tube), stomach, pancreas (probably), kidney, bladder, uterus, cervix, colorectum and ovary (mucinous), and from acute myeloid leukemia (see chapter 8). In 2014, tobacco use is estimated to contribute to at least 30% of all 585,720 US cancer deaths, or 175,716 smoking-related deaths, of which 126,260 are from lung cancer and over 50,000 involve other anatomic sites.

Cigarette smoking is by far the most flagrant cause of preventable respiratory disease and death, but as cigarette use diminishes in high-income countries, including the USA, sales and usage of other tobacco products is steadily growing, both those that are smoked [pipes, cigars and nicotine-containing e-cigarettes (see chapter 23)] and those that are smokeless ([snuff, chewing tobacco and 'spitless' powders [4] (see also chapters 21 and 22)]). The health consequences of various tobacco products differ to some extent, but all possess malignant potential.

Chronic Obstructive Pulmonary Disease

Recent Developments
There have been dramatic advances in our understanding of COPD in the last 2 decades. Perhaps the most important is the recognition that COPD is a complex, multisystem, multicomponent disease, not just a single organ disease of the lungs [21]. This change in focus is important as it affects diagnosis and management. The defining feature of COPD in the past was that it causes airflow obstruction or airflow limitation, and is best identified and quantified by the forced expiratory volume in 1 s (FEV_1). As our understanding of COPD deepens, better tools to identify and quantify COPD are emerging to help clinicians manage patients with COPD better. Many risk factors are now known to play a role in the pathogenesis of COPD, but cigarette smoking and other forms of tobacco remain the most common cause of this increasingly prevalent condition.

Definitions
Along with changes in our understanding of COPD have come changes in the definition and in our recommendation of which diseases should be included in the term 'COPD'. The current definition of COPD that is used most widely is the definition recommended by the Global Initiative on Chronic Obstructive Lung Disease (GOLD) [21], which has undergone several revisions since GOLD started in 2002. The major changes that have been introduced are to stress that COPD is a *preventable and treatable disease* and that COPD encompasses a group of diseases characterized by an abnormal inflammatory response. GOLD defines COPD as: 'a common preventable and treatable disease characterized by persistent airflow limitation that is usually progressive and associated with an enhanced inflammatory response in the airways and the lung to noxious particles or gases. Exacerbations and comorbidities contribute to the overall severity in individual patients'.

Prevalence and Mortality
There is now considerable information about the prevalence of COPD in countries at all levels of economic development – thanks to several large studies spanning the globe – that have paid meticulous attention to quality control. The largest of these are the Burden of Obstructive Lung Disease (BOLD) Study [22] (data now from 32 countries) and the PLATINO Study [23] (data from 5 Latin American countries). Both of these large studies used the same protocol, same quality control and same definition for COPD, so it is acceptable to compare data across both studies.

The data on mortality from COPD are sobering. The Global Burden of Disease [24] has reported the most recent data from 187 countries and provided projections for mortality up to 2020. COPD is already the third leading cause of death worldwide and is one of the fastest growing causes of death, thanks to the changing global demographics with a larger proportion of people in all countries living into the COPD age range and the increase in tobacco smoking, particularly in resource-poor countries. However, as noted below, risk factors for COPD in medium- and low-income countries are likely to differ from those in high-income countries; mortality from COPD is high in both low- and middle-income countries, whereas the prevalence of smoking is still quite low, especially in women [25].

Pathophysiology
The chronic airflow limitation that characterizes COPD is caused by both *small-airway disease* and *parenchymal destruction*, both of which are a result of an abnormal inflammatory response [21]. The small-airway disease results in a narrowing of the *bronchioles*, whereas the parenchymal disease is a destruction of the lung parenchyma that leads to loss of alveolar attachments to the small airways and loss of lung elastic recoil called *emphysema*. The mix of both airway and/or parenchymal involvement varies from person to person and is likely an individual gene-environment response; this means that the environmental component (risk factor) and the genetic makeup of the individual interact to determine the pathologic outcome in any given person.

Cigarette smoking greatly increases the risk of COPD in α_1-antitrypsin-deficient patients, leading to severe, early-onset emphysema due to destruction of alveolar septa in the lung as a consequence of the protease-antiprotease imbalance [26].

Chronic bronchitis used to be included in COPD but it is more usually separated out now as it does not necessarily cause chronic airflow limitation and is primarily a clinical definition, defined by chronic cough and sputum [21]. Chronic bronchitis is common in smokers, with or without chronic airflow obstruction, and is the reason for the troubling cough that many smokers report and that has a significant effect on their quality of life.

Chronic Obstructive Pulmonary Disease – A Multisystem, Multicomponent Disease

Until recently, COPD was thought of as a single organ disease or condition. We now recognize that it is part of a multisystem disorder involving many organs and complex systems; these include bones, including bone marrow, cardiovascular system, skeletal muscles, adipose tissue, mental health and probably many more [21]. Smoking is, as mentioned, by far the most common and important risk factor for all of these manifestations, and precisely how they are connected is gradually being clarified.

As noted above, the pathologic changes seen in COPD result from an abnormal inflammatory process involving airways, leading both to small-airway fibrosis and scarring, and to lung parenchymal destruction, resulting in emphysema. Subsequent air trapping causes progressive airflow limitation. The chronic inflammation causes an influx of inflammatory cell types, predominantly polymorphonuclear neutrophils. Smoking cessation does not always reverse this process for reasons that are not clearly understood [21].

Risk Factors

Risk in humans can be considered as the particular outcome of the interplay between genetic and environmental influences. Until recently, smoking was considered the only *causative* risk factor for COPD, meaning that other risk factors (such as occupational exposures) could *contribute* to the development of COPD but could not *cause* COPD by themselves. This thinking is now outdated. There is no question that tobacco smoking remains, and always has been, the *most important* risk factor for COPD globally, but evidence accumulated over the past 2 decades has helped to broaden our understanding of risks for COPD [27]. Conceptually, the model that is most helpful when thinking about risk for COPD is that inhaled particles (and some gases) incite an inflammatory response in the airways and the net response in any individual is determined by interaction between the inhaled substances and the genetic makeup of the individual. Because all particles are not equal, size and composition are key determinants of the outcome. Particles come in a wide range of size with only the smallest particles (<2.5 μm) being able to penetrate far into the lungs. Cigarette smoke, as discussed earlier in this chapter, comprises a mixture of particles and gases which also include powerful carcinogens and potent toxins (see also chapter 4).

Causative Risk Factors

Smoking. Smoking was the first *causative* risk factor to be etiologically related to COPD; in other words, a factor for which there is high-level evidence that it can cause COPD. Globally, smoking is without doubt the most important risk factor. Large well-designed and executed worldwide prevalence surveys, such as BOLD [22] and PLATINO [23], discussed above, have again confirmed the strong link between smoking and COPD. However, the picture has become more complicated as additional information about smoking habits has accumulated [22, 23]. At present, smoking is uncommon in women in much of the developing world, but in men, although smoking is common, the total pack-years of exposure is modest compared with rich-country levels, but is steadily increasing in several resource-poor nations. The dose-response relationship is not linear and understanding the precise relationship between dose and outcome is complex as dose is hard to quantify accurately, methods of inhalation vary widely, and the geometry of the airways is affected by many factors, including sex, disease and an individual's genes.

Passive smoking is exposure to tobacco smoke (see also chapters 9 and 10), and has a clear-cut linkage with lung cancer. By contrast, it is uncertain whether secondhand smoke, by itself, is *causal* for COPD and is best thought of as an important risk factor that adds to the particulate and chemical burden in the lungs and that has a similar composition as mainline tobacco smoke [28–30].

Occupational Exposures. The strength of the evidence linking occupational exposures to COPD has increased over the past few years and has now reached the level at which some occupational exposures are considered as *causative* for COPD [27]. These exposures are especially important in countries in which occupational environmental controls are weak. They may be from particles and/or gases, and the outcome will depend on the composition of the material, the dose, the distribution of the particles or gases and the individual's genetically determined susceptibility.

Associated Risk Factors

Associated risk factors are those for which there is evidence that they are *associated* with COPD but the level of evidence for *causation* is not yet adequate. Below are brief comments about several important associated risk factors for COPD; asthma and pre- and postnatal exposure factors are discussed later.

Sex. Whether women or men are at greater risk for COPD remains controversial. Women are more likely to develop severe early-onset COPD, but this is probably a phenotypically different form of the disease [21, 25]. If the dose and exposure of the inhaled risk factors are the same, it is not clear that there is a clear sex-related susceptibility.

Age. COPD is a disease that tends to progress with age. Age, therefore, has a strong association with COPD, yet is not *causal* in the absence of other risk factors [21].

Outdoor Air Pollution. The dramatic, historic outdoor air pollution episodes in urban areas, such as London fogs in the 1950s, will always be associated with chronic bronchitis. Whether outdoor air pollution *causes* COPD is still controversial and presumably depends on the composition of the air pollution, its dose and deposition, other concomitant inhaled risk factors and, once again, the individual's genes [27]. Currently, urban areas with very high levels of air pollution – such as Beijing, Jakarta and other megacities – are noted for a high prevalence of chronic cough and sputum, but the next step of demonstrating that this *causes* chronic airflow limitation, in the absence of other risk factors, is missing.

Indoor Air Pollution. Fifty-two percent of the world's population uses some form of biomass fuel, which includes wood, coal, crop waste and dung, for cooking and heating. The WHO has reported that indoor air pollution causes 1.6 million deaths annually, more than half are children 5 years or younger [31]. These dramatic reports have stimulated a global initiative (Clean Cookstove Initiative) to introduce 200 million clean cookstoves by 2020; this is a worthy initiative that will doubtless decrease the burden of respiratory disease among the affected populations. The problem we are addressing is to summarize the strength of the evidence linking indoor air pollution as *causing* COPD, which is presently inadequate. Again, it is likely that the risk relates to the composition of the exposure, the dose, the presence of other inhaled risk factors and the individual's genetic makeup [25, 27]. Because the use of biomass fuels for heating and cooking is so widespread in developing countries, understanding the link between biomass fuel use and COPD is an urgent priority.

Tuberculosis. There is now strong evidence that chronic airflow limitation is more common in individuals who have had tuberculosis than in those without lung involvement. The mechanism is almost certainly the result of structural changes in the airways and lung parenchyma caused by the disease [32].

Poverty. Socioeconomic deprivation has many elements. The consequences may start in utero and continue during childhood and into adult years. In order to develop a successful strategy to prevent the adverse consequences of poverty, its components must be identified and correct-

ed. Smoking adds to the burden of poverty, and in rich countries it is more prevalent in lower than in higher socioeconomic groups, whereas the reverse is true in poor countries. The growing body of information that COPD mortality is high in developing countries yet the smoking rates are still low, especially in women, highlights the urgent need to better understand the link between poverty and COPD.

Diet. The evidence linking COPD with diet is currently very slim. The mechanism is likely to be related to the antioxidant properties [33] of specific dietary components, but *when* this is important or crucial in the whole life span is not yet known.

COPD in Nonsmokers. Although smoking is the causative factor most closely related to COPD, COPD also occurs commonly in nonsmokers, especially in developing countries, as noted above [30]. This is an important public health message for clinicians and the responsible risk factors are beginning to be teased out.

Diagnosis

Spirometry is required to confirm the presence of airflow limitation [21] in order to avoid misclassification and to direct management. Since FEV_1 has a poor correlation with disease severity, there is mounting interest in developing and evaluating other diagnostic and predictive tests that are more useful clinically and take the multisystem nature of COPD into account. The ones that have had the most attention are the BODE (body mass index, FEV_1, dyspnea and exercise capacity) [34]; ADO (age, dyspnea and FEV_1), and the DOSE (dyspnea, FEV_1, smoking status and frequency of COPD exacerbations) Indices [35]. New high-tech imaging methods are also being evaluated as a clinical tool; when drugs are developed that are able to target small airways and lung parenchyma, imaging is likely to become an even more viable clinical tool [21].

Clinical Perspective

Direct-to-public advertising is helping to encourage the term 'COPD' and clinicians are encouraged to do this, too. A key component in the message to clinicians about COPD is that the diagnosis should be verified by spirometry to avoid misclassification and inappropriate treatment and management. In several large prevalence surveys carried out in many countries worldwide, the problem of misclassification has been documented repeatedly. This misclassification goes in both directions: many individuals with normal lung function are being called COPD and many who have COPD are not being identified. Both of these clinical errors are important: the overdiagnosis because it leads to overtreatment or inappropriate treatment, the underdiagnosis because it results in withholding treatment for conditions that have some degree of reversibility. Whether spirometric measurements reveal expiratory airflow obstruction or not, everyone should be encouraged to stop using tobacco. As shown many years ago, stopping smoking slows the decline in FEV_1, the earlier the more successful (fig. 3) [36].

The clinical implications of COPD being part of a multisystem disorder are that clinicians need to consider diagnostic approaches to identifying all systems that may be involved in an individual patient, rather than just focusing on one system. Of course, this applies both to primary-care health care professionals and specialists, as there is ample evidence that many individuals with COPD at all its stages are undiagnosed and untreated, and perhaps misclassified as, for example, single organ heart disease.

Prevention

In the US and other rich countries, aggressive, multitargeted 'never smoke' and 'stop smoking' campaigns are slowly reducing the countrywide prevalence of cigarette smoking; by contrast, as shown in figure 4, the prevalence of low- and middle-income smokers is steadily rising [37]. Thus, owing to the steadily lengthening worldwide life expectancy, and the increased prevalence of smokers in population-rich low- and middle-income countries, tobacco-related sickness and death are predicted to relentlessly increase [8].

The focus for prevention must continue to emphasize tobacco control: discouraging smoking during pregnancy, infancy and early childhood, and in the adolescent years in particular. Other avenues of prevention and control include the elimination of hazardous occupational exposure and reduction of outdoor and indoor air pollution. The other important risk factor, poverty, is hard to fit into a prevention strategy, as the components of poverty are so diverse.

Interstitial Lung Diseases

For over half a century, accumulating clinical, functional, radiographic and pathological findings have conclusively documented that tobacco smoke underlies the pathogenesis of most cases of COPD; today, the same cascade of evidence has shown that tobacco smoke causes a substantial percentage of patients with pulmonary fibrosis, which, as discussed

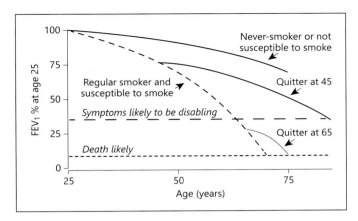

Fig. 3. Schematic diagram of the decline in lung function with age in nonsmokers, smokers and those who quit. Note that stopping smoking slows the rate of decline of lung function [with permission from ref. 36].

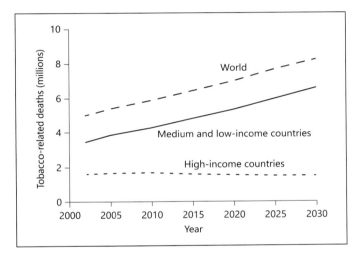

Fig. 4. Projected numbers of tobacco-related deaths for the world and for high- and middle- plus low-income countries from 2002 to 2030 (modified from Mathers and Loncar [37]).

in this section, occurs primarily in the form of ILDs. The common denominator – tobacco smoke – creates the familiar and distinct phenotypes of COPD and pulmonary fibrosis, which, as postulated by Morse and Rosas [38], share some common pathogenic features but derive from 'unique individual susceptibilities'. To strengthen the interrelationships among the three chief tobacco-related lung diseases, the presence of COPD is a well-established risk factor for lung cancer, with an effect independent of cigarette smoking [39], and a similar partnership appears to link lung cancer and fibrosis in ILDs [40].

Smoking-Related Interstitial Lung Diseases

ILDs are receiving increasing attention owing to their growing prevalence and clinical importance, their greatly improved diagnostic characterization and the fact that smoking tobacco is now widely believed to play a primary pathogenic role in particular ILDs [41]; most notably *respiratory bronchiolitis-associated ILD* [42], *desquamative interstitial pneumonia* [43] and *adult pulmonary Langerhans cell histiocytosis* [44]; to this trio should now be added a relative newcomer, *combined pulmonary fibrosis and emphysema* [45], which has all the features of closely associated *smoking-related interstitial fibrosis* [46].

The three long-confirmed smoking-related ILDs have impressive cigarette smoking backgrounds: a 95% association with respiratory bronchiolitis-associated ILD; a 60–90% association with desquamative interstitial pneumonia, and a 95–97% association with adult pulmonary Langerhans cell histiocytosis [41]. Nearly all but not quite 100% of these specific diseases appear to be caused by tobacco smoke as a direct pathogenic factor; the uncommon but well-documented occurrence of never smokers in each of these classic smoking-related entities appears to be attributable to unknown determinants, such as environmental exposures or genetic factors.

In addition, after the appearance of occasional case reports, the first comprehensive review of combined pulmonary fibrosis and emphysema was published in 2005 [45]. All 61 patients were smokers, all but 1 was male, and all had distinguishing characteristics that included CT-defined 'significant' upper-lobe emphysema and lower-lobe pulmonary fibrosis. Striking functional findings included normal total lung capacities, moderately low FEV/FEV$_1$ values and markedly reduced diffusing capacities for carbon monoxide; about half the patients had or developed pulmonary hypertension and survival was poor. Completely different results were recently reported in an analysis of 2,416 patients who had high-resolution CT scans, 8% of which revealed the presence of 'interstitial lung abnormalities' that were associated with reduced total lung capacities and lower percentages of emphysema [47].

Other Interstitial Lung Diseases

The risk of tobacco smoking clearly augments the risk of developing other specific ILDs, including acute *eosinophilic pneumonia* and *pulmonary hemorrhage syndromes*, but identical disorders may occur in never smokers. An international cohort of expert clinicians, radiologists and pathologists recently met in a failed effort to identify a specific phenotype for a smoking-related ILD [48]; this group concluded that tobacco smoking is 'strongly associated with ILD', but it proved difficult to distinguish clinical, physiologic, radiographic and pathologic features between smokers and nonsmokers unless a smoking history was known. To complicate matters further, at least two diseases, *hypersensitivity pneumonitis* and *sarcoidosis*, are known to be less prevalent in smokers compared with nonsmokers [41].

Asthma

Definition

There is no uniformly accepted definition of asthma, which poses problems in both communication and collection of data. The operational designation for asthma includes the presence of underlying chronic airway inflammation associated with reversible airway obstruction, which is characterized by recurrent episodes of wheezing and breathlessness. Ancillary features include, atopy (the genetic predisposition to IgE-dependent responses to common inhaled antigens); bronchial hyperresponsiveness, and inflammatory cell infiltration of airways (eosinophils, basophiles, neutrophils and mast cells). Other quasi-specific terms such as late-onset, exercise-induced, intrinsic and extrinsic, occupational and cardiac asthma attempt to subdivide asthma into special categories, not always successfully. 'Severe asthma', according to the European Respiratory Society-American Thoracic Society [49] is defined as 'asthma which requires treatment with high-dose inhaled corticosteroids (ICS) … plus a second controller (and/or systemic corticosteroids)' to achieve optimum control: treatment is paramount, pathogenesis is ignored.

The Global Initiative for Asthma affirms that asthma is one of the most common chronic diseases in the world and affects around 300 million children and adults [50]. Moreover, as the global population continues to grow, and more and more people adopt western lifestyles and move from rural areas to cities, asthma is projected to increase substantially. The Centers for Disease Control and Prevention recently reported that 6.8 million, or 9.3%, of US children have asthma [51], making it the most prevalent chronic disease in those under 18 years. Asthma disproportionately affects Americans with incomes below the poverty level; in addition, African-Americans have considerably higher rates of emergency department visits and hospitalizations for asthma than Caucasians, and death rates are nearly twice as high.

Chapter 8

Loddenkemper R, Kreuter M (eds): The Tobacco Epidemic, ed 2, rev. and ext.
Prog Respir Res. Basel, Karger, 2015, vol 42, pp 85–96 (DOI: 10.1159/000369368)

Cardiovascular and Other (Except Respiratory) Disorders Related to Smoking Tobacco

Joaquin Barnoya[a, b] · Jose C. Monzon[b]

[a]Division of Public Health Sciences, Department of Surgery, School of Medicine, Washington University in St. Louis, St. Louis, Mo., USA; [b]Research Department, Unidad de Cirugia Cardiovascular de Guatemala, Guatemala City, Guatemala

Abstract

Smoking is the leading cause of preventable death and disease worldwide. In addition to local harmful effects of tobacco smoke, it exerts dramatic systemic effects in the entire body. In this chapter, we summarize the evidence of the diseases caused by smoking, with particular emphasis on cardiovascular diseases (for respiratory diseases, see chapter 7). The cardiovascular system is particularly sensitive to the effects of tobacco smoke. Within minutes of exposure, the effects of smoking on blood vessels become manifest and grow over time. In addition to causing cancer in the respiratory tract, smoking is also causally linked with 13 additional cancer sites. Together, smoking accounts for 30% of all cancers. As with cardiovascular diseases, the increased risk is dose dependent (cigarettes/day and years of smoking). Osteoporosis, periodontal disease, age-related macular degeneration and other diseases are also causally linked to smoking. In conclusion, smoking affects the entire body, not only the respiratory system. Every patient should, therefore, be advised to quit smoking, regardless of their condition or disease.   © 2015 S. Karger AG, Basel

Tobacco-induced disease kills more than 5 million people every year worldwide, and if no effective interventions are implemented by 2030, this number will total 8 million, 80% of them in low- and middle-income countries [1] (see fig. 4 in chapter 7). If current smoking trends continue, tobacco will kill 1 billion people this century [1] (see chapter 2).

Smoking and Cardiovascular Disease

Smoking is the leading cause of preventable cardiovascular disease (CVD). Smoking causes coronary heart disease (CHD; also know as ischemic heart disease) and leads to angina pec-toris and acute myocardial infarction (AMI; table 1) [2]. Almost a third of all smoking-induced deaths are due to CVD (see fig. 1 in chapter 2), most (66%) from CHD [2]. Smoking increases the risk of dying from CHD by a factor of 2–3 [3]. Smoking also causes stroke, sudden cardiac death (SCD), abdominal aortic aneurysm, heart failure and peripheral artery disease (table 1) [2]. Of all cardiovascular deaths, smoking causes more than 20% in North America and 11% worldwide [4]. Heavy smokers (≥20 cigarettes/day) are at higher risk than light smokers (<10 cigarettes/day), but even occasional smokers experience a substantially increased risk of cardiovascular death compared to nonsmokers (relative risk, RR, 1.5, 95% confidence interval, CI, 1.0–2.3) [2, 5]. The dose-response relationship is highly nonlinear with most of the risk appearing at even the lowest levels of cigarette consumption (fig. 1) [6]. Therefore, light and intermittent (nondaily) smokers – not just heavy smokers – should be advised to quit and assisted in doing so.

CVD is responsible for a third of all deaths attributed to active smoking [7]. The RR of dying from CHD in smokers compared to nonsmokers is higher for younger people because the baseline risk of heart disease increases with aging [2, 8]. While smoking increases the risk of an ST-elevation myocardial infarction by a factor of 3.4 in the general population, in those aged 18–34 years this risk is increased by a factor of 11.4 [9]. The risk of nonfatal AMI progressively increases with the number of cigarettes smoked daily, however, the dose-response relationship is highly nonlinear (fig. 1) [5, 6]. Despite the much lower dose of exposure, light smoking (4–7 cigarettes/day) has approximately 70% of the effect of heavy smoking (≥23 cigarettes/day) [6]. Similarly, the risk of CHD

Table 1. Health consequences causally linked to smoking [adapted from ref. 7]

Cancers
    Lung
    Larynx
    Oro- and hypopharynx
    Esophagus
    Stomach
    Liver
    Pancreas
    Colon/rectum
    Kidney and ureter
    Cervix
    Bladder
    Acute myeloid leukemia
Chronic diseases (other than respiratory)
    Coronary heart disease
    Stroke
    Atherosclerotic peripheral vascular disease
    Aortic aneurysm
    Sudden cardiac death
    Heart failure
    Blindness, cataracts or age-related macular
    degeneration
    Periodontitis
    Osteoporosis (hip fractures)
    Reproductive disturbances (premature birth/
    reduced fertility)
    Erectile dysfunction
    Diabetes mellitus
    Altered immune function

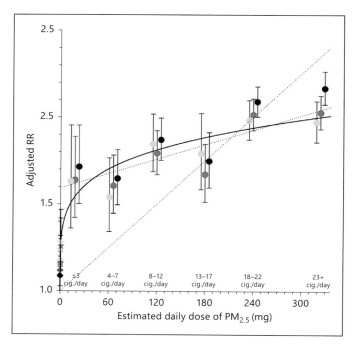

Fig. 1. Adjusted RR and 95% CIs of ischemic heart disease (light gray), cardiovascular disease (dark gray) and cardiopulmonary disease (black) mortality plotted over baseline estimated daily dose of $PM_{2.5}$ (particulate matter with an aerodynamic diameter ≤2.5 μm) from different increments in current cigarette (cigs) smokers (relative to never smokers). Diamonds represent comparable mortality risk estimates for $PM_{2.5}$ from air pollution. Stars represent comparable pooled RR estimates associated with exposure from the 2006 Surgeon General's Report and from the INTERHEART study. The solid and dotted lines are fitted linear and nonlinear lines illustrating alternative monotonic exposure-response relationships (from Pope et al. [6] with permission).

among 35- to 39-year-old men and women who consume 1–4 cigarettes/day is almost three times higher compared to that of nonsmokers (RR 2.74 in men and 2.94 in women) [5, 10]. The RR of dying after an AMI has been shown to be lower in smokers than in nonsmokers *(the smokers' paradox)* [11, 12]. This has been ascribed to the lower prevalence of other AMI risk factors in smokers (younger, less likely to have diabetes, hypertension or hyperlipidemia and less complex lesions) although some studies suggest that there are other factors, including enhanced response to antiplatelet, anticoagulation and revascularization therapies among smokers or the added benefit of smoking cessation after AMI [11–13]. In this regard, cessation is always beneficial and should always be strongly encouraged, either before or after treatment initiation, to reduce the risk of death or subsequent disease [12].

Smokers have a higher risk of SCD than nonsmokers [14, 15]. Retrospective analysis of SCD victims yields that current smoking is more common than hypertension among these subjects, as opposed to the reference population where prevalence is similar [16]. Epidemiological studies show that smokers have a higher RR for SCD than for AMI or CHD [17]. After quitting, the SCD risk drops rapidly [15, 18, 19]. These facts suggest that the acute triggering effects of exposure to tobacco smoke may be a more important mechanism than atherosclerosis in smoking-related SCD.

Smoking is the third most important risk factor for heart failure (after CHD and diabetes, both of which are also caused by smoking [7]), increasing the risk by about 60% (population-attributable risk of 17.1%) [20]. Cardiac remodeling and reduced ventricular function, traditional features of heart failure, are also caused by smoking [21–23]. Therefore, patients at high risk of developing heart failure should be strongly advised to quit smoking [24].

Smoking causes extracardiac vascular diseases, including ischemic stroke and subarachnoid hemorrhage, abdominal aortic aneurysms and peripheral artery disease. Smokers have a two- to fourfold increase in the risk of stroke compared to nonsmokers, an increase that drops months after quitting [7]. Smoking causes abdominal aortic aneurysms and increases the rupture risk [7, 25]. One-time screening is recommended for men between 65 and 75 years of age who have ever smoked and only selectively in never smokers (data are not yet conclusive to make such recommendations for women) [26].

In women, smoking acts synergistically with hormonal contraceptives to increase the risk of CHD. The combined risk of smoking and using hormonal contraceptives is larger than the sum of the separate risks. Indeed, most of the increased risk of hormonal contraceptives appears to be limited to smokers [27]. Although most studies have shown significant increases in the AMI risk with the combination of smoking and hormonal contraceptives [27], estrogen doses have since decreased [28], but data with currently used doses of estrogens are limited [29]. Nevertheless, guidelines recommend against using hormonal contraceptives (oral, injected, patch or ring) in smokers above age 35 (particularly those smoking ≥15 cigarettes/day) [29]. In addition to the increased risk of AMI, smoking in women taking hormonal contraceptives increases the risk of deep vein thrombosis and pulmonary emboli [27].

Low-Tar ('Light') Cigarettes
Starting in the 1950s, cigarette manufacturers reengineered their product to reduce tar yields as measured by cigarette smoking machines, marketing these cigarettes as a 'healthier' alternative to 'full flavor' [30] (see also chapter 1); 'ultralight', 'light' and 'full-flavor' terms were often used to describe machine tar yields per cigarette (1–6, 7–15 and >15 mg, respectively) [31]. The reported tar and nicotine yields are measured by a machine with fixed smoking patterns, which does not accurately reflect smoking by real people, who adjust how they smoke to get the amount of nicotine necessary to satisfy their addiction [32, 33]. Furthermore, smokers tend to compensate any reduced nicotine delivery per puff by altering their smoking pattern taking deeper puffs, more puffs per cigarette or smoking more cigarettes per day [31, 34].

Although evidence regarding the different risks between smokers of cigarettes with different yields is still developing, smoking even low-tar cigarettes carries excess risk compared to not smoking. A pooled analysis of three case-control studies revealed that smokers of low-tar (<10 mg) cigarettes have an odds ratio (OR) of 2.70 (95% CI 2.01–3.63) for

Table 2. Tobacco smoke and cardiovascular disease: mechanisms

Endothelial dysfunction
Platelet activation
Arterial stiffness
Dyslipidemia
Inflammation
Oxidative stress
Hemodynamic effects

AMI compared to nonsmokers [35]. Therefore, low-tar cigarettes should not be recommended as a cardiovascular risk reduction strategy. The important point is that these cigarettes are not safer than 'regular' cigarettes, particularly in terms of CVD, where even low levels of smoke exposure confer substantial risks.

Pathophysiology of Tobacco Smoke and Cardiovascular Disease

Smoking affects the cardiovascular system through multiple biological mechanisms (table 2). Rather than isolated, these mechanisms can interact with each other and have a multiplier effect on CVD risk.

Of the more than 7,000 components of tobacco smoke (see chapter 4), acrolein [36–39], cadmium [40], lead [41–43], particulate matter [44, 45], carbon monoxide [18], benzo[a]pyrene [46], crotonaldehyde [45], 1,3-butadiene [45] and polycyclic aromatic hydrocarbons [47] have been identified to induce one or more of these mechanisms.

Smoking causes atherosclerosis [7], the underlying pathophysiologic process in CHD, peripheral vascular disease and stroke. The mediating processes include oxidative stress, inflammation, platelet activation, endothelial dysfunction and dyslipidemia (decreased high-density lipoprotein cholesterol, HDL, and increased low-density lipoprotein) [2]. Carotid artery intima-media thickness (a noninvasive quantitative measure of atherosclerosis and predictor of AMI and stroke [48]) and the number of atherosclerotic plaques are increased in current and former smokers compared to never smokers [49]. In addition, smoking causes and interacts with diabetes, leading to more atherosclerotic damage [50].

Endothelial dysfunction is strongly and independently associated with cardiovascular events [51]. Under normal conditions, the endothelium is a source of nitric oxide (NO) produced by endothelial NO synthase using L-arginine as the primary substrate. NO regulates vasodilation and vasoconstriction to maintain normal coronary (and other) blood flow and inhibit inflammation and platelet aggregation [52]. As blood speeds up through a vessel, the resulting increased shear stress stimulates normal endothelium to secrete NO which, in turn, leads to vasodilation. This so-called flow-mediated dilation is a clinical marker of endothelial control of the vasomotor tone in arteries [53]. In addition, the endothelium secretes several factors that have anti-aggregatory effects on platelets or have anticoagulatory or fibrinolytic properties [54], and prevents platelet interaction with subendothelial connective tissue [45]. Smoking interferes with this process leading to endothelial dysfunction, a decrease in the anticoagulatory potential of the endothelium, an increase in procoagulatory modulators (e.g. tissue factor and plasminogen activator inhibitor [54]) and a reduction in endothelium (NO)-dependent vasodilation. These effects result in atherosclerosis, plaque rupture, inflammation, platelet activation and decreased blood flow due to thrombosis and vasospasm.

The effects of smoking on the endothelium manifest shortly after exposure [45]. In a group of smokers, endothelial function was significantly impaired immediately after smoking a cigarette and remained significantly lower after 20 min compared to a measurement before smoking [55].

Platelet activation and subsequent thrombosis are also key factors in the development of CVD [56] and triggering of acute coronary events. The imbalance of prothrombotic and fibrinolytic factors produced by cigarette smoke produces a prothrombotic state, increasing the risk of AMI and SCD. This prothrombotic state explains why smokers are generally younger and have less risk factors and CHD than nonsmokers at the time of their first AMI [11]. At autopsy, smokers are more likely than nonsmokers to have acute thrombosis rather than stable plaques [2].

Another mediating mechanism leading to an increased risk of CVD is the effect of smoking on arterial stiffness [57, 58]. Smoking 1 cigarette increases arterial stiffness within 5 min [59]. At the 6-year follow-up of 2,000 healthy Japanese, pulse wave velocity (arterial stiffness) was increased in all subjects due to aging, but the increase was significantly higher in smokers (mean ± SD 11.0 ± 1.9 cm/s/year) than in never smokers (5.5 ± 0.6 cm/s/year) [58]. In addition, chronic smoking appears to sensitize the arterial response to acute smoking [60].

Smoking also leads to a more atherogenic lipid profile. In smokers (and chewers), total cholesterol levels were 17% higher compared to levels in nonsmokers [61]. In addition, smokers have lower concentrations of HDL and higher tri-glyceride levels compared with nonsmokers in a dose-dependent manner [62, 63]. Higher total low-density lipoprotein and very low-density lipoprotein cholesterol levels have also been documented [2].

The presence of the metabolic syndrome predicts CVD. The metabolic syndrome is defined as the combination of abdominal obesity with two or more of the following conditions: high triglycerides, low HDL levels, hypertension and raised fasting plasma glucose [64]. Smoking is associated with an increased risk of the metabolic syndrome that appears to be higher in male and heavy smokers [65]. In a sample of nearly 5,000 Chinese individuals, current smokers had a significantly higher risk of the metabolic syndrome compared to nonsmokers (OR 1.61, 95% CI 1.13–2.50) [66]. In addition to low HDL and high triglycerides, other components (glucose intolerance [67] and abdominal obesity [68–70]) are also associated with tobacco use.

Inflammation, a key step in atherosclerosis and CVD development, is also more pronounced among smokers [7, 71]. Levels of inflammatory markers are higher in current than former smokers, which are, in turn, higher than in never smokers [71]. In addition, white blood cell counts have been found to be independently associated with pack-years, carbon monoxide and the Fagerström test for Nicotine Dependence, indicating a dose-response relationship (higher inflammation with higher smoking frequency and intensity) [72].

Oxidative stress results when the body is unable to detoxify reactive oxygen species (ROS) and free radicals. Oxidizing agents can initiate the inflammatory cascade as well as be produced by an inflammatory process [44]. Cigarette smoke delivers oxides of nitrogen, free radicals and other oxidizing chemicals to smokers [18] and can increase ROS production directly, thus damaging cardiomyocytes [73]. Smokers are exposed to an estimated 10^5 oxidative free radicals per puff [74]. Plasma 8-isoprostane, a surrogate marker of lipid oxidation [75], and oxidized proteins [76] are increased in smokers compared to nonsmokers. Although not yet conclusive, tobacco smoke constituents related to increased oxidative stress include particulate matter [44], heavy metals, particularly lead and cadmium [45], and possibly nicotine [77].

Smoking also affects the autonomic nervous system [78]. Decreased heart rate variability is a marker of autonomic dysfunction and a predictor of CHD, heart failure, CVD death, and death and arrhythmic complications after AMI [79, 80]. Compared to nonsmokers, smokers have decreased heart rate variability, and the effects appear within the first 5–10 min of smoking [81, 82].

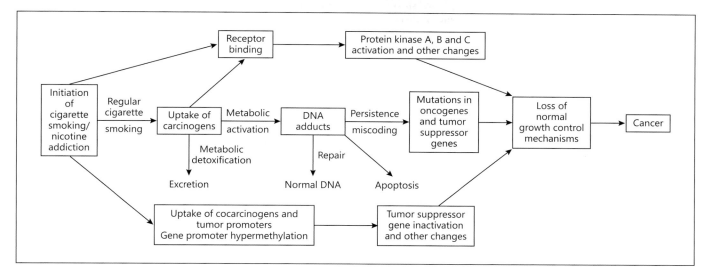

Fig. 2. Pathway for causation of cancer by carcinogens in tobacco (source: [7]; printed with corrections, January 2014).

Smoking and Cancers Outside the Respiratory System

Cigarette smoking is responsible for nearly 30% of all cancer deaths, including cancers of the lung (see chapter 7), oral cavity, larynx, esophagus, bladder, stomach, pancreas, kidney, uterine cervix and liver (table 1).

Mechanisms of Disease
Exposure to carcinogens, metabolism to reactive intermediates and DNA damage leading to critical gene mutations have been established as major mechanisms by which tobacco smoke causes cancer (fig. 2). Tobacco smoke contains more than 7,000 chemicals, and at least 69 are recognized carcinogens [7] (see chapter 4). These chemicals are foreign to the human body and, consequently, are acted upon by detoxifying metabolizing enzymes. However, during this process, certain reactive compounds may be formed as intermediates and bind covalently to nucleophilic sites in the DNA to form adducts. During DNA replication, these adducts are critical in the carcinogenesis process if they are not fixed by DNA repair enzymes. If not repaired, they cause DNA miscoding and modify the normal growth control mechanisms, leading to uncontrolled proliferation, further mutations and ultimately cancer [7].

The presence of DNA adducts has been found to be higher in smokers compared to nonsmokers, while many of these remain unidentified, specific carcinogen-DNA adducts in the tissue of smokers [83]. Furthermore, epigenetic changes (nonsequence DNA changes) are also an integral part of cancer progression. Since cigarette smoke induces oxidative damage and gene promoter methylation, this may also play a role in cancer development [7].

Breast Cancer
In 2005, the California Environmental Protection Agency concluded that 'the epidemiological studies, the biology of the breast and the toxicology of tobacco smoke constituents together, the data provide support for causal association between active smoking and breast cancer risk' [84]. As of 2014, the Surgeon General's Report on smoking and cancer concluded that the evidence was suggestive (one step below causal) that smoking is a cause of breast cancer [7]. Analysis of the risk separately for genetic subgroups and women within higher exposure categories accounts for this difference between the California Environmental Protection Agency and the Surgeon General's Report. Early age of smoking initiation, smoking before the first pregnancy, highest total years of smoking and total pack-years, and the effect on risk estimates for active smoking after controlling for passive smoking have all been found to yield higher and significant estimates of the breast cancer risk [85]. In 2014, the Surgeon General's Report also concluded that there is enough evidence to identify the mechanisms by which smoking may cause breast cancer [7]. Furthermore, there are 20 identified mammary carcinogens in tobacco: benzene, benzo[a]pyrene, dibenz[a,h]anthracene, dibenzo[a,e]pyrene, dibenzo[a,h]pyrene, dibenzo[a,i]pyrene, dibenzo[a,l]pyrene, N-nitrosodiethylamine, N-nitrosodi-n-butylamine, acrylamide, acrylonitrile, 1,3-butadiene, iso-

prene, nitromethane, propylene oxide, urethane, vinyl chloride, 4-aminobiphenyl, nitrobenzene, o-toluidine) [84, 86].

Women seeking breast cancer care or screening should be advised to quit smoking as breast cancer patients who smoke have been found to have the worst prognosis (increased risk of recurrence and all-cause mortality) compared to their nonsmoking counterparts [87]. This increased risk of recurrence and all-cause mortality was observed even in former smokers [87].

Cervical Cancer

The 2001 Surgeon General's Report on women and smoking confirmed the association between smoking and cervical cancer [27]. Nicotine, cotinine and the tobacco-specific carcinogen NNK [4-(methylnitrosamino)-1-(3-pyridyl)-1-butanone] have been found in cervical secretions of smokers [2]. The most important confounder is infection with the human papilloma virus (HPV). HPV has been recognized as the main cause of cervical cancer worldwide, and the extent to which the association of smoking and cervical cancer is independent of HPV infection remains unknown [27]. A study conducted in the United States that adequately controlled for HPV infection found smoking to be a risk factor among both HPV-positive and HPV-negative women (RR 2.4, 95% CI 1.4–4.3, and RR 3.2, 95% CI 2.0–5.0, respectively) [88]. In addition, higher HPV DNA load has been documented in smokers, with no dose-response relationship indicating a possible low threshold for the effect of smoking on viral load [89].

Stomach Cancer

Stomach cancer, mostly prevalent in Asia and Latin America, is also causally linked to smoking [7, 90]. The risk for stomach cancer for men who smoke ≥15 cigarettes/day has been found to be approximately 1.4 times higher than the risk of a nonsmoker (increases to 1.7 with ≥35 cigarettes) [91]. One biologic mechanism by which smoking might cause stomach cancer is by increasing the infectivity or acting synergistically to increase the carcinogenic properties of *Helicobacter pylori*, the bacteria causing gastric cancer [2, 92]. Eradication, through antibiotics, of *H. pylori* may reduce the long-term risk of gastric cancer [92]. This eradication might be less effective in smokers as it has been found that failure rates of treatment for *H. pylori* are almost twice those observed in nonsmokers [93].

Leukemia

Smoking has been causally linked, in a dose-dependent manner, with acute myeloid leukemia [7]. This has been confirmed both epidemiologically and biologically. Current

smokers have been found to have an RR of 1.40 (95% CI 1.22–1.60) of developing acute myeloid leukemia compared to nonsmokers [94]. Even among ever smokers, RR was significant (1.2, 95% CI 1.15–1.36). The risk is dose dependent, ranging from 1.27 to 1.77 among smokers of <10 to >30 cigarettes/day, respectively (p for trend 0.001) [94]. Furthermore, leukemia patients who are current smokers have lower overall survival and worst outcomes compared to nonsmoking leukemia patients [95, 96].

From a biological standpoint, a likely biologic mechanism for this increased risk of leukemia is the fact that cigarette smoke contains benzene and polonium-210. These agents are known causes of human leukemia. Among other sources of benzene, cigarette smoke is the main source of exposure in the United States, accounting for almost 90% of the exposure in smokers [2]. In addition, specific chromosomal abnormalities have been found among smokers with leukemia [2].

Liver Cancer

The 2014 Surgeon General's Report concludes that 'the evidence is sufficient to infer a causal relationship between smoking and hepatocellular carcinoma' [7]. Given the role of the liver as a primary site for metabolism of several carcinogens, it is biologically plausible for this causal association. From a biological standpoint, chronic hepatitis B (HBV) and C virus (HCV) infection and alcohol ingestion (chronic) are recognized as causal agents of liver cancer; therefore, studies of smoking and liver cancer need to be adjusted for such infection [97, 98]. In a meta-analysis, current smoking increased the risk of hepatocellular carcinoma by approximately 70% after controlling for alcohol consumption, HBV and HCV infections [7]. Furthermore, a synergistic effect has been found between HBV and HCV and smoking [99]. Therefore, all carriers of HBV and HCV should be strongly advised to quit smoking.

Ovarian Cancer

According to the Surgeon General, the available evidence is inadequate to infer the presence or absence of a causal relationship between smoking and ovarian cancer [2]. However, data suggest that the risk for some types of ovarian cancer might be increased in current smokers [100–102]. A 2006 systematic review and meta-analysis concluded that the risk of ovarian cancer in smokers might depend on the histological type of ovarian cancer given that they arise from different pathways. Current smokers have twice the risk of mucinous ovarian cancer than never smokers (RR 2.1, 95% CI 1.7–2.7). This increased risk appears to be dose dependent

ciations, it may be difficult to disentangle the effects of intra-uterine and early post-natal smoke exposure, and perhaps also associated adverse factors such as low socio-economic status and pollutants. Be that as it may, the association between the SIDS risk and passive smoke exposure is well established [15, 16]. Crucially, however, as the proportion of smoke-free homes has fallen, so has the prevalence of SIDS [17]. This North American study suggested that over the 12-year study period, 4,402–6,406 excess deaths from SIDS (95% confidence intervals) could be attributed to passive smoke exposure. This amounts to around 20% of total SIDS cases. Although the authors could not disentangle the effects of ante- and post-natal exposure, the structural changes described in animal models of nicotine exposure in pregnancy and the cord blood immunological changes mediating susceptibility to infection in the babies of smoking mothers (below) suggest that antenatal exposure cannot be acquitted. The mechanisms of this effect are unclear. A study of the lungs of SIDS victims whose mothers smoked in pregnancy revealed increases in inner airway wall thickness and airway smooth muscle [18, 19]. Whether this is a direct effect of smoke, and if so whether ante- or post-natal, or related to another factor which caused the sudden death, is still conjectural.

Smoking in Pregnancy

That maternal smoking damages the foetus, has lifelong effects and is a *bad thing*, is indisputable. The effects of smoking may be divided into four categories (text box 2). Recent work has highlighted the structural effects of foetal exposure to nicotine in particular. This is particularly relevant regarding the question of safety of electronic cigarettes in pregnancy (which of course contain nicotine, as well as numerous other chemicals, whose consequences are unknown, http://www.newscientist.com/article/dn25319-dont-let-vaping-obesity-and-boozing-become-norms.html#.UzXZ9Y8sHNQ), which is discussed in chapter 23 in this volume.

Effects on Lung Structure

One important model is the subcutaneous administration of nicotine to timed pregnant rhesus monkeys. One study showed that this increased airway wall dimensions, and the expression of type 111 collagen mRNA and protein, as well as elastin, probably via the α_7 nicotinic acetylcholine receptor [20]. Nicotine exposure in vitro (bronchial epithelial cells) and in vivo (same antenatal nicotine exposure model) led to increased MUC5AC and mucin expression [21]. In another animal study [22], pregnant mice were exposed to nicotine on gestation days 7–21, gestation day 14 to postnatal day 7 and postnatal days 3–15. Post-natal lung function measurements showed that pre-natal nicotine exposure between gestation day 14 and postnatal day 7 led to a decrease in forced expiratory flow in the offspring modulated through the α_7 nicotinic acetylcholine receptor. Pathologically, there was increased airway length and decreased diameter. Adult mice exposed to pre-natal nicotine exhibit an increased response to methacholine challenge, even in the absence of allergic sensitisation; the question of antenatal programming and smoking will be discussed in a subsequent section. Collagen expression was also increased. There were no effects seen in α_7 nicotinic acetylcholine receptor knockout mice. It should be noted that these are nicotine-driven changes; thus, although nicotine-containing medications (patches, gum and electronic cigarettes) may be safer than actual cigarettes in pregnancy, there use cannot be considered to be safe. They should be considered the lesser of evils. Finally, one factor preventing airway collapse is the phenomenon of interdependence, whereby alveolar attachments to the airway help to hold it open. The offspring of smoke-exposed guinea pigs have reduced numbers of alveolar attachment points to the airway [23]. This is likely to result in a reduction in airway stability and increased collapsibility.

In summary, there is clear-cut evidence of structural changes in the foetus caused by nicotine exposure, which leads to airflow obstruction in the infant. Below I demonstrate that this has lifelong effects.

Effects on Foetal Immunological Responses

There are numerous studies showing that maternal smoking may have immunological as well as physiological and structural effects [24]. For example, maternal smoking leads to lower cord blood IL-4 and IFN-γ [25], and also increased cord blood mononuclear cell proliferation to house dust mite [26]. Other cord blood studies showed that maternal smoking was associated with increased IL-13 and reduced IFN-γ mRNA responses by stimulated cord blood cells [27]. The Perth group [28] investigated the effects of maternal smoking on foetal Toll-like receptors (TLRs) and their signalling. Smoking during pregnancy was associated with reduced TLR2-mediated IL-6, IL-10 and TNF-α production. TLR3- and TLR4-mediated signalling of TNF-α, but not IL-6, IL-10 and IL-12, was reduced in the infants of mothers who smoked. In terms of TLR9 responses, there were attenuated IL-6 and increased IFN-γ responses in the infants of smoking mothers. There is an important functional read-out of immunological changes in cord blood. The COAST study showed that cord blood IFN-γ responses were inversely related to the frequency of viral infections [29]. The same group showed that respiratory syncytial virus (RSV)-induced wheeze was associated with reduced phytohaemagglutinin-induced cord blood cell IL-13 responses, and median IL-13 responses diminished in non-wheezing children in the 1st year of life. Children with at least two episodes of wheeze had lower phytohaemagglutinin-induced IFN-γ responses and were less likely to have rhinovirus-induced IFN-γ responses at birth. Children with measurable cord blood IFN-γ responses to RSV were less likely to wheeze in the 1st year of life [30]. The long-term implications of childhood lower respiratory tract infections are discussed below.

Priming of Future Adult Responses

The hypothesis that in utero events can reprogram an individual for immediate adaptation to gestational disturbances but with adverse consequences for later responses to adverse events, known as the Developmental Origins of Health and Disease hypothesis, has been supported by observations in many different contexts. This hypothesis has been studied in animal models in respiratory diseases [31]. Relevant to this chapter is the effect of in utero smoke exposure leading to enhanced responses to post-natal allergen and fungal exposure [32]. The extent and relevance of these mechanisms to human foetal tobacco exposure require further study. However, indirectly smoking can lead potentially to long-term programming by its effects on inducing premature birth (below). In murine models, hyperoxia may affect adult cardiovascular function and lifespan [33] and alter pulmonary oxidative stress and immune responses [34, 35]. The mechanism may be epigenetic through DNA methylation [36, 37].

Timing of Delivery and Birth Weight

Maternal smoking is causal of prematurity, low birth weight and small-for-gestational-age births. Poor intrauterine growth, but not poor post-natal growth, increased the risk of adult asthma, particularly if the family came from a back-ground of low socio-economic status [38]. In a longitudinal birth cohort study of 5,390 men and women born full term and prospectively followed to adulthood [39], adult FEV_1 and forced vital capacity (FVC) increased linearly with higher birth weight in both men and women with no apparent threshold. The lowest spirometry was in adults with lower birth weight who were smokers, led a sedentary lifestyle or were overweight. The Aberdeen cohort, albeit a smaller study (n = 381), confirmed this finding [40].

It is known that extreme prematurity per se, even without the need for intensive care, is associated with long-term airflow limitation in survivors, and this is worse in those requiring prolonged ventilation. It should also be noted that the nature of chronic lung disease of prematurity is changing with changes in neonatal intensive care unit practice, such that current long-term follow-up studies may not be relevant to today's preterm survivors. However, in mid-childhood, there is evidence of airflow obstruction with bronchodilator responsiveness in these children [41]. The airway disease is not characterised by asthmatic-type eosinophilic inflammation [42–44], but there is evidence of increased oxidative stress [34]. High-resolution CT scans show evidence of structural changes in the lung, including bullous destruction [45, 46]. There is some evidence that there may be improvement in airway obstruction at follow-up to adult life [47, 48], however, this is by no means the case in all studies [49]. However, in small-for-gestational-age babies, only birth weight remained a strong predictor of spirometry at age 20–22 years. In adult life, the survivors of preterm birth also have evidence of impaired exercise tolerance and increased morbidity from respiratory disease. Although it is clear that treatment strategies are getting better at minimising chronic lung disease of prematurity [50], the problem is not about to disappear imminently.

Importantly, it should be noted that 'late-preterm' infants (gestational age 33–34 weeks), who rarely need intensive care, also have long-term spirometric abnormalities [51]. There is an increased risk of an asthma diagnosis even in early-term babies (37–38 weeks of gestation) [52], although the exact nature of the airway disease is not known, as well as an increased risk of admission to hospital [53]. This last is still present in adults born prematurely [54]. There are, of course, many more late-preterm and early-term than extreme-preterm babies, which makes this finding particularly concerning. It should be noted that these babies are at increased risk of death in early adult life; in one study [55], late-preterm birth was associated with a 31% (13–50%) increase in young adulthood mortality. Finally, the extrapulmonary complications of extreme prematurity in particular should be considered, such as neurodevelopmental handicap, which, although important, are beyond the scope of this chapter.

Finally, it is gratifying to see that one of the effects of the tobacco control legislation in Belgium has been a parallel reduction in premature births. Over a period from January 2002 to December 2011, comprising 606,877 deliveries [56], there was a stepwise decline in preterm deliveries as a result of successive tobacco control interventions in Belgium (banning smoking in the workplace, then in restaurants and then in bars serving food). Whether the effect is due to reduced exposure of pregnant women to the tobacco smoke of others, or due to reduced numbers of mothers smoking, cannot be determined. It should be stated that a meta-analysis suggests that passive smoke exposure alone is unrelated to preterm birth [57], although this is controversial [56]. Although causality cannot be proven, the internal consistency of the results makes this a very convincing conclusion. Whatever the mechanism, the long-term health benefits of this reduction will be incalculably huge.

Transgenerational Risk

Adverse effects of smoking on the foetus may commence even before the *mother* of the foetus was born. There are worrying data suggestive of a transgenerational effect of smoking. Li et al. [58] performed a case-control study involving 338 children who had been given an asthma diagnosis within the first 5 years of life and 570 controls. The expected associations between maternal smoking in pregnancy and foetal outcomes were seen, but worryingly, if the grandmother had smoked while pregnant, her daughter's children had an increased asthma risk, even if she herself did not smoke. The putative mechanism is by epigenetic transgenerational modification of DNA. The same group demonstrated [59] that DNA methylation patterns on buccal scrapes were seen in children (a) whose mothers smoked and (b) who carried the common GSTM1 genotype, i.e. were unable to detoxify tobacco metabolites. Two of eight genes (AXL and PTPRO) could be validated as showing significant increases in methylation. Limitations of the study included that these genes are not relevant to asthma; the changes described in buccal cells may not be relevant to the airway, and that environmental exposures were determined retrospectively. However, taken together, the study results serve as proof of concept that passive smoking causes epigenetic changes which may be transgenerational.

Passive Smoking, Normal Development and Wheezing Syndromes

Normal and Abnormal Lung Growth

Understanding the adverse long-term effects of smoking requires knowledge of normal lung development, which is discussed in detail elsewhere [8–10]. Briefly, airway branching is determined in the first 16 weeks of pregnancy, and, thereafter, airways increase in size but not number; thus, the second half of pregnancy is a key time in which passive smoke exposure may lead to airflow obstruction. Post-natally, the evolution of spirometry has been best described by the Global Lung Initiative (http://www.lungfunction.org/); in summary, FEV_1 rises to a plateau at age 20–25 years, and then steadily declines through the aging years. A series of overlapping birth and other cohort studies of normal and wheezing individuals has established that (for the most part) the standard deviation score for spirometric indices is established for the individual in the preschool years, and thereafter tracks, with no evidence of catch-up growth [60–63]. The possible exception is survivors of chronic lung disease of prematurity, in whom some catch-up growth has been suggested (above). Thus the three key requirements for normal lung development are (a) being born with normal lung function; (b) having normal growth of lung function as a child and young adult, and (c) having a normal rate of decline of lung function from the 3rd decade (the effects of smoking in later life are discussed in chapter 7 in this volume). Impairment in any of these requirements means that the threshold for respiratory symptoms and disability is crossed prematurely, or, in other words, the subject has premature airflow obstruction. Smoking has adverse effects on all three areas.

The multiple factors affecting airway development are beyond the scope of this chapter. However, given the interaction between smoking and asthma, it should be noted that asthma may adversely impact on childhood airway development, irrespective of treatment. The CAMP study compared the effects of prophylactic inhaled budesonide or nedocromil with no prophylaxis; around 30% of children showed a drop-off in spirometric growth, independent of the treatment arm [64]. The mechanism of this is as yet unknown.

There is much less information on alveolar development, because of the lack (until recently) of reliable non-invasive methods of measuring this. Previously, it was thought that alveolar numbers were virtually completely laid down by about 2 years of age. Studies using hyperpolarised helium suggest that in fact alveolar numbers continue to increase until the late teenage years and that there may be catch-up in alveolar numbers after preterm birth [65, 66]. This catch-up is obviously beneficial, but increases the window of vulnerability of the developing lung to tobacco smoke.

The important principle is that the role of apparently small deficits in lung function must not be underestimated; although they may be insufficient to cause symptoms, their effects become magnified during development and aging, and may lead to early-onset airflow obstruction in particular.

Maternal Smoking and Lung Function at Birth
Numerous studies have demonstrated that maternal smoking in pregnancy leads to airflow obstruction soon after birth, prior to any likely effects of post-natal exposure [67–69]. Low lung function at birth is a risk factor for asthma in mid-childhood [70]. The dominant effect of antenatal over post-natal smoking in fact persists in mid-childhood in terms of lung function, wheezing and physician diagnosis of asthma [71, 72].

Maternal Smoking and Childhood Atopy
This effect has been more controversial, and indeed Strachan and Cook [4] could not find an association. However, more recent studies [73] have suggested an association between maternal smoking and food allergy, and a recent meta-analysis confirmed an association with atopy [74]. A mechanistic study related lower cord blood regulatory T cells with stable FOXP3 expression to genetic (atopic family history) and environmental factors (maternal smoking in pregnancy) to the subsequent development of atopic dermatitis [75]. Taken together, these studies strongly suggest that maternal smoking in pregnancy does increase the likelihood of some atopic diseases in the baby, and given the well-known associations between atopic dermatitis and food allergy, and subsequent asthma, this is likely another mechanism whereby smoking impacts adversely on long-term respiratory outcomes.

Maternal Smoking and the Microbiome
We know that maternal smoking primes the baby's immune system (above). A fruitful area of research will be the effect of this on the airway microbiome. Although conventional wisdom is that the lower airways are sterile, and that viruses not bacteria cause wheeze, as with much conventional wisdom, both are wrong [76]. Conventional culture techniques isolate only around 1% of bacteria; if molecular techniques are deployed, then the lower airways are found to have a diverse flora, which is necessary for normal immunological development [77]. Furthermore, early bacterial isolation from the upper airways is associated both with an abnormal immunological profile in the upper airways [78], neonatal respiratory symptoms [79], neonatal bronchiolitis and pneumonia [80], and an increased likelihood of subsequent wheeze [81], although in these studies there was no association with maternal smoking. However, active and passive smoking certainly can affect upper airway cultures [82–84]; whether the lower airway microbiome is affected by passive smoke exposure in children remains to be seen. Nonetheless, there is likely still much to be learned about the interactions between smoking in pregnancy, the foetal immune responses, the microbiome and viral infections.

Childhood Respiratory Infections: Bronchiolitis
International comparisons of bronchiolitis are confounded by the different definitions used in different parts of the world. The issues for all childhood respiratory viral infections are both the interactions between passive smoke exposure and susceptibility to viral infections, and the long-term consequences of infections. Susceptibility may be determined antenatally (impaired lung function/altered foetal immunology) and post-natally (effects on host defence, although these are more controversial). Acute RSV bronchiolitis is the commonest reason for admission to hospital in the 1st year of life. A study from Tennessee of 101,245 infants showed that 20% had one or more health care visits for bronchiolitis [85]. They showed that both maternal asthma and maternal smoking during pregnancy (a shocking 25% of all mothers!) were independently associated with the risk of bronchiolitis in otherwise normal-term infants. Smoking alone increased the risk by 14%, maternal asthma alone by 39% and both risk factors in the same mother by 47%. An accompanying editorial [86] highlighted that other risk factors for bronchiolitis were not considered, and that the particular viruses causing the symptoms could only be inferred. It should also be pointed out that such studies cannot disentangle the effects of smoking in pregnancy from antenatal effects of smoke exposure, nor is it possible to determine the relative contributions of ante- or post-natal mechanisms.

Not merely the prevalence but also the severity of bronchiolitis is affected by tobacco smoke exposure [87]. A prospective study of 206 hospitalised infants showed unsurprisingly that the younger an infant was, the more severe the infection tended to be as measured by the lowest oxygen saturation. However, infants exposed to post-natal, but not pre-natal cigarette smoke from the mother also had a lower oxygen saturation than those not exposed. The failure to detect an effect of pre-natal smoke may relate to the relatively small numbers studied, but this and other studies underscore that it is never too late for a parent to benefit a child by stopping smoking.

A study from Perth [88] showed that infants hospitalised for bronchiolitis had pre-morbid airway obstruction, and this tracked into mid-childhood; around 20% of infants were born to mothers who smoked. The COAST study showed altered cord blood responses in babies who would go on to develop RSV or rhinovirus wheezing lower respiratory illness (see the section on foetal responses). Likely, there are multiple pathways whereby smoke exposure increases susceptibility to respiratory virus infections.

Passive Smoking and Preschool and Childhood Wheeze
The morbidity, sometimes even mortality, and fiscal cost together make preschool viral infections an important public health issue, but the long-term implications are also of potential importance. There is no doubt that tobacco exposure increases the number and severity of viral-induced wheezing episodes in children. The effects are not confined to preschool children, who might be expected to be more vulnerable to parental smoking. A study from Cape Town, South Africa, enrolled 368 cases and 294 controls on the basis of reported asthma diagnosis or symptoms [89]. They found an exposure-response relationship between the urinary cotinine/creatinine ratio and asthma or wheeze. Among the predictors of asthma in a multivariate analysis were maternal smoking in pregnancy (odds ratio, OR = 1.87; 95% confidence interval, CI = 1.25–2.81), and each additional household smoker (OR = 1.15; 95% CI = 1.01–1.30). This study suggests that maternal smoking in pregnancy and current household exposure are independent contributors to this effect.

The major long-term controversy is whether respiratory infections are causal of asthma and other long-term health issues, or merely a marker of other adverse underlying events. So, for example, is RSV bronchiolitis a cause of asthma [90] or do the symptoms gradually regress [91]? The COAST study has been pivotal in describing the effects of viral infection in the first 6 years of life. The group showed that rhinovirus infection in the first 3 years of life was associated with a tenfold increased risk of asthma at age 6, much greater than RSV (2.6-fold) [92]. However, the group concluded that it was aeroallergen sensitisation which predisposed to viral infections, rather than the reverse [93]. Nonetheless, episodic viral wheeze is associated with long-term consequences; the Aberdeen group showed that in middle age, infants who had had what was then called 'wheezy bronchitis' (which we would now call episodic viral

wheeze) had an accelerated rate of decline in lung function [94]. However, an independent role of viral infections, and hence whether the long-term adverse effects of passive smoke exposure operate through the pathway of increasing susceptibility to childhood viral infections, will await an intervention study.

In summary, there is no doubt that one effect of the tobacco epidemic is increasing the prevalence and severity of childhood viral infections; whether there is a long-term effect of viruses per se, or the long-term effects are related to factors which predispose to viral infections, such as altered foetal immunology, remains unclear.

Cui Bono: Does Smoke-Free Legislation Help Children?
It might be thought that banning smoking in the workplace would not impact children much, given that they go to school but do not work. However, there is absolutely clear evidence that asthma severity and hospitalisations have been reduced dramatically by legislation [94–98]. This alone should put an end to the self-serving expostulations of the industry about the freedom of the individual; does any individual have the right to harm others, least of all children, by their behaviour? In this context, the recent example of the UK parliament to follow Australia by banning smoking in cars in which children are travelling is particularly welcome, and further health benefits can confidently be expected [99, 100].

Long-Term Effects of Parental Smoking

Bad though the immediate effects of smoking on childhood are, the long-term consequences are even more concerning. Smoking in pregnancy reduces long-term lung function directly and also indirectly via an effect on birth weight. It is difficult to disentangle the effects of maternal smoking during pregnancy from those in early childhood when considering long-term effects of passive smoke exposure, since virtually all mothers who smoke during pregnancy will continue to do so after birth. Stein et al. [101] related birth weight to lung function at age 38–59 years in 286 Indians from Mysore. They found that mean FEV_1 fell with decreasing birth weight, falling by 0.09 litres per pound (454 g) decrease in birth weight in men (95% CI) 0.01–0.16 and by 0.06 (95% CI –0.01 to 0.13) in women. Mean FVC fell by 0.11 litres (95% CI 0.02–0.19) per pound decrease in birth weight in men and by 0.08 litres (95% CI 0.002–0.16) in women. Upton et al. [102] conducted a prospective assessment of risk factors against adult lung function in 2,195 adult offspring (age 46–64 years) of couples who participated in a population-based study. They looked at the effects of a history of personal smoking, and maternal and paternal smoking on lung function tests and COPD prevalence. They demonstrated a reduction in FEV_1 by 0.053 litres and FVC by 0.062 litres for every 10 cigarettes smoked by the mother per day, and also an increase in prevalent COPD by 1.7 (95% CI 1.2–2.5).

The effect of childhood respiratory infections on the rate of decline of lung function in adult life is controversial. As above, childhood respiratory infection is one of the five risk factors for later COPD [13]. The Aberdeen cohort [92] reported an accelerated rate of lung function decline in adults who had had 'wheezy bronchitis' as young children, but this was not confirmed by the findings of the 1958 British birth cohort [103]. It is clear from many studies, however, that patients with COPD do not necessarily have an accelerated rate of lung function decline [104–106].

A recent cohort study from Brisbane reported the 14-year follow-up of 1,129 subjects, 237 of whose mothers smoked in pregnancy (n = 92 reported current smoking) [107]. Maternal smoking in pregnancy was associated with reduced lung function, an asthma diagnosis and altered immune function, but not with atopy or increased bronchial hyper-responsiveness. The ongoing risk of pregnancy smoking was clear, but some of the underlying mechanisms were not; there is clearly more to tobacco harm than just reducing airway calibre and effects on atopic disease.

Double Whammy: Interactions between Smoking by Parents and Their Children
Finally, a recent report from Tucson has shown a synergistic interaction between parental smoking and the effect of the child taking up active smoking [108]. There were 519 sibling parent pairs available for study. At 26 years of age, participants exposed to parental and active smoking had pre-bronchodilator FEV_1/FVC levels that were 2.8% (0.9–4.8%; p = 0.003) lower than participants who were not exposed to parental or active smoking. Young adults who themselves smoked, but whose parents did not, had normal spirometry. Between the ages of 11 and 26 years, participants with exposure to parental and active smoking had the steepest decline in spirometry.

Summary: Maternal Smoking and the Child's Respiratory Tract
There are multiple mechanisms whereby passive smoke exposure affects the child's airway, even disregarding the effect of parental smoking on the likelihood of the child tak-

ing up smoking. The particularly dangerous period is antenatally and also probably in the immediate post-natal period. The key messages are that there is no recovery or compensation for damage done at that time, and although the effects seem relatively trivial, they are magnified during the aging process, whereby the legacy of COPD, or, strictly, premature airflow obstruction, comes back to strike the child.

Smoking and Upper Airway Disease

There is an increased prevalence of otitis media with effusion, snoring, adenoidal hypertrophy, sore throats and tonsillitis in children of parents who smoke. The effect is seen even with smoking in pregnancy [109–112]. The Norwegian Mother and Child Study [113] studied 32,077 children born between 2000 and 2005 with questionnaire data on tobacco smoke exposure and acute otitis media up to 18 months of age. After adjusting for postnatal exposure and covariates, the relative risk for acute otitis media for infants aged 0–6 months when exposed to maternal smoking in pregnancy was 1.34, (95% CI 1.06–1.69); the risk tailed off by a year of age. There was also a slightly increased risk of recurrent acute otitis media in children exposed both pre- and post-natally (relative risk 1.24, 95% CI 1.01–1.52). Smoke exposure affects the response to surgery [114]. Maternal smoking was associated with an importantly increased risk of recurrent acute otitis media (OR 4.15, 95% CI 1.45–11.9) after the insertion of tympanostomy tubes in 217 children aged 1–4 years. Parents thus need to be encouraged to stop smoking even after the insertion of tympanostomy tubes in their children.

There may be as much as a doubling of the performance of tonsillectomy in such children. A meta-analysis showed that for a child living with a smoker there was an increased risk of middle ear disease (OR 1.62, 95% CI, 1.33–1.97) for maternal post-natal smoking and 1.37 (95% CI, 1.25–1.50) for any household member smoking [115]. Paternal and pre-natal maternal smoking did not carry a risk. The strongest effect was on the risk of surgery for middle ear disease, for both maternal and paternal smoking. Per year, 130,200 of childhood episodes of the middle ear in the United Kingdom and 292,950 of child frequent ear infections in the United States are directly attributable to tobacco smoke exposure in the home. An estimate of the morbidity in terms of hearing loss would be of interest. Finally, as the percentage of smoke-free homes increased in the USA, the prevalence of significant otitis media decreased, although in fair-

other removal processes may decrease the concentration of SHS airborne constituents, alter the size distribution of suspended particles and chemically modify some of the more reactive constituents of SHS (table 1) [7].

The term *third-hand smoke* is a neologism coined by a research team from the Dana-Farber/Harvard Cancer Center [8]. The 'third-hand' component of the term is a reference to the remnants on surfaces after 'second-hand smoke' has cleared out. The term *first-hand smoke* refers to what is inhaled into the smoker's own lungs, while *SHS* is a mixture of exhaled smoke and other substances leaving the smouldering end of the cigarette that enters the atmosphere and can be inhaled by others; third-hand smoke is contamination on the surfaces of objects that remains after SHS has cleared.

Smoking inside Households
SHS is a common indoor pollutant at home, making passive smoking a serious health risk for both those who smoke and those who do not. Tobacco smoke inside a room tends to hang in mid-air rather than disperse (fig. 1). Hot smoke rises, but tobacco smoke cools rapidly, which stops its upward climb. Since the smoke is heavier than the air, the smoke starts to descend. A person who smokes heavily indoors causes a permanent low-lying smoke cloud that other householders have no choice but to breathe. Children are at particular risk of serious health effects from SHS (for details, see chapter 9). The other places where children in particular are exposed to SHS are playgrounds, parks, school campuses, private vehicles and beaches.

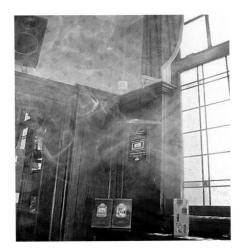

Fig. 1. Tobacco smoke in an Irish pub before a smoking ban came into effect on March 29, 2004.

Table 1. Carcinogens in SS and SHS from cigarettes

Constituent	Emissions in SS/ cigarette	Amount in SHS/m³
Benzene, µg	163–353	4.2–63.7
Benzo(a)pyrene, ng	45–103	0.37–1.7
NNK, ng	201–1,440	0.2–29.3
4-Aminobiphenyl, ng	11.4–18.8	
2-Naphthylamine, ng	63.1–128	
1,3-Butadiene, µg	98–205	0.3–40
Formaldehyde, µg	233–485	143

NNK = 4-Methylnitrosaminol-1-(3-pyridyl)-1-butanone. Table adapted with permission from [7].

Measurement of Second Hand Smoke

Multiple approaches can be used to measure SHS, including administering questionnaires, observing smoking behaviour, measuring components of tobacco smoke in the air and measuring components of tobacco smoke in the human body. A brief overview of some of these approaches is described below [9].

Self-Report or Observation
One can collect information on SHS exposure by administering self-report questionnaires or by collecting observational data. The information gathered complements the other methods used to monitor SHS exposure and is often used simultaneously.

Observational Monitoring. This method is broad and can be tailored to meet specific goals. In general, this method re-

lies on inspecting the environment of interest for the presence of smoking and smoke-free polices. Sentinel observations can include counting smokers or cigarette butts, and looking for no smoking signs and/or sale of tobacco products.

Questionnaires. Participants are asked to recall settings where they were exposed to SHS over some period of time.

Levels in the Environment
SHS levels in the air can be determined by measuring concentrations of tobacco components: toxic, airborne gases such as nicotine, arsenic, carbon monoxide and cyanide or PM <2.5 µm in diameter ($PM_{2.5}$) capable of penetrating deep into the lungs.

Air Nicotine Monitoring. This method typically uses a passive air nicotine monitor, which is a small, lightweight, circular plastic badge containing a filter. As air passes through it, nicotine in the air is absorbed into the filter. Laboratory analysis can be conducted to determine the amount of nicotine collected. Results are reported in milligrams of nicotine per cubic meter of air.

$PM_{2.5}$ Air Monitoring. This method uses a TSI AM 510 SidePak Personal Aerosol Monitor (or other similar devices) to measure respirable suspended particles. The SidePak uses a pump to draw air inside to measure the real-time concentration of air PM with aerodynamic diameter <2.5 μm. $PM_{2.5}$ is measured because particles of this size are easily inhaled deeply into the lungs.

Levels in the Human Body

Biological markers or 'biomarkers' are substances measured as indicators of human exposure. Several different components of tobacco smoke have been measured in biological samples, such as blood, saliva, hair and toenails. Two of the most widely measured tobacco-related compounds are nicotine, the addictive component of tobacco, and cotinine, a metabolite of nicotine.

Hair Bio-Monitoring. This method measures nicotine concentrations in the hair as a biomarker for personal exposure to SHS in the environment. It can be used to measure long-term, cumulative exposure. Because human hair grows at approximately 1 cm per month, even a small amount of hair – 2 or 3 cm from the scalp – can potentially represent tobacco smoke exposure for several months.

Saliva Bio-Monitoring. Cotinine, a metabolite of nicotine, is measured in the saliva. Salivary cotinine is a particularly useful biomarker to measure short-term exposure, but it is not a good marker for long-term exposure to tobacco.

The conclusions drawn on the US Surgeon General Report in 2006 [2] in relation to assessing exposure to SHS are listed in the following.

Conclusions of the US Surgeon General Report

Building Designs and Operations
Current heating, ventilating and air conditioning systems alone cannot control exposure to SHS.

The operation of a heating, ventilating and air conditioning systems can distribute SHS throughout a building.

Exposure Models
Atmospheric concentration of nicotine is a sensitive and specific indicator for SHS.

Smoking increases indoor particle concentrations.

Models can be used to estimate concentrations of SHS.

Biomarkers of Exposure to SHS
Biomarkers suitable for assessing recent exposures to SHS are available.

At this time, cotinine, the primary proximate metabolite of nicotine, remains the biomarker of choice for assessing SHS exposure.

Individual biomarkers of exposure to SHS represent only one component of a complex mixture, and measurements of one marker may not wholly reflect an exposure to other components of concern as a result of involuntary smoking.

What Is a Safe Level of Second-Hand Smoke?

SHS is classified as a 'known human carcinogen' (cancer-causing agent) by the US Environmental Protection Agency [1], the US National Toxicology Program and the WHO International Agency for Research on Cancer [10]. Even low levels of SHS can be harmful. The only way to fully protect non-smokers from SHS is to completely eliminate smoking in indoor spaces. Separating smokers from non-smokers indoors, cleaning the air and ventilating buildings cannot completely eliminate exposure to SHS. Protection from SHS in other situations (open and semi-open settings) is now under consideration because SHS as a class A carcinogen has no safe level. Smoke-free playground in public parks and sports stadia are becoming common in Europe. In Ireland, funding for playgrounds is withheld by government unless they are smoke free. Some beaches in the USA are also smoke free. It seems likely that any country contemplating a 'tobacco endgame' will need to ban smoking in all public places.

Harmful Health Effects of Passive Smoking in Adults

SHS virtually affects all parts of a human body (fig. 2).

Evidence of the health risks of involuntary smoking comes from epidemiological studies, which have directly assessed the associations of SHS exposure levels with disease outcomes (table 2). Judgments about the causality between SHS exposure and health outcomes are also based upon extensive evidence derived from the biological and toxicological investigation of the health consequences of active smoking.

The literature on SHS and health has been periodically reviewed [6, 11]. One review was completed in 2005 by the California Environmental Protection Agency [12] and another review in 2006 by the Office of the US Surgeon General [2]. Causal conclusions were reached as early as 1986, when involuntary smoking was found to be a cause of lung

Table 2. Adverse health effects to SHS exposure published in major reports

Health effect	SGR 1984	SGR 1986	EPA 1992	Cal EPA 1997	UK 1998/2004	WHO 1999	IARC 2004	Cal EPA¹ 2005²	SGR 2006
Increased prevalence of chronic respiratory symptoms	yes/a	yes/a	yes/c	yes/c	yes/c	yes/c		yes/c	yes/c
Decrement in pulmonary function	yes/a	yes/a	yes/a	yes/a	yes/a*	yes/c		yes/a	yes/c
Increased occurrence of acute respiratory illnesses	yes/a	yes/a	yes/a	yes/c		yes/c		yes/c	yes/c
Increased occurrence of middle ear disease		yes/a	yes/c	yes/c	yes/c	yes/c		yes/c	yes/c
Increased severity of asthma episodes and symptoms		yes/c	yes/c			yes/c		yes/c	yes/c
Risk factor for new asthma		yes/a	yes/c					yes/c	yes/c
Risk factor for sudden infant death syndrome				yes/c	yes/a	yes/c		yes/c	yes/c
Risk factor for lung cancer in adults		yes/c	yes/c	yes/c	yes/c		yes/c	yes/c	yes/c
Risk factor for breast cancer for younger, primarily premenopausal women								yes/c	
Risk factor for nasal sinus cancer								yes/c	
Risk factor for coronary heart disease in adults				yes/c	yes/c			yes/c	yes/c

SGR = US Surgeon General's Report; EPA = US Environmental Protection Agency; Cal EPA = California Environmental Protection Agency; IARC = International Agency for Research on Cancer; UK = United Kingdom Scientific Committee on Tobacco and Health; yes/a = association; yes/c = cause.
¹ Added in 2004. ² Only effects causally associated with SHS exposure are included.
Table adapted from US Department of Health and Human Services (2006) and from ASHRAE (Environmental Tobacco Smoke, position document, page 9, table 1) (2005).
©American Society of Heating, Refrigerating and Air-Conditioning Engineers, Inc.

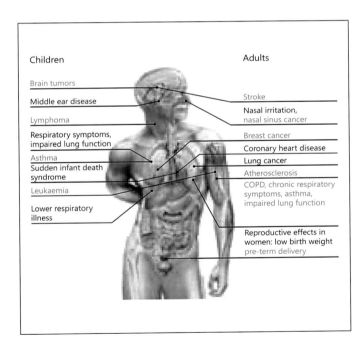

Fig. 2. Harmful health effects of passive smoking in both adults and children. Health effects with suggestive evidence of causation are in blue and those with sufficient evidence of causation are in black.

cancer in non-smokers by the International Agency for Research on Cancer [10], the US Surgeon General [6] and the US National Research Council [11]. Each of these reports interpreted the available epidemiologic evidence in the context of the deep understanding of active smoking and lung cancer. In spite of somewhat differing approaches for reaching a conclusion, the findings of the three reports were identical: involuntary smoking is a cause of lung cancer in non-smokers. This and subsequent causal conclusions have had broad public health impact.

Cardiovascular Disease
Exposure to SHS has immediate adverse effects on the cardiovascular system and can cause coronary heart disease and stroke [2, 13, 14].
- SHS causes nearly 34,000 premature deaths from heart disease each year in the United States among non-smokers [13].
- Non-smokers who are exposed to SHS at home or at work increase their risk of developing heart disease by 25–30% [15].
- SHS increases the risk for stroke by 20–30% [13].
- SHS exposure causes more than 8,000 deaths from stroke annually [13].

- Breathing SHS can have immediate adverse effects on your blood and blood vessels, increasing the risk of having a heart attack [2, 13].
- Breathing SHS interferes with the normal functioning of the heart, blood and vascular systems in ways that increase the risk of having a heart attack [13].
- Even brief exposure to SHS can damage the lining of blood vessels and cause your blood platelets to become stickier. These changes can cause a deadly heart attack [13].

Lung Cancer

SHS causes lung cancer in adults who have never smoked [13].
- Non-smokers who are exposed to SHS at home or at work increase their risk of developing lung cancer by 20–30% [2].
- SHS causes more than 7,300 lung cancer deaths among US non-smokers each year [13].
- Non-smokers who are exposed to SHS are inhaling many of the same cancer-causing substances and poisons as smokers [2, 13].
- Even brief SHS exposure can damage cells in ways that set the cancer process in motion [13].
- As with active smoking, the longer the duration and the higher the level of exposure to SHS, the greater the risk of developing lung cancer [13].

Respiratory Health Effects

Several cross-sectional studies have investigated the association between respiratory symptoms in adult non-smokers and involuntary exposure to tobacco smoke. These studies have primarily considered exposure outside the home. Consistent evidence of an effect of passive smoking on chronic respiratory symptoms in adults has not been found [16, 17], although the small particles in SHS would be anticipated to reach the airways and alveoli and potentially cause injury. Several studies suggest that passive smoking may cause acute respiratory morbidity (i.e. illnesses and symptoms) [18, 19].

People with asthma and chronic obstructive pulmonary disease (COPD) may be at increased risk from SHS exposure. However, experimental studies have not clearly demonstrated a role of SHS in exacerbating asthma in adults. The acute responses of asthmatics to SHS have been assessed by exposing persons with asthma to tobacco smoke in a chamber. This experimental approach cannot be readily controlled because of the impossibility of blinding subjects to exposure to SHS. However, suggestibility does not appear to underlie physiological responses of asthmatics of SHS [20]. Of the earlier studies involving exposure of unselected

Table 3. Potentially relevant exposure periods for reproductive and perinatal outcomes

Outcome	Relevant exposure periods		
	before conception	pre-natal	post-natal
Fertility (female)	X		
Spontaneous abortion	X	X	
Low birth weight, small for gestational age, intrauterine growth retardation	X	X	
Congenital malformations	X	X	
Infant death (including sudden infant death syndrome)	X	X	X
Cognitive development	X	X	X
Childhood behaviour	X	X	X
Height/growth	X	X	X
Childhood cancer	X	X	X

Table adapted with permission from [2].

asthmatics to SHS, only one showed a definite adverse effect [21]. One study recruited 21 asthmatics who reported exacerbation with exposure to SHS [22]. With challenge in an exposure chamber at concentrations much greater than typically encountered in indoor environments, 7 of the subjects experienced a more than 20% decline in the forced expiratory volume in 1 s.

In cross-sectional investigations, exposure to SHS has been associated with reduction in several lung function parameters [2]. One observational study found that after adjusting for known risk factors, increased SHS exposure in non-smokers was associated with increased COPD prevalence and concluded that SHS exposure in multiple settings could have an effect comparable to smoking up to 14 cigarettes per day [23]. However, the findings have not been consistent and methodological issues constrain interpretation of the findings. Thus, a conclusion cannot yet be reached on the effects of SHS exposure on lung function in adults, but there is reasonable evidence that SHS influences onset of respiratory symptoms in patients with α_1-antitrypsin deficiency [24].

Recent evidence indicates associations of SHS with tuberculosis [25, 26] and meningococcal infections [27].

Effects on Reproduction

SHS exposure may have adverse effects potentially throughout the reproductive and developmental processes (table 3).

The conclusions drawn on the US Surgeon General Report published in 2006 [2] are described in the following.

Fertility

In contrast to first-hand smoking, the evidence is inadequate to infer the presence or absence of a causal relationship between maternal exposure to SHS and female fertility or fecundability. No data were found on paternal exposure to SHS and male fertility or fecundability.

Pregnancy (Spontaneous Abortion and Perinatal Death)

The evidence is inadequate to infer the presence or absence of a causal relationship between maternal exposure to SHS during pregnancy and spontaneous abortion.

Infant Deaths

The evidence is inadequate to infer the presence or absence of a causal relationship between exposure to SHS and neonatal mortality.

Sudden Infant Death Syndrome

The evidence is sufficient to infer a causal relationship between exposure to SHS and sudden infant death syndrome.

Preterm Delivery

The evidence is suggestive but not sufficient to infer a causal relationship between maternal exposure to SHS during pregnancy and preterm delivery.

Low Birth Weight

The evidence is sufficient to infer a causal relationship between maternal exposure to SHS during pregnancy and a small reduction in birth weight.

Childhood Cancer

The evidence is suggestive but not sufficient to infer a causal relationship between pre- and postnatal exposure to SHS and childhood cancer.

Global Burden of Second-Hand Smoke Exposure among Adults

Two major more recent reports have been published in Europe: ASPECT (Analysis of the Science and Policy in Europe for the Control of Tobacco) in 2005 [28] and Lifting the smokescreen – 10 reasons to go smokefree by the Smoke Free Partnership in 2006 [29]. Both dealt with the extent of the health effects of SHS in European countries and the economic considerations. The Smoke Free Partnership Report estimated 79,449 deaths in adults alone due to SHS in EU-25 (25 Member States) for the year 2002 and also estimated mortality for each

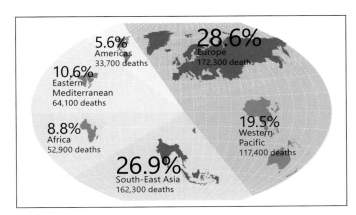

Fig. 3. Distribution of global deaths from exposure to SHS by WHO regions in 2004 [47].

Table 4. Total deaths: including lower respiratory tract infections (LRI) and ischaemic heart disease (IHD), and disability adjusted life years (DALYs) from SHS by outcome, 2004 [30]

Health outcome	Deaths		DALYs	
	children	adults	children	adults
LRI	165,000	NA	5,939,000	NA
Otitis	<100	NA	24,900	NA
Asthma	1,100	35,800	651,000	1,246,000
Lung cancer	NA	21,400	NA	216,000
IHD	NA	379,000	NA	2,836,000
Total	166,000	436,000	6,616,000	4,297,000

NA = Not applicable.

separate Member State. Numbers of deaths induced by SHS exposure according to WHO regions are shown in figure 3.

A recent study in *The Lancet* in 2011 reported that SHS exposure was estimated to have caused 379,000 deaths from ischaemic heart disease, 165,000 from lower respiratory infections, 36,900 from asthma and 21,400 from lung cancer in 2004 (table 4); 603,000 deaths were attributable to SHS in 2004, which was about 10% of worldwide mortality. In addition, 47% of deaths from SHS occurred in women, 28% in children and 26% in men (fig. 4) [30].

Protecting Adults from SHS Exposure

Exposure to SHS is almost entirely preventable, but it is not always easy to achieve (fig. 5). Only 5% of the world population had 100% smoke-free policies in place in 2008. However,

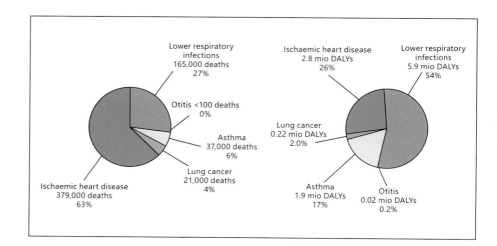

Fig. 4. Distribution of total deaths and disability adjusted life years (DALYs) attributable to SHS exposure in 2004. Percentage of total deaths/DALYs attributable to SHS: total = 100% [30].

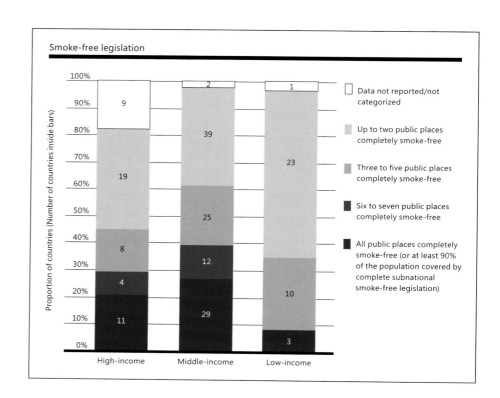

Fig. 5. Comprehensive smoke-free legislation is the most widely adopted measure, with 1.1 billion people covered [48].

MPOWER 2013 reported that comprehensive smoke-free legislation was by then the most widely adopted measure, with 1.1 billion people covered, which is a great improvement.

The WHO and the European Commission (EC) have declared that through Article 8 of the Framework Convention for Tobacco Control (FCTC) [31] and the EC through a Council Recommendation that people have the right to be protected from SHS in public and how this can be achieved (see also chapter 13). To this end, they have pointed out that they recognise the harmful effects of SHS and that comprehensive legislation is needed to prevent harm and that since there is no safe level of exposure, SHS being a class A carcinogen, that mechanical ventilation solutions are unacceptable. Many countries have now enacted comprehensive legislation since Ireland introduced their Smoke-Free Law in March 2004 (see also chapter 12). These laws protect adults in the workplace and entertainment venues. Although children may also benefit from legislation in general, the laws do not prevent exposure in utero or in the home or in private vehicles. Playgrounds in public parks are also increasingly smoke free in Ireland and in New York City. Legislation to achieve smoke-free private housing may not be feasible or considered appropriate at present, but education and strong encouragement and advice should be offered.

Emerging Market of Novel Tobacco Products
Blanket bans on waterpipes similar to smoke-free policies are not in place in nations where waterpipe smoking is prevalent and is culturally and socially acceptable (see chapter 22). Protecting adults from SHS attributable to newer tobacco products, such as electronic cigarettes, is also uncertain at this stage. Evidence to date in relation to e-cigarettes is inadequate. A recent trial in *The Lancet* reported that e-cigarettes may be used as smoking cessation aids [32]. However, another study demonstrated that vapours from e-cigarettes contain toxic and carcinogenic carbonyl compounds [33] (see chapter 23).

Nonetheless, there is debate around this especially when issues such as 'renormalizing' the habit of smoking through 'vaping' cannot be adequately addressed. The UK Medicines and Healthcare products Regulatory Agency is considering regulating e-cigarettes as medicinal products while the EU Parliament may consider this as conventional tobacco product in 2016 through its Tobacco Products Directive (2014/40/EU). The US Food and Drug Administration has authority to regulate e-cigarettes as tobacco or medicinal products, and such regulation is expected to be announced and in May 2014 the FDA proposed new e-cigarette regulation. The WHO has released its recommendations in a report to the Conference of the Parties recommending strong regulation [34]. The worrying trend, however, is that there is doubling of the usage of e-cigarettes among youths in the US in recent years and similar trends may follow elsewhere. This problem is partly attributable to unregulated marketing of this product over social network sites. In addition, the fast growing of this market has rocketed into a USD 3 billion industry selling more than 250 brands of e-cigarettes, with the venturing in of the Big Tobacco into this lucrative market!

Health Benefits of Smoke-Free Legislation

Respiratory Health Benefits
There is considerable experience and knowledge of the beneficial effects of comprehensive smoke-free legislation. Early studies from California [19] showed that there were early respiratory health benefits in bar workers. The introduction of the Irish smoke-free legislation and subsequently the Scottish and other national legislation has allowed the opportunity to measure health benefits on an individual and population basis. Various studies have confirmed the California results showing significantly reduced respiratory symptoms and improved spirometry. This was accompanied by a reduction in cotinine and exhaled breath carbon monoxide in the Irish studies [35, 36] which also found a significant improvement in gas exchange in the lung. These significant effects were seen in non-smokers and former smokers but did not reach statistical significance in current smokers. It is also of importance to note that these subjects were not patients and that they were in full-time employment with pulmonary function in the normal range and yet had significant improvements 1 year after the ban.

A recent Irish study reported a 38% reduction in COPD (RR: 0.62; 95% CI: 0.46–0.83) mortality after the smoking ban [37]. The COPD mortality reductions were seen at ages ≥65 years, but not 35–64 years, and multivariate analysis showed a gender effect (RR: 0.47; 95% CI: 0.32–0.70) for females.

Figure 6 reports the health benefits of the comprehensive smoke-free legislation in Ireland.

Cardiovascular Health Benefits
There was consistent evidence in support of the cardiovascular health benefits of comprehensive smoke-free legislations from different population settings. Studies in patients in the US [38, 39], Italy [40] and Scotland [41] showed definite reductions in acute myocardial infarctions varying from 17% in Scotland to 11% in Italy. A couple of meta-analyses were also published recently in support of this [42]. A recent English study shows a definite but lesser (2.5%) reduction [43]. However, a recent Irish study [37] reported a 26% reduction in ischaemic heart disease (RR: 0.74; 95% CI: 0.63–0.88) and a 32% reduction in stroke (RR: 0.68; 95% CI: 0.54–0.85).

Reproductive Health Benefits
Smoke-free legislation has the potential to reduce the substantive disease burden associated with SHS exposure in relation to reproductive health and adverse birth outcomes. A recent systematic review and meta-analysis in *The Lancet* [44] in 2014 reported that smoke-free legislation was associated with reductions in preterm birth (1,366,862 individuals; –10.4%; 95% CI –18.8 to –2.0) but no significant effect on low birth weight was identified (>1.9 million individuals: –1.7%; 95% CI –5.1 to 1.6; p =

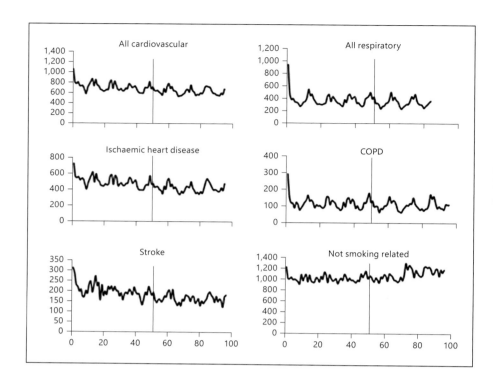

Fig. 6. Observed monthly mortality in the Republic of Ireland, 2000–2007 [37].

0.31). This systematic review included two studies – one from Ireland [45] and one from Scotland [46]. The Irish study also reported a significant decline in both very small-for-gestational-age births and rates immediately after the ban [(–5.3%; 95% CI –5.43 to –5.17%, p < 0.0001) and (–0.45%; 95% CI: –0.7 to –0.19%, p < 0.0007)], respectively. Figure 7 clearly demonstrates this.

Future of Tobacco Control in Protecting Adults from Second-Hand Smoke Exposure

Research

The controversies around electronic cigarettes are to be adequately addressed especially in terms of their safety. Research must also focus on the potential of reducing harm employing modified tobacco products. In addition, evidence is essential to support further expansion of smoke-free policies among vulnerable population groups, such as mental health patients, prisoners and nursing homes (see also chapters 16 and 17).

Policy Considerations

Further expansion of smoke-free policies is crucial to curb the tobacco epidemic. Smoke-free housing units and smoke-free households are important to reduce childhood

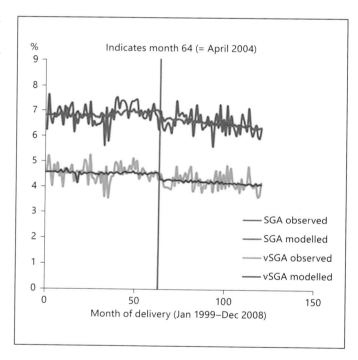

Fig. 7. Monthly observed and modelled (expected) small-for-gestational-age (SGA) and very SGA (vSGA) rates in Ireland by month of delivery, January 1999 to December 2008 (the bar indicates month 64 = April 2004) [45].

exposure to SHS. SHS exposure in pregnancy is hugely detrimental and protection from exposure should be coupled with tailored anti-smoking interventions (see chapter 20). Smoke-free private vehicles, smoke-free playgrounds and parks, and smoke-free beaches must be considered if nations are moving towards tobacco-free futures. Regulation of electronic cigarettes is also mandatory simply because of the inherent 'renormalization' of cigarette smoking. Funding of global tobacco control is crucial to keep the momentum going in the war on tobacco – the battle has begun but not won yet. The next logical step would be to plan the tobacco endgame.

Key Points

- The term *first-hand smoke* refers to what is inhaled into the smoker's own lungs, while *second-hand smoke (SHS)* is a mixture of exhaled smoke and other substances leaving the smouldering end of the cigarette which can be inhaled by others;

third-hand smoke, is contamination on the surfaces of objects that remains after SHS has cleared.
- SHS is a complex mixture of gases and some 4,000 particulate phase chemicals (of which ≥250 are known to be toxic or carcinogenic) generated during the burning and smoking of tobacco products. SHS is a class A carcinogen and therefore has no safe level and adversely affects virtually all parts of the human body.
- Current heating, ventilating and air conditioning systems alone cannot control exposure to SHS, and the operation of a heating, ventilating or air conditioning system can distribute SHS throughout a building.
- The Smoke Free Partnership Report estimated 79,449 deaths in adults alone due to SHS in EU-25 for the year 2002 and also estimated mortality for each separate Member State.
- There is doubling of the usage of e-cigarettes among youths in the US in recent years and similar trends are emerging in Europe with unknown consequences.
- There are proven respiratory, cardiovascular and reproductive health benefits of smoke-free legislation, which was first introduced on a national basis in Ireland in 2004, but only 5% of the world population has 100% smoke-free policies in place in 2008.

References

1 US Environmental Protection Agency: Respiratory Health Effects of Passive Smoking: Lung Cancer and Other Disorders. Smoking and Tobacco Monograph No 4. Washington, US Environmental Protection Agency, Office of Health and Environmental Assessment, Office of Research and Development, 1992.

2 US Department of Health and Human Services: The Health Consequences of Involuntary Exposure to Tobacco Smoke: A Report of the Surgeon General. Atlanta, US Department of Health and Human Services, Centers for Disease Control and Prevention, Coordinating Center for Health Promotion, National Center for Chronic Disease Prevention and Health Promotion, Office on Smoking and Health, 2006.

3 Report on Carcinogens, ed 11. Washington, US Department of Health and Human Services, National Institutes of Health, National Institute of Environmental Health Services, National Toxicology Program, 2005, http://ntp.niehs.nih.gov/ntp/roc/eleventh/profiles/s176toba.pdf.

4 Baker RR: Product formation mechanisms inside a burning cigarette. Progress in energy and combustion. Science 1981;7:135–153.

5 Claxton LD, Morin RS, Hughes TJ, Lewtas J: A genotoxic assessment of environmental tobacco smoke using bacterial bioassays. Mut Res 1989;222:81–99.

6 US Department of Health and Human Services. The Health Consequences of Involuntary Smoking: A Report of the Surgeon General. DHHS Publ No 87-8398. Atlanta, US Department of Health and Human Services, Public Health Service, Centers for Disease Control, 1986.

7 Gibson GJ, Loddenkemper R, Sibille Y, Lundbäck B (eds): European Lung White Book. Respiratory Health and Disease in Europe. Sheffield, European Respiratory Society, 2013, www.erswhitebook.org.

8 Matt GE, Quintana PJ, Destaillats H, et al: Thirdhand tobacco smoke: emerging evidence and arguments for a multidisciplinary research agenda. Environ Health Perspect 2011; 199:1218–1226.

9 Secondhand Smoke Monitoring, Johns Hopkins Bloomberg School of Public Health. http://www.shsmonitoring.org/.

10 International Agency for Research on Cancer: Tobacco Smoke and Involuntary Smoking. IARC Monographs. Lyon, IARC, 2004, vol 83.

11 National Research Council, Committee on Passive Smoking: Environmental Tobacco Smoke: Measuring Exposures and Assessing Health Effects. Washington, National Academy Press, 1986.

12 California Environmental Protection Agency (Cal EPA), Office of Environmental Health Hazard Assessment: Health Effects of Exposure to Environmental Tobacco Smoke. Sacramento, Cal EPA, 1997.

13 US Department of Health and Human Services: The Health Consequences of Smoking – 50 Years of Progress: A Report of the Surgeon General. Atlanta, US Department of Health and Human Services, Centers for Disease Control and Prevention, National Center for Chronic Disease Prevention and Health Promotion, Office on Smoking and Health, 2014.

14 Institute of Medicine: Secondhand Smoke Exposure and Cardiovascular Effects: Making Sense of the Evidence. Washington, National Academy of Sciences, Institute of Medicine, 2009.

15 US Department of Health and Human Services: Let's Make the Next Generation Tobacco-Free: Your Guide to the 50th Anniversary Surgeon General's Report on Smoking and Health. Atlanta, US Department of Health and Human Services, Centers for Disease Control and Prevention, National Center for Chronic Disease Prevention and Health Promotion, Office on Smoking and Health, 2014.

16 Kauffmann F, Dockery DW, Speizer FE, Ferris BG Jr: Respiratory symptoms and lung function in relation to passive smoking: a comparative study of American and French women. Int J Epidemiol 1989;18:334–344.

17 Hole DJ, Gillis CR, Chopra C, Hawthorne VM: Passive smoking and cardiorespiratory health in a general population in the west of Scotland. BMJ 1989;299:423–427.

18 Leuenberger P, Schwartz J, Ackermann-Liebrich U, et al: Passive smoking exposure in adults and chronic respiratory symptoms (SAPALDIA Study). Swiss Study on Air Pollution and Lung Diseases in Adults, SAPALDIA Team. Am J Respir Crit Care Med 1994;150:1222-1228.

19 Eisner MD, Smith AK, Blanc PD: Bartenders' respiratory health after establishment of smoke-free bars and taverns. JAMA 1998;280:1909–1914.

20 Urch RB, Silverman F, Corey P, Shephard RJ, Cole P, Goldsmith LJ: Does suggestibility modify acute reactions to passive cigarette smoke exposure? Environ Res 1988;47:34–47.

21 Dahms TE, Bolin JF, Slavin RG: Passive smoking. Effects on bronchial asthma. Chest 1981;80:530–534.

22 Stankus RP, Menon PK, Rando RJ, Glindmeyer H, Salvaggio JE, Lehrer SB: Cigarette smoke-sensitive asthma: challenge studies. J Allergy Clin Immunol 1988;82:331–338.

23 Hagstad S, Bjerg A, Ekerljung L, Backman H, Lindberg A, Rönmark E, Lundbäck B: Passive smoking exposure is associated with increased risk of COPD in never smokers. Chest 2014;145:1298–1304.

24 Mayer AS, Stoller JK, Vedal S, Ruttenber AJ, Strand M, Sandhaus RA, Newman LS: Risk factors for symptom onset in PI*Z alpha-1 antitrypsin deficiency. Int J Chron Obstruct Pulmon Dis 2006;1:485–492.

25 Slama K, Chiang CY, Enarson DA, Hassmiller K, Fanning A, Gupta P, Ray C: Tobacco and tuberculosis: a qualitative systematic review and meta-analysis. Int J Tuberc Lung Dis 2007;11:1049–1061

26 Lindsay RP, Shin SS, Garfein RS, Rusch ML, Novotny TE: The association between active and passive smoking and latent tuberculosis infection in adults and children in the United States: results from NHANES. PLoS One 2014;9:e93137.

27 Murray RL, Britton J, Leonardi-Bee J: Second hand smoke exposure and the risk of invasive meningococcal disease in children: systematic review and meta-analysis. BMC Public Health 2012;12:1062.

28 European Commission: Tobacco or Health in the European Union: Past, Present and Future – The ASPECT Consortium. Luxembourg, European Commission, 2004, http://ec.europa.eu/health/ph_determinants/life_style/Tobacco/Documents/tobacco_fr_en.pdf.

29 Smoke Free Partnership: Lifting the smokescreen – 10 reasons to go smokefree. http://www.smokefreepartnership.eu/Lifting-the-smokescreen-10-reasons.

30 Oberg M, Jaakkola MS, Woodward A, Peruga A, Prüss-Ustün A: Worldwide burden of disease from exposure to second-hand smoke: a retrospective analysis of data from 192 countries. Lancet 2011;377:139–146.

31 World Health Organization: Framework Convention on Tobacco Control. Geneva, WHO, 2003, http://www.who.int/fctc/cop/art%208%20guidelines_english.pdf.

32 Bullen C, Howe C, Laugesen M, McRobbie H, Parag V, Williman J, Walker N: Electronic cigarettes for smoking cessation: a randomised controlled trial. Lancet 2013;382:1629–1637.

33 Kosmider L, Sobczak A, Fik M, Knysak J, Zaciera M, Kurek J, Goniewicz ML: Carbonyl compounds in electronic cigarette vapors – effects of nicotine solvent and battery output voltage. Nicotine Tob Res 2014;16:1319–1326.

34 Conference of the Parties to the WHO Framework Convention on Tobacco Control. Sixth Session, Moscow, Russian Federation, 13–18 October 2014, http://www.who.int/fctc/cop/sessions/cop6/en/.

35 Goodman P, Agnew M, McCaffrey M, Paul G, Clancy L: Effects of the Irish smoking ban on respiratory health of bar workers and air quality in Dublin pubs. Am J Respir Crit Care Med 2007;175:840–845.

36 Goodman PG, Haw S, Kabir Z, Clancy L: Are there health benefits associated with comprehensive smoke-free laws. Int J Public Health 2009;54:367–378.

37 Stallings-Smith S, Zeka A, Goodman P, Kabir Z, Clancy L: Reductions in cardiovascular, cerebrovascular, and respiratory mortality following the national Irish smoking ban: interrupted time-series analysis. PLoS One 2013;8:e62063.

38 Sargent RP, Shepard RM, Glantz SA: Reduced incidence of admissions for myocardial infarction associated with public smoking ban: before and after study. BMJ 2004;328:977–980.

39 Juster HR, Loomis BR, Hinman TM, Farrelly MC, Hyland A, Bauer UE, Birkhead GS: Declines in hospital admissions for acute myocardial infarction in New York State after implementation of a comprehensive smoking ban. Am J Public Health 2007;97:2035–2039.

40 Barone-Adesi F, Vizzini L, Merletti F, Richiardi L: Short-term effects of Italian smoking regulation on rates of hospital admission for acute myocardial infarction. Eur Heart J 2006;10:2468–2472.

41 Pell JP, Haw S, Cobbe S, Newby DE, Pell AC, Fischbacher C, et al: Smoke-free legislation and hospitalizations for acute coronary syndrome. N Engl J Med 2008;359:482–491.

42 Meyers DG, Neuberger JS, He J: Cardiovascular effect of bans on smoking in public places: a systematic review and meta-analysis. J Am Coll Cardiol 2009;54:1249–1255.

43 Sims M, Maxwell R, Bauld L, Gilmore A: Short term impact of smoke-free legislation in England: retrospective analysis of hospital admissions for myocardial infarction. BMJ 2010;340:c2161.

44 Been JV, Nurmatov UB, Cox B, Nawrot TS, van Schayck CP, Sheikh A: Effect of smoke-free legislation on perinatal and child health: a systematic review and meta-analysis. Lancet 2014;383:1549–1560.

45 Kabir Z, Daly S, Clarke V, Keogan S, Clancy L: Smoking ban and small-for-gestational age births in Ireland. PLoS One 2013;8:e57441.

46 Mackay DF, Nelson SM, Haw SJ, Pell JP: Impact of Scotland's smoke-free legislation on pregnancy complications: retrospective cohort study. PLoS Med 2012;9:e1001175.

47 Eriksen M, Mackay J, Ross H: The Tobacco Atlas, ed 4. Atlanta, American Cancer Society/New York, World Lung Foundation, 2012, http://www.tobaccoatlas.org.

48 World Health Organization: Tobacco Free Initiative (TFI): WHO Report on the Global Tobacco Epidemic 2013: Enforcing Bans on Tobacco Advertising, Promotion and Sponsorship. Geneva, WHO, 2013, http://apps.who.int/tobacco/global_report/2013/en/.

Prof. Luke Clancy, BSc, MB, MD, PhD, FRCPI, FRCP (Edin), FFOMRCPI, Director General
TobaccoFree Research Institute Ireland
PO Box 12489, DIT Focas Building, 8 Camden Row
Dublin 8 (Ireland)
E-Mail lclancy@tri.ie

Loddenkemper R, Kreuter M (eds): The Tobacco Epidemic, ed 2, rev. and ext.
Prog Respir Res. Basel, Karger, 2015, vol 42, pp 121–135 (DOI: 10.1159/000369436)

Economics of Tobacco Use and Control

Joy Townsend

Department of Social and Environmental Health Research, London School of Hygiene and Tropical Medicine, London, UK

Abstract

The six largest tobacco companies have a turnover of some USD 350 billion and profits of USD 35 billion, so for good reason are called Big Tobacco. Nearly 20% of the world's adult population smoke, and smoking diseases account for 1 in 10 of all deaths globally. Tobacco is a huge public health problem and a major cause of inequalities in health and mortality. Evidence-based tobacco control policies are highly cost-effective and more so than most medical and surgical treatments; many are cost saving. A 10% price rise via a tax increase is estimated to be the most cost-effective at USD 18–457 per disability-adjusted life year (2013 prices) plus substantial tax revenue benefits: compared to USD 523–2,799 for cessation support and USD 212–4,228 for other effective policies. In all cases, interventions are far more cost-effective in low- and middle-income countries than in high-income countries. Price differences account for much of the differences in countries' smoking rates, which tend to be highest where prices are lowest. Raising cigarette prices by 10% would save 10 million smoking-attributable deaths globally in the long run. The effects of electronic cigarettes need to be studied, as a significant switch to these products may significantly reduce mortality and morbidity. Evidence-based policies to reduce smoking and its harm are in place in many countries, but are frequently hampered by inadequate government action and the hostile influence of the transnational tobacco companies including foreign investment. Addressing these with serious action across the world will save lives and strengthen economies.   © 2015 S. Karger AG, Basel

The Smoking Epidemic

Smoking tobacco as cigarettes developed through the first half of the 20th century (see chapter 1) and proved to be far more dangerous than the previous pipes, snuff or cigars as the smoke was inhaled; cigarettes were socially acceptable and very cheap, and so were smoked not as the occasional one or two, but as twenty or so a day. The introduction and growth of cigarette smoking was followed roughly 30 years later by a parallel shadow of lung cancer (fig. 1) [1]: from the 1930s physicians began to relate lung cancer to tobacco use in case-control studies [2, 3].

But it was the results of the huge definitive longitudinal studies of smokers and non-smokers [2, 4, 5] that clearly established the relationship, not only with cancer but also with cardiovascular disease, chronic obstructive pulmonary disease and a host of other diseases (see chapters 7–10). It is one of the biggest causes of premature death [6], causing nearly 6 million deaths annually, which represents 10% of all deaths. Tobacco kills up to half of its users and someone dies from tobacco use every six seconds. There are wide differences in smoking rates for men (ranging from 8% in Nigeria to 67% in Indonesia) and for women (ranging from less than 1% in a number of countries to 45% in Austria; see chapter 2).

A Brief Economic History of Tobacco

Economics and tobacco are inextricably linked. The tobacco industry is one of the largest and most politically powerful industries in the world. It has grown from the initial cultivation of tobacco in Central America 8 millennia ago as a hallucinogenic brew or chew and its introduction to the west by Christopher Columbus. Early on, it was condemned in the west as a satanic practice, but became used medicinally and then smoked in pipes and cigars and used as snuff. As its use

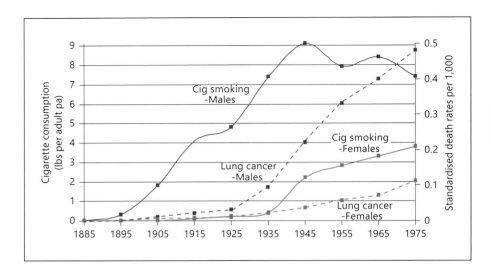

Fig. 1. Cigarette consumption and lung cancer (UK) [1].

grew, heads of state saw it as a valuable source of taxation. In the mid-19th century, Philip Morris, a small tobacconist in London, began selling hand-rolled Turkish cigarettes called Oxford Ovals. Through the 20th century with automation of the industry, cigarette consumption escalated supported by huge advertising. Up to 80% of industry profits were invested in advertising [7].

China is now by far the largest grower of tobacco leaves, producing 43% of the world's tobacco, followed by Brazil, India, USA, Malawi, Indonesia and Argentina [8]. The value of the industry relates mainly to cigarettes (USD 610 billion), but also to cigars (USD 20 billion), smokeless tobacco (USD 14 billion) and other tobacco products (USD 20 billion). Huge profits from the marketing and manufacturing of tobacco products drive the supply side; prices, taxes, advertising and other pressures modify demand. The major exporting country is Germany (181 billion sticks per annum), followed by the Netherlands (115 billion sticks), Poland (89 billion sticks), USA (60 billion sticks), and Indonesia (57 billion sticks).

The international tobacco industry is concentrated in a few companies, each with a turnover greater than the gross domestic product of many countries. With a turnover of USD 346 billion, the industry is one of the largest in the world and one of the most profitable with profits of over USD 35 billion annually. In the USA alone, advertising and promotion expenditure reached USD 9.9 billion in 2008, while USD 17 million was used to directly influence political decisions. The industry also exerts influence through associations with other organisations, including the hospitality industry, convenience stores and advertising and farmer associations.

It operates to minimise tobacco control measures in every country and wherever and however it can, by strongly lobbying governments to keep tobacco taxes low and taxation structures that suit its interest (see chapter 3). It argues against smoke-free policies, advertising bans and warnings on packs, and often works through other organisations and even other countries, as shown in its action against Australia's introduction of plain packages, where it has persuaded three countries to object to the World Trade Organisation.

Uruguay has some of the strongest tobacco control laws in the world, including graphic health warnings that cover 80% of cigarette packages, and a policy of one package per brand, which was adopted to deter the tobacco industry's use of packages with colours and other symbols to substitute for misleading descriptors such as 'light' and 'low-tar' cigarettes. In February 2010, Philip Morris International filed for arbitration at the World Bank's International Centre for Settlement of Investment Disputes, claiming that the use of a single presentation of a brand, as well as graphic health warnings that cover 80% of tobacco packages, posed a risk to its investments. This lawsuit is a legal manoeuvre designed to force the Government of Uruguay to weaken its tobacco control laws, and therefore to no longer effectively protect its citizens from the deadly consequences of tobacco use (see chapter 3).

Shirane et al. [9] have investigated the influence of the tobacco industry in Bulgaria, Poland and the Czech Republic. With regard to excise level changes resulting from Bulgaria's EU accession, they demonstrate that transnational tobacco companies (TTCs) primarily lobbied for derogation and were greatly concerned to prevent any significant increase in excise duties with accession, and acted to ensure that any increase would be only gradual. They worked collectively to prevent and postpone excise increases, and lobbied successfully for derogation of excise level increases in accession countries. As a result of derogations and rising incomes, cigarettes became more affordable in some accession countries. There are many similar examples. Although the international tobacco industry, consisting of a few huge TTCs, is mostly based in Europe, it markets aggressively to the developing world. As British American Tobacco has written there are '…strong areas of growth particularly in Asia and Africa … it is an exciting prospect'. This is bad news for developing countries, which are expecting to experience a doubling in smoking and smoking deaths in the next quarter century. Into these impoverished economies, the tobacco industry is expanding and marketing tobacco by association with glamour, sport and modern living – methods they claimed to have given up 30 years ago.

Smoking in Africa increased 50% between 1995 and 2000 and is now rising by 4.3% per year, with some 29% of men and 7% women now smoking; some rates are much higher, for example in Uganda, where a third of 13- to 15-year-old teens are smokers. Cancers, cardiovascular disease and tuberculosis ensue. Tobacco tax is low in most African countries – mostly due to tobacco industry advice to governments. The World Bank estimates that a 10% rise in tobacco tax across sub-Saharan Africa would result in three million smokers giving up the habit, and some 700,000 lives being saved, but this is not happening, mainly because tobacco companies persuade governments that it is not in their interest.

As many of these tobacco companies are based in Europe, European governments need to take responsibility for the policies. The International Monetary Fund is also responsible, having promoted the lifting of trade restrictions on tobacco and private state-owned tobacco industries as part of its loan conditions. This has led to increased marketing, reductions in excise taxes, falls in prices and overall increased cigarette consumption. Foreign investment by tobacco companies has done great harm to public health. The profits leave the country of investment, which is left with the health effects and household poverty. The Framework Convention on Tobacco Control (FCTC) guidelines contain no provision covering tobacco industry investments, and this is seen by some as a serious omission [10].

Estimates of Costs of Smoking

In their book on the economic evaluation of smoking control policies, Goel and Nelson [11] stated that to their knowledge there have been no studies on the costs of smoking. This is not entirely true, but measuring costs is complex and problematic, and for good reason not often undertaken. In considering costs, the perspective needs to be decided – whether the costs are to society, government, the health service or the individual; the period of costs needs to be decided, as smoking has a long shadow with lags of decades between smoking initiation and some costs, and costs and savings need to be related to other realistic alternative use of resources. Externalities relating to extra health care, premature mortality and fires may be borne by nonsmoking members of society or by members of other societies, and cause third-party costs and smoking-related mortality.

However, estimates of costs have been made. Shafey et al. [12] have estimated the cost of tobacco to the world economy at some USD 500 billion annually in lost productivity, health care costs, deforestation, pesticide/fertiliser contamination, fire damage, cleaning costs and discarded litter, and to reduce individual national income by as much as 3.6%.

It is estimated that about a half the direct health care costs of respiratory disease in the EU are attributable to smoking at a cost of approximately EUR 27.4 billion per year [13].

Smoking-related health problems were estimated to cost the UK National Health Service GBP 9.5 billion in 2008, equal to 4.6% of UK health care costs [14]. There is also a recent estimate of annual costs of smoking in Germany of EUR 48 billion with direct costs of EUR 18 billion [Effertz, unpubl. data].

Costs to Individuals and Their Families

But it is individual smokers and their families who pay the most heavily in terms of direct costs, reduced income from smoking diseases and loss of income for other urgent family needs. In Albania, for example, it is estimated that the average smoker spends 2 months' wages (USD 436) per year on cigarettes. Viscusi and Hersch [15] have estimated that the private mortality costs of smoking in terms of value of life should add USD 222 to each packet of cigarettes for men and USD 94 for women. Based on 2012 data, WHO estimates that increasing tobacco taxes by 50% would reduce the number of smokers by 49 million within the next 3 years and ultimately save 11 million lives. It calls on countries to raise taxes to encourage users to stop. Efroymson et al. [16] show that 'If poor people did not smoke… potentially 10.5 million fewer people would be malnourished in Bangladesh'. 'Each tobacco user represents one or more people – whether the smoker or his or her spouse or child – who is needlessly go-

Table 1. Case study of EU 2002--2007

Problem	High smoking rates and smoking disease across EU Highly diverse tax structures and levels across EU Need to harmonise EU-15 and then new EU member states
Policies	Directives requiring structural move to harmonisation Minimum tax rates increased Average tax rates increased 33%
Result	2002–2007 smoking fell by 12% Tax revenue receipts rose 15% Fine cut for roll-your-own cigarettes increased from low level Problem of smuggling from EU eastern border increased

Table 2. Case study of UK: plan to reduce smoking prevalence

Problem	Early 1990s, high smoking rates of 28% and high rates of smoking disease Late 1990s, rapidly increasing smuggling of cigarettes and fine-cut tobacco into the UK
Policies	Raise tax 3% above inflation 1993–1996; 5% above inflation 1997 After smuggling problem, tax increased in line with inflation 2001–2008 To reduce smuggling: large increase in staff and scanners; fiscal marks and covert markings introduced, new supply chain legislation, new marketing strategy, memoranda of understanding with tobacco companies After 2008, when smuggling reduced, tax raised above inflation each year
Result	Smoking prevalence fell: from 28 to 21% for adults and from 13 to 6% for children 11–15 years Smuggling reduced from 23 to 10% of consumption Tobacco tax revenue rose and then steadied; the increased tax revenue was ten times the cost of the anti-smuggling operations At least 1.2 million lives saved from premature death in the long run

ing hungry'. Tobacco expenditure could have bought an additional 800 calories a day, which could make an enormous difference to the nutritional status and health of children and others in households that suffer from severe malnutrition in Bangladesh and elsewhere.

Tobacco Control Measures

Research into the costs of smoking is rare, probably because it is not possible to make very useful or meaningful estimates. More useful perhaps is to look at the cost-effectiveness of policy instruments to reduce smoking, and the costs and benefits of change (tables 1, 2). Following the initial publication of the research which established the lethal effects of smoking, there was surprisingly little policy response around the world. Slowly this changed: initially through the pressure from doctors and pressure groups, including an early banning of tobacco advertising on television in the UK in 1965.

Evidence of the effects of and rationale for different tobacco control measures is discussed below. These were introduced gradually across the world over the past 50 years, culminating in the World Health Organisation (WHO) FCTC, which came into force in 2005 and is now signed by 174 countries committed to a wide range of policies, including banning advertising and promotion, smoke-free workplaces, cessation support, warnings on packets, increases of taxation, control of smuggling and avoidance of influence of the tobacco industry on policies (for details see chapter 13) [17, 18]. The rationale is clear and fairly uncontroversial for most policies, although strongly opposed by tobacco companies. Taxation, on the other hand, is sometimes more controversial, particularly to free-market economists who consider there should be no interference with the workings of the market and that tax will reduce the welfare of smokers. It is useful to consider the arguments for taxation.

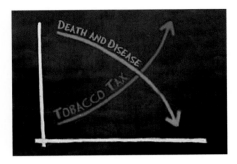

Fig. 2. Association between tax increases and morbidity/mortality.

Rationale for Tobacco Taxation

All governments need to raise tax revenue. The economic justifications for taxes are therefore primarily to raise necessary revenue, but also to adjust for externalities and as a sumptuary tax to reduce the effects of harmful products [19, 20]. Tobacco fulfils all these criteria well. It is also in the unique position of being a popular tax in many countries at least in Europe [21]. Tobacco tax is a relatively efficient vehicle for raising tax as it has a high elasticity of total revenue with respect to the tax rate compared to other products. Also, as the price elasticity of demand for cigarettes is low, the dead weight welfare loss or excess burden (loss of satisfaction to the consumer, less the gain to the government in revenue) is minimised. So, on the grounds of economic efficiency alone, there is a case for shifting taxes from other commodities to tobacco. There is also the serious issue that most smokers begin smoking as minors, become addicted and the majority regret being smokers and wish to give up the habit. Tax is often the trigger to make this happen. A meeting of economists from the US and the UK concluded that the value of increased taxation in discouraging children from becoming addicted to nicotine was potentially the most powerful argument supporting increased taxes [20] (fig. 2).

As Hanson and Kysar [22] have put it, 'Our awe …may sometimes cause us to overlook less desirable aspects of the market system. Put differently, the fact that all manner of fresh fruits and vegetables can be purchased year-round at extremely low prices truly is a marvel. The fact that 3,000 (US) children are convinced every day to purchase and ignite a combination of chemicals that may well addict them, enfeeble them, and ultimately kill them is a tragedy. And it remains a tragedy even if accomplished efficiently'.

Tobacco Taxation and Price Increase

A first principle of economics is that the demand for a normal good is related negatively to its price, and the extent of this decrease can be assessed by a unit-free measure, price elasticity. Many studies from countries around the world have confirmed the important role of price in determining whether and how much people smoke. These studies have demonstrated that a 10% increase in the real price of cigarettes would result in a decrease of about 2.5–5% in cigarette consumption and vice versa [23, 24] in high-income countries. Half the effect is likely to be from a reduction in prevalence and half from a reduction in the amount smoked by the remaining smokers. These elasticity estimates are mainly from higher-income countries; earlier research has shown higher price response in lower-/middle-income countries [25], but recent evidence is more mixed showing price response more similar to that in high-income countries. As an illustration of smokers' response to price changes, figure 3 shows price in real terms against demand for cigarettes in Italy from 1970 to 2003.

Tax has been singled out by the WHO, the World Bank and others as the most effective means of tobacco control and the most productive and cost-effective means for reducing the demand for tobacco [25]. It also has a low administrative burden [19, 25]. Ranson et al. [26] have estimated that a 10% price increase could have the hugely beneficial effect of averting 5–16 million premature deaths worldwide, 90% in low-/middle-income countries, and predominantly of those now young, at a cost of only USD 4–102 (adjusted to 2013 prices) per disability-adjusted life year (DALY) in the short run. Several studies have estimated that the reduction in demand would be twice as much in the long run as in the short run, requiring a continuous increase in real price to keep pace with inflation.

Most governments impose tobacco taxes to raise revenue and this is insisted on by the International Monetary Fund for certain countries in budget deficit. Increasing tax rates will almost always raise extra government revenue, and, as well as being the most effective tobacco control measure, is a necessary adjunct to the effects of other tobacco control measures which, by decreasing demand for tobacco, will also decrease tax revenues. The WHO calculates that if all countries increased tobacco taxes by 50% per pack, governments would earn an extra USD 101 billion in global revenue and that, 'These additional funds could – and should – be used to advance health and other social programmes'.

Countries such as France and the Philippines have already seen the benefits of imposing high taxes on tobacco. Between the early 1990s and 2005, France tripled its infla-

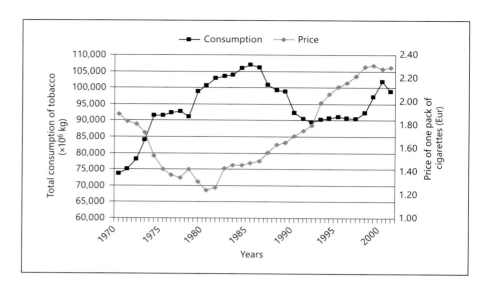

Fig. 3. Price and demand for cigarettes in Italy from 1970 to 2003 (source: Gallus et al. [24]).

tion-adjusted cigarette prices and sales fell by more than 50%. A few years later, the number of young men dying from lung cancer in France started to go down. In the Philippines, one year after increasing taxes, the Government has collected more than the expected revenue and plans to spend 85% of this on health services. Tobacco companies globally try to mislead governments into thinking that tobacco tax revenues will fall if taxes are raised.

The Tax Rate Elasticity of Tax Revenue

It is important to know just how tax revenue changes with changes in the tobacco tax rate.

The tax rate elasticity for tax revenue is positive and equal to $1 + (T/P) \times e$, where T/P is the share of tax in price, and e is the elasticity of demand [23].

Tax revenue will increase with a tax rate increase (tax elasticity >0)

if $T/P \times e < -1.0$ that is if $e < -P/T$.

As T/P is typically 0.4–0.8 (tax is usually 40–80% of the price of a packet of cigarettes).

So P/T will typically be between 1.25 and 2.5 and no estimates of (– e) have been as high as 1.25 (typically 0.25–0.5).

Tax revenue will therefore rise with a rise in tax rate and the tax elasticity will be typically 0.68–0.86, meaning that a 10% rise in tax rate will result in a rise of 6.8–8.6% in tax revenue, other things being equal.

There is now published research from many countries reporting increases in government tax revenue following to-bacco tax rate increases, and also falls following reductions in the real tax rate. Figure 4 shows how tobacco revenue increased when tobacco tax rates were increased from 29 to 59% of the retail price in Poland between 1996 and 2007 [27].

Tobacco industry officials frequently argue that a reduction in tobacco consumption may result in increased unemployment and so damage the economy. The manufacture of cigarettes is highly capital intensive, i.e. uses little labour; few other industries are as capital intensive [28] and most job losses in the industry have been due to increased capitalisation. When the consumption of tobacco products falls, the money previously spent on tobacco is spent on other products, and creates jobs elsewhere [25] from more labour-intensive goods or services. One study predicts a net increase of almost 100,000 jobs in the UK if income spent on tobacco were shifted to other luxury items [28].

Smoking Prevalence and Price in Europe

In comparing prices, it is useful to use a common currency that allows for differences in affordability; WHO uses USD PPP, which is US dollars in terms of purchasing power parity. Cigarette prices vary hugely across the WHO European region from 1.03 USD PPP in Kazakhstan to 9.51 USD PPP in Ireland for the 'most sold' cigarettes [6]. This represents a 9-fold difference. Even greater variations are evident in the prices of the 'cheapest' cigarettes sold in each country, which vary more than 20-fold from 0.4 USD PPP in Kyrgyzstan to 8.62 USD PPP in Ireland.

Townsend

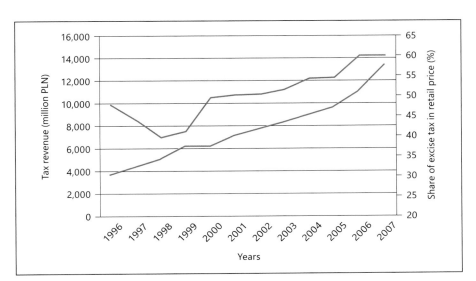

Fig. 4. Tax and tax revenue (million PLN) in Poland from 1996 to 2007 [27]. Red line = Percentage share of excise tax in retail price; blue line = tobacco excise tax revenue.

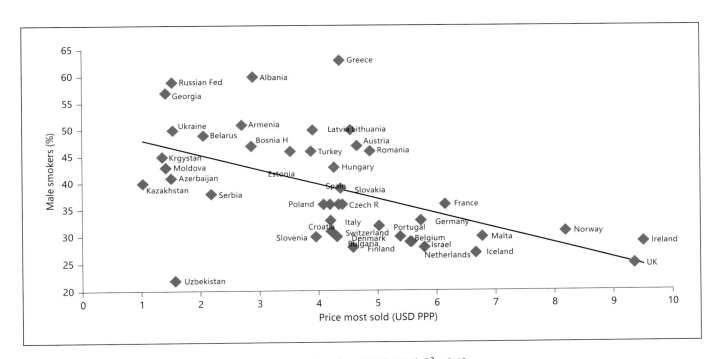

Fig. 5. Price most sold (USD PPP) by percent male smokers (data from WHO 2011). $R^2 = 0.40$.

Price has a major influence at least for men, as can be seen in figure 5 above, although not the only factor influencing the variation in smoking between European countries. The relationship between cigarette price and prevalence of smoking by men in the countries of the WHO European Region is highly significant, and price alone explains 40% of the variation ($R^2 = 0.40$), with log prevalence = 0.53 (0.024) – 0.0314 (0.0061) log price (p = 0.000007) + error term (standard errors in parentheses and author's calculations).

This implies that every one US dollar decrease in price between countries in Europe is associated with a 3% higher prevalence of men smoking. The price elasticity of demand across the region is estimated at about –0.35. For the Russian

Federation, it would mean that by raising the price of cigarettes even to the average European price of about 5.5 USD PPP would reduce smoking by about one third and save possibly over 100,000 Russian lives in the long term.

Women and Price

For cultural reasons, the price/prevalence relationship is different for women in Europe. Smoking prevalence is very low in some countries, particularly in the former Soviet Union, even though prices are low in Russia, Ukraine, Kazakhstan, Belarus, Georgia, Republic of Moldova, Uzbekistan, Kyrgyzstan and Albania. 'Within country' time series analyses suggest that adult women are more sensitive than men to price increases [29, 30]. A recent study has also shown that women who smoke are at greater risk than men from heart disease [31], so are likely to benefit even more than men from smoking cessation.

Tobacco Tax Structure

The structure of tobacco tax affects prices, and is partly responsible for the low tax in former Soviet Union countries and the wide differences in cigarette prices between countries. Tobacco companies act to minimise the tax impact whatever the structure and have most control when the tax is entirely or mainly levied as an ad valorem tax (i.e. as a percentage of the final price), as keeping the 'before tax' price low yields a low tax and a low price. Ad valorem taxes were common in southern European countries; they tend to result in a wider range of prices and make it easier for smokers to trade down to cheaper brands. A high specific or minimum tax (tax as a fixed monetary sum) allows the least manipulation from the industry and is generally considered the best for tobacco control. It requires regular adjustment in line with inflation and income changes. The ideal structure is a high specific or minimum tax with an additional high ad valorem tax, so that higher priced or longer cigarettes also get appropriately taxed.

Fine-cut tobacco used for roll-your-own cigarettes is taxed at a much lower rate than manufactured cigarettes in all European countries; even the EU minimum tariff for fine-cut tobacco is much lower than for manufactured cigarettes. This again provides an option for smokers, particularly low-income smokers, to trade down to a cheaper product and bypass raised taxes, as was the case in Hungary over the short period from 2000 to 2006. Due to the increasing

divergence in price of manufactured cigarettes, roll-your-own cigarettes have also become used to a much higher extent in the UK, France and Finland [21]. Increasing tobacco prices is particularly effective in encouraging young people in their 20s to give up smoking, but has not been shown to be a significant factor in initiation of smoking by adolescents [32, 33].

Illicit Trade

Illicit trade and cross-border smuggling reduce the average price paid and so increase the demand for tobacco with subsequent increase in health problems. Cross-border smuggling may increase if tobacco prices are raised in one country making a significant difference in price across the border. Harmonising tobacco tax upwards between countries is therefore in the interest of the health and revenue of all countries.

Price and tax differences have been shown not to be the main cause of smuggling. An empirical analysis for European countries estimated that price increases led to increased revenue even when smuggling was increasing [34]. Corruption, organised crime and distribution networks for illicit goods are of greater importance than price, and little relationship has been shown between the extent of smuggling of tobacco and its price or tax [35].

Parties to the FCTC negotiated a Protocol for a universal system for counteracting illicit trade in tobacco formally agreed in 2012. The main elements are tracing (the re-creation of the route of seized illicit cigarettes) based on unique, secure and non-removable markings on all unit packets and packages and on outside packaging of cigarettes within five years (and of other tobacco products within 10 years) of entry into force of the Protocol. Licensing of all those involved in manufacturing, distribution and retailing of tobacco is also required. Resources are needed to monitor and enforce the agreement and the illicit production of cigarettes, but these should be more than repaid by the increase in tax revenue available to governments from the fall in illicit trade. A study by West et al. [36] found that eliminating the illicit cigarette trade in the UK would reduce cigarette consumption by 5.0–8.2% and lower the tobacco death toll by 4,000–6,560 premature deaths per year. A later study by Joossens et al. [37] concluded that the revenue lost globally to governments by illicit trade was about USD 40.5 billion a year and cost 164,000 premature deaths a year from 2030 onwards; this burden currently falls disproportionately on low- and middle-income countries.

Table 3. Cost adjusted to 2013 USD per DALY for different policies (Ranson et al. [26])

Policy options	Low- and middle-income countries	High-income countries including most western and northern European countries	World
Price increase of 10%: low-[a] to high-end estimates[b], USD	4–102	121–4,046	18–457
Publicly provided cessation support with NRT (0.5–2.5 effectiveness) low-[c] to high-end estimates[d], USD	408–1,270	1,095–10,521	523–2,799
Combination of other (non-price) effective measures (2–10% effectiveness) low-[e] to high-end estimates[f], USD	52–1,037	1,016–20,329	212–4,228

[a] Calculations based on: intervention cost of 0.005% of gross national product (GNP), high elasticity (–1.2 for low-/middle-income regions, –0.8 for high-income regions), benefits (DALYs saved) distributed over 30 years and discounted at 3%.

[b] Calculations based on: intervention cost of 0.02% of GNP, low elasticity (–0.4 for low/middle-income regions, –0.2 for high-income regions), benefits (DALYs saved) distributed over 30 years and discounted at 10%.

[c] Calculations based on: effectiveness of 2.5%, intervention cost of 0.005% of GNP (plus drug costs), benefits distributed over 30 years and discounted at 3%.

[d] Calculations based on: effectiveness of 0.5%, intervention cost of 0.02% of GNP (plus drug costs), benefits distributed over 30 years and discounted at 10%.

[e] Calculations based on: effectiveness of 10%, intervention cost of 0.005% of GNP and repeated annually over 30 years and discounted at 3%, benefits (DALYs saved) distributed over 30 years and discounted at 3%.

[f] Calculations based on: effectiveness of 2%, intervention cost of 0.02% of GNP and repeated annually over 50 years and discounted at 10%, benefits (DALYs saved) distributed over 50 years and discounted at 10%.

Cost-Effectiveness of Tobacco Control Measures

Many tobacco control policies cost very little. Tax increases can often be implemented simply by legislative action where there is effective tax administration. Ranson et al. [26] have estimated the cost-effectiveness of different tobacco control measures in terms of cost per DALY saved based on highly conservative assumptions of effectiveness and assuming maximum costs, and are therefore likely to understate cost-effective. Their estimates are adjusted to 2013 values in table 2.

Price increases, including administrative costs but excluding the increases in tax revenue, were found to be the most cost-effective form of tobacco control, particularly for low- and middle-income countries. In addition, there would be huge additional benefit to governments in terms of extra tax revenue, so that for governments, tax increases are not only cost-effective but highly cost saving. Even with deliberately conservative assumptions, tax increases that would raise the real price of cigarettes by 10% worldwide would prevent between 5 and 16 million tobacco-related deaths and could cost USD 3–70 per DALY saved in low- and middle-income regions. Nicotine replacement therapy (NRT) and a package of non-price interventions other than NRT are also cost-effective in low- and middle-income regions, at

USD 280–870 and 36–710 per DALY, respectively, as shown in table 3. In high-income countries, price increases were found to have a cost-effectiveness of USD 83–2,771 per DALY, NRT USD 750–7,206 DALY and other non-price interventions USD 696–13,924 per DALY.

Tobacco control policies, particularly tax increases on cigarettes, are cost-effective relative to other health interventions. The estimates are subject to considerable variation in actual settings, so local cost-effectiveness studies are required to guide local policy.

Hurley and Matthews [38] estimated that the Australian National Tobacco Campaign cost AUD 10 million and saved AUD 740.6 million in net health care costs alone, taking into consideration the later health care costs of survivors who would have died earlier, but not including their pension costs. The campaign was reported to be highly cost saving, paying for itself 70 times over. It was followed by a substantial reduction in mortality from heart disease from 1995 to 2006 of 42% and in cerebral vascular disease of 36%. Another Australian study [39] assessed the impact of televised anti-smoking advertising and other tobacco control policies on adult smoking prevalence over the years 1995–2006, reporting a 0.3% reduction in prevalence from weekly televised advertisements and a similar reduction for each 0.3% increase in price. There was no detectable effect of sales of

NRT or smoke-free restaurant laws. They concluded that their findings 'suggest that increased tobacco taxation, implementation of comprehensive smoke-free laws and broad reach mass media campaigns provided large and particularly rapid returns on investment'.

Mass Media Campaigns

Lawrence et al. [40] have recently stressed the importance of population-based approaches to smoking cessation using mass media campaigns, noting that these tend to be neglected, and so important tobacco control opportunities have been missed. Good mass media campaigns raise awareness and change attitudes about the risks of using tobacco and the benefits of quitting [41, 42]. They can be effective in preventing young people from starting to smoke and can increase cessation rates of both youth and adults, especially when combined with other interventions [43]. A youth-targeted anti-tobacco multimedia campaign in Norway reported that non-smoking youth in the intervention counties were less likely to start smoking than those in the control counties [41]. Forty years ago, Hamilton [44] reported for the US that the broadcasting of anti-smoking advertisements in 1968/1970 reduced cigarette smoking by 14% per year and was a much greater deterrent from smoking than advertising was an encouragement, and that this was clearly appreciated by the tobacco companies. Campaigns need to be sustained with appropriately targeted messages for the intended population [45]. Widespread media reporting of research findings showing the harmful effects of tobacco have been particularly effective where knowledge of the health consequences of tobacco use is low, as is often the case in emerging economies [25]. Media reporting was very effective in the 1960s in the USA and the UK [46] and may also be an important strategy for some European countries.

Advertising and Promotion Bans

Advertising bans were the very first tobacco control measures. The effects of bans are not easy to measure as their full effect may take place over many years. Three main types of analysis have been used: correlation of year-by-year fluctuations; cross-sectional comparisons between countries, and analyses of cigarette consumption before and after banned tobacco advertising. The latter present the most direct measure. The tobacco advertising ban in New Zealand [47] was estimated to have reduced consumption by 5.5%, in Canada

by 4% [48], Finland by 7% [49] and in Norway by 16% [50]. A cross-sectional study of 22 member countries of the Organisation for Economic Co-Operation and Development reported a significant effect of different levels of advertising restriction scored from 1 to 10, with each point associated with a 1.5% decrease in consumption [50]. A time series study suggested that a ban would reduce consumption by 7.5% [51]. On average, it is estimated that bans reduce smoking by some 7%.

A study by Saffer and Chaloupka [52] reported that partial bans have little or no effect on smoking, as the tobacco industry simply re-channels its marketing to other media. In Switzerland in1993, an initiative to ban all direct and indirect advertising of tobacco products was voted down by an unusually large majority because the tobacco industry enlisted the support and influence of other stakeholders, including media, sports industry and cultural activity planners, many of whom relied on tobacco advertising revenue [53].

Warning Labels

Warning labels on cigarette packs are recommended by the FCTC and are a requirement for EU countries. They have been shown to be effective in some cases. A study in the US reported that teenagers considered warning labels (not graphic) on cigarette packets 'uninformative and irrelevant' [54]. However, in Canada, 90% of surveyed smokers reported that they had noticed the highly graphic warning labels on cigarette packages, 43% had become more concerned about the health risks, and 44% felt more motivated to quit [12]. To increase the potential for effectiveness, it has been recommended that warning labels be prominent, placed on the largest surfaces (front and back) of the packages and be very distinct graphically from the rest of the package design [55]. Hammond [56], in a recent systematic review of 87 studies, concludes that health warning on packages are among the most direct and prominent means of communicating with smokers, a source of health information to both smokers and non-smokers, and that larger warnings with pictures that elicit strong emotional response are the most effective, including among the young, and may prevent smoking initiation.

Australia has recently passed laws requiring plain packaging of cigarettes, as the pack 'has been used for years to generate luxury, freedom, glamour, status, masculinity, femininity, and false comfort about health effects' [57]. Cases against it are in progress with the World Trade Organisation via three countries. Uruguay is also facing law suits. New Zealand and the UK are considering bills for plain packaging, as is the Indian Health Ministry.

Smoke-Free Environments

An early systematic review of interventions for preventing smoking in public places concluded that such restrictions in workplaces reduced the prevalence of smoking by almost 4% [58] and may yield reductions of up to 10% [59, 60]. In a more recent review of 37 studies of smoke-free policies in worksites or communities from 1976 to 2005, 21 reported reduced prevalence of 3.4% (1.4–6.3) and a further 11 studies reported increased cessation of 6.4% (1.3–7.9) [43]. Four of the studies demonstrated economic benefits. However, a time series analysis of 21 countries or states, which had implemented comprehensive smoke-free legislation, reported that the legislation had increased the rate at which prevalence was declining in some locations, but in the majority had no measurable impact on existing trends [61]. Other countries have reported reductions in heart disease deaths following smoke-free legislation, and this legislation is generally considered to be highly successful.

Cessation Support

Physician advice to patients to quit smoking has long been demonstrated to be among the most cost-effective interventions [62] (see also chapter 20) compared to other common secondary prevention, including drug therapies for hypertension and high blood cholesterol [63]. Individual counselling by a cessation specialist and group therapy have also been shown to be effective [64].

A comparative cost-effective modelling study estimated the incremental cost per quality-adjusted life year of various cessation interventions over and above the non-intervention control rate of quitting (see also chapters 18–20). Brief opportunistic advice from a general practitioner with telephone or self-help material (A) was the most cost-effective, next was opportunistic advice alone from a general practitioner or hospital nurse (B), and, lastly, opportunistic advice plus NRT (C) was still cost-effective but at four times the cost of B and eight times the cost of A [65]. The more effective methods, being relatively expensive, are not the more cost-effective and there is debate as to whether NRT works at a population level. Another UK study of NRT use for smoking reduction or temporary abstinence concluded that

the use of NRT for smoking reduction does not appear to be associated with lower cigarette consumption relative to smoking reduction without NRT [66].

A particularly important area for cessation relates to pregnant women. Smoking during pregnancy increases the risk of miscarriage, premature birth, low birth weight, still birth and sudden infant death syndrome [67] in addition to the usual smoking risks. It is estimated that it costs the British National Health Service GBP 20–87.5 million per year to treat mothers and infants under a year old with problems caused by smoking in pregnancy. Interventions to assess pregnant women, and advice and referral for cessation are particularly important. A UK study estimated that spending GBP 14–37 per pregnant smoker on low-cost smoking cessation interventions would be cost saving [68]. Smoking by pregnant women in the UK is now at its lowest level on record.

Youth and Tobacco Control

Smoking by youth is reducing in some countries, but increasing elsewhere. Most smokers start smoking as adolescents, with a peak at the age of 15 years in Europe, and the initiation age is rapidly reducing. It may therefore seem obvious to aim tobacco control measures directly and specifically to them (see also chapter 14). Policies directed specifically at youth include school education and health promotion, and age restrictions and access; school health education has resulted in a high level of awareness of the risks of smoking and has influenced children's attitudes, and undoubtedly is essential (see chapter 14). However, evaluations have failed to show an effect of information on adolescents' decisions to start smoking, although there is some evidence that it may delay uptake. Anti-smoking programmes for youth are consistently evaluated as less effective than programmes to adults, due also to the long-term consequences of smoking, to which youth do not easily relate. It is known that young people are most likely to smoke if their parents smoke or if their parents have a liberal attitude towards their smoking. Many adolescent smokers, in particular, underestimate their risk of addiction to nicotine.

There is evidence that multimedia campaigns can prevent young people from starting, and persuade them and adult smokers to stop [69]. Müller-Riemenschneider et al. [70] reported the results of a literature review of 33 studies on behavioural interventions to prevent smoking in children and youth. They reported some evidence for the effect of community-based and multi-sectoral interventions but not for school-based programmes. Restrictions on youth access have generally been reported as non-effective and difficult to implement, although a study in England, where there was a rise in the legal age of sale from 16 to 18 years in 2007, reported a relative fall in prevalence of 4.7% (odds ratio 1.36, p = 0.024) in 16/17-year-olds [71].

Hublet et al. [72] report for 29 European countries using data for 2005/2006 that boys but not girls smoked less where there were restrictions on vending machines (odds ratio 0.7, p = 0.2) or a price policy (odds ratio 0.97, p = 0.05). Many studies have confirmed the effects of price rises in reducing youth smoking; Kostava et al. [73] conclude that cigarette prices are very important to adolescent smoking with a total price elasticity of cigarette demand of –2.11. Emery et al. [74], looking at whether young people's decision to experiment with cigarettes was influenced by price, concluded that it was not, as they were typically 'given' cigarettes at this early experimental stage. They reported that price was important for more established smoking behaviour, and so may reduce progress to established smoking. In the Public Health Research Consortium systematic review of 45 studies of adolescent smoking, price increases do appear to reduce smoking participation, prevalence, level of smoking, increases in quit rates and smoking initiation [68]. 'Price increases are 2–3 times more effective in reducing tobacco use among young people than among older adults', says Dr. Douglas Bettcher, Director of the Department for Prevention of Non-Communicable Diseases at WHO. 'Tax policy can be divisive, but this is the tax rise everyone can support. As tobacco taxes go up, death and disease go down.' Chaloupka demonstrates that price does have a clear negative effect on the prevalence of smoking amongst youth in the US [75].

In conclusion, it seems clear that the most effective means of reducing youth smoking is to reduce adult smoking, via the mechanism of price increases, smoke-free policies and of good well-directed multimedia programmes.

Smoking and Poverty, Inequalities and Smoking by Socio-Economic Group

Smoking prevalence tends to be highest among adults of poor socio-economic circumstances (see chapters 16 and 18). The decline in smoking in many western European countries over the last decades has been lowest amongst low-income smokers [76, 77]. Smoking is one of the major causes of inequalities in health and mortality in many countries, being particularly high amongst those in lower socio-economic groups, unemployed and lone parents [78, 79].

Adults in families with low incomes tend to have the highest smoking rates in both high- and low-income countries. They suffer the highest morbidity and mortality from lung cancer and heart disease and high sickness absence, and they spend a disproportionately large share of their income on tobacco. Smoking, therefore, not only directly harms their health, but also decreases resources available to them more generally for food, education and health care [16].

It has been shown in the UK, that whereas smokers from all socio-economic groups are equally likely to try to quit smoking, those in higher grades (professional and managerial) are twice as likely to be successful as those in the lowest groups (unskilled manual workers) (see chapters 16 and 18). The triggers for trying to quit differ, with those in higher grades being concerned about future health, and those of lower grades more concerned about cost and present health problems [80], suggesting that smoking cessation programmes need to be tailored and targeted differentially. There is evidence that pregnant women are more likely to be smokers if they are of lower socio-economic status or of low educational attainment.

There is concern that tobacco tax is regressive and this is stressed by the tobacco industry in their arguments to governments to reduce taxes. This is a complex issue, as increases in tax are also the most effective means by which poorer people are released from addiction to smoking, and the heavy risk of poor health and premature death. Studies from the US and the UK have shown that on average tobacco tax increases are in fact progressive as poor smokers are most likely to reduce their smoking or quit in response to price rises [81, 82] and so on average reduce their tax spend. However, for those who do continue to smoke and do not cut down, the tax they pay will increase with tax increases. It is important that this is addressed so that poor smokers in particular are offered good cessation support and targeted social welfare, and services, education and health programmes need to be used to offset any regressivity. There is evidence of widespread popular support for tobacco tax revenues to go towards such costs. Poor smokers are more likely to use fine-cut tobacco for roll-your-own and discounted cigarette brands. Effective tobacco tax structures and policy, including equal taxation on all tobacco products, can be useful in nudging low-income smokers to quit, and need to be supported by the provision of good cessation support and mass media campaigns to reduce health inequalities.

Electronic Cigarettes

The increased use of e-cigarettes, which provide inhalation of nicotine without the other dangerous ingredients of tobacco, needs to be watched, and if there is a significant switch by cigarette smokers to these products, there may be a resultant major reduction in harm. There are concerns that the industry is using e-cigarettes and advertising to re-normalise smoking (see chapter 23).

Conclusions

Smoking takes a huge toll of life and health globally. In addition, it costs economies heavily in terms of health care costs, reduced productivity and fires caused by smoking. Effective tobacco control measures have reduced tobacco use in some (particularly in higher-income) countries, but the overall level of smoking is still high and the death rate from smoking appalling. Tobacco control measures, especially good tax measures, mass media programmes, smoke-free policies, advertisement and promotion bans, and well-run smoking cessation support have been shown to be cost-effective and in many cases cost saving. Smoking cessation is central to reduce smoking and for countries to reap the economic benefits. Some countries are aiming for an 'endgame' to apply tobacco control policies to reduce cigarette use to negligible levels by a given date and to create a tobacco-free generation.

The huge price discrepancy between countries with different taxation levels is a major problem. Low prices keep smoking levels and deaths high and deprive governments of tax revenue, as well as cause problems of cross-border cheap trade. There is an urgent need for taxes to be raised, to be predominantly specific, or a high minimum, with equivalent taxes on all products, and these should be increased annually at least in line with and preferably above inflation and income levels. This policy would provide governments with more tax revenue, reduce smoking, lower health and productivity costs, and reduce inequalities in health and youth smoking. A portion of the tax revenue should be made available for tobacco control purposes, particularly cessation support.

There are still huge gaps between countries in the levels of other tobacco control measures; most countries fail to use good mass media campaigns, and many lack adequate bans on advertising, smoke-free policies, warnings on packs or cessation programmes.

Smoking by youth is decreasing in some countries, but is increasing elsewhere. There are two important issues here: to protect children from taking up smoking and to protect them from others' smoke. The evidence is clear that initiation is most affected by reducing adult smoking, by increasing mass media campaigns and by reducing advertising and promotions. To protect them from others' smoke, full smoke-free policies are required. In parts of the world, smoking by women is still very low, but tobacco companies see them and young people as promising potential markets to be exploited; action needs to be taken to prevent these developments.

Tobacco companies, particularly TTCs, have pernicious influence in presenting misinformation to governments to undermine tobacco control and to keep taxes low. There is good evidence that direct foreign investment by TTCs has resulted in increased advertising, low taxes, holding back other tobacco control measures and serious misinformation to governments, at the cost of the health of the recipient countries. Evidence-based policies to reduce smoking and its harm are in place in many countries, but are frequently hampered by inadequate government action and the hostile influence of TTCs including foreign investment. Addressing these with serious action across the world will save lives and strengthen economies.

Key Points

- The six largest tobacco companies have an annual turnover of USD 350 billion and profits of USD 35 billion.
- Evidence-based tobacco control policies are highly cost-effective and more cost-effective than most medical and surgical treatments.
- A 10% price rise via a tax increase is estimated to be the most cost-effective at USD 18–457 per disability-adjusted life year (2013 prices) plus substantial tax revenue benefits.
- Raising cigarette prices by 10% would save 10 million smoking-attributable deaths globally in the long run.
- Price differences account for much of the difference in countries' smoking rates, which tend to be highest where prices are lowest.
- Evidence-based policies to reduce smoking and its harm are frequently hampered by inadequate government action and the hostile influence of the transnational tobacco companies including foreign investment.

References

1 Townsend J: Smoking and lung cancer: a cohort data study of men and women in England and Wales 1935–70. J R Stat Soc A 1978;141:95–107.

2 Doll R, Hill AB: Lung cancer and other causes of death in relation to smoking. Br Med J 1956;ii:1071–1081.

3 Wynder E, Hultberg S, Jacobson F, et al: Environmental factors in cancers of the upper alimentary tract. Cancer 1957;10:470–487.

4 Hammond E: Smoking in relation to the death rates of one million men and women. Natl Cancer Inst Monogr 1966;19:127–204.

5 Kahn H: The Dorn study of smoking and mortality among U.S. veterans: report on eight and one-half years of observation. Natl Cancer Inst Monogr 1966;19:1–125.

6 World Health Organization: Smoking Statistics. Geneva, WHO, 2011.

7 Huber GL, Pandina RJ: The economics of tobacco use; in Bolliger CT, Fagerström KO (eds): The Tobacco Epidemic. Prog Respir Res. Basel, Karger, 1997, vol 28, pp 12–63.

8 Eriksen M, Mackay J, Ross H: Tobacco Atlas. Atlanta, American Cancer Society/New York, World Lung Foundation, 2012.

9 Shirane R, Smith K, Ross H, et al: Tobacco industry manipulation of tobacco excise and tobacco advertising policies in the Czech Republic: an analysis of tobacco industry documents. PLoS Med 2012;9:e1001248.

10 Lo CF: FCTC guidelines on tobacco industry foreign investment would strengthen controls on tobacco supply and close loopholes in the tobacco treaty. Tob Control 2010;19:306–310.

11 Goel RK, Nelson MA: Global Efforts to Combat Smoking: An Economic Evaluation of Smoking Control Policies. Aldershot, Ashgate, 2008.

12 Shafey O, Eriksen M, Ross H, Mackay J: Tobacco Atlas. Atlanta, American Cancer Society, 2009, p 42.

13 Gibson GJ, Loddenkemper R, Sibille Y, Lundbäck B: The European Lung White Book. Sheffield, European Respiratory Society, 2013, p 24.

14 Public Health Research Consortium Report: Tobacco Control, Inequalities in Health and Action at the Local Level in England. Final Report. York, York University, 2011.

15 Viscusi WK, Hersch J: The mortality cost to smokers. J Health Econ 2008;27:943–958.

16 Efroymson D, Ahmed S, Townsend J, Alam SM, Dey AR, Saha R, Dhar B, Sujon AI, Ahmed KU, Rahman O: Hungry for tobacco: an analysis of the economic impact of tobacco consumption on the poor in Bangladesh. Tob Control 2001;10:212–217.

17 World Health Organization: WHO Report on the Global Tobacco Epidemic, 2008: The MPOWER Package. Geneva, WHO, 2008.

18 World Health Organization: Framework Convention on Tobacco Control. Geneva, WHO, 2005.

19 Townsend J: Price and consumption of tobacco. Br Med Bull 1996;52:132–142.

20 Warner K, Chaloupka F, Cook P, Manning W, Joseph P, Townsend J: Criteria for determining an optimal cigarette tax: an economist's perspective. Tob Control 1998;4:380–386.

21 Currie L, Townsend J, Leon Roux M, Godfrey F, et al: Policy Recommendations for Tobacco Taxation in the European Union: Integrated Research Findings from the PPACTE Project. Dublin, the PPACTE Consortium, 2012.

22 Hanson JD, Kysar DA: Joint failure of economic theory and legal regulation; in Slovic P (ed): Smoking, Risk, Perception and Policy. Thousand Oaks, Sage, 2001, p 27.

23 Townsend J: Tobacco Price and the Smoking Epidemic, Smoke-Free Europe 9. Copenhagen, WHO, 1997.

24 Gallus S, Fernandez E, Townsend J, et al: Price and consumption of tobacco in Italy over the last three decades. Eur J Cancer Prev 2003;12:333–337.

25 Jha P, Chaloupka FJ: Curbing the Epidemic: Governments and the Economics of Tobacco Control. Washington, World Bank, 1999.

26 Ranson MK, Jha P, Chaloupka FJ, Nguyen SN: Global and regional estimates of the effectiveness and cost-effectiveness of price increases and other tobacco control policies. Nicotine Tob Res 2002; 43:311–319.

27 Poland Ministry of Finance : Demand for Cigarettes in Poland, 2008.

28 Buck D, Godfrey C, Raw M, Sutton M: Tobacco and Jobs. Society for the Study of Addiction and the Centre for Health Economics. York, University of York, 1995.

29 US Department of Health and Human Services: Women and Smoking: A Report of the Surgeon General. Atlanta, US Department of Health and Human Services, Public Health Service, Center for Disease Control and Prevention, National Center for Chronic Disease Prevention and Health Promotion, Office of Smoking and Health, 2001.

30 Townsend JL, Roderick P, Cooper J: Cigarette smoking by socio-economic group, sex, and age: effects of price, income, and health publicity. Br Med J 1994;309:923–926.

31 Huxley RR, Woodward M: Cigarette smoking as a risk factor for coronary heart disease in women compared with men: a systematic review and meta-analysis of prospective cohort studies. Lancet 2011;378:1297–1305.

32 Lewit EM, Coate D, Grossman M: The effects of government regulation on teenage smoking. J Law Econ 1981;24:545–569.

33 Grossman M, Chaloupka FJ: Cigarette taxes. The straw to break the camel's back. Public Health Rep 1997;112:290–297.

34 Merriman D, Yurekli A, Chaloupka F: How big is the worldwide cigarette-smuggling problem? in Jha P, Chaloupka F (eds): Tobacco Control in Developing Countries. Oxford, Oxford University Press, 2000.

35 Joosens L, Chaloupka FJ, Merriman D: Issues in the smuggling of tobacco products; in Jha P, Chaloupka F (eds): Tobacco Control in Developing Countries. Oxford, Oxford University Press, 2000.

36 West R, Townsend J, Joossens L, Arnott D, Lewis S: Why combating tobacco smuggling is a priority. BMJ 2018;337:a1933.

37 Joossens L, Merriman D, Ross H, Raw M: The impact of eliminating the global illicit cigarette trade on health and revenue. Addiction 2010;105:1640–1649.

38 Hurley S, Matthews J: Cost-effectiveness of the Australian National Tobacco Campaign. Tob Control 2009;17:375–384.

39 Wakefield MA, Durkin S, Spittal MJ, et al: Impact of tobacco control policies and mass media campaigns on monthly adult smoking prevalence. Am J Public Health 2008;98:1443–1450.

40 Lawrence D, Mitrou F, Zubrick R: Global research neglect of population-based approaches to smoking cessation: time for a more rigorous science of population health interventions. Addiction 2011; 106:1349–1354.

41 WHO: Regional Office for Europe's Health Evidence Network (HEN). Which are the most effective and cost-effective interventions for tobacco control? Geneva, WHO, 2003.

42 Flay BR: Mass media and smoking cessation: a critical review. Am J Public Health 1987;77:153–160.

43 Hopkins DP, Razi S, Leeks KD, Priya Kalra G, Chattopadhyay SK, Soler RE; Task Force on Community Preventive Services: Smoke-free policies to reduce tobacco use. A systematic review. Am J Prev Med 2010;38(2 suppl):S275–S289.

44 Hamilton JL: The demand for cigarettes: advertising, the health scare and the cigarette advertising ban. Rev Econ Stat 1972;54:401–410.

45 Lantz PM, Jacobson PD, Warner KE, et al: Investing in youth tobacco control: a review of smoking prevention and control strategies. Tob Control 2000;9:47–63.

46 Atkinson AB, Skegg JL: Anti-smoking publicity and the demand for tobacco in the UK. Manchester Sch Econ Soc Stud 1973;41:265–282.

47 Toxic Substances Board: Health or Tobacco? Summary and Recommendations. An End to Tobacco Advertising and Promotion. Wellington, Department of Health, 1989.

48 Department of Health Economics and Operational Research Division: Effect of Tobacco Advertising on Tobacco Consumption. London, Department of Health, 1992.

49 Pekurinen M: The demand for tobacco products in Finland. Br J Addict 1989;84:1183–1192.

50 Laugeson M, Meads C: Tobacco advertising restrictions, price, income and tobacco consumption in OECD countries. 1960–1986. Br J Addict 1991;86:1343–1354.

51 McGuiness T, Cowling K: Advertising and the aggregate demand for cigarettes. Eur Econ Rev 1975;6:311–328.

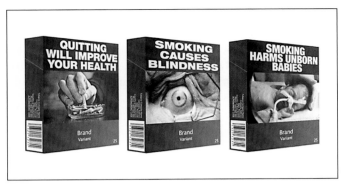

Fig. 8. Examples of plain cigarette packaging in Australia (Australian Government Department of Health and Aging, 2012).

those who smoked branded packs, smokers who used plain packs believed their cigarettes to be of lower quality, were more likely to think about quitting every day, rated quitting as a higher priority in their lives and found their cigarettes less satisfying than the year before [29]. Other observed behavioural changes included hiding cigarette packs in social situations, smoking less around others, smoking fewer cigarettes overall and a 78% increase in calls to Quitline, the national cessation service. Furthermore, cigarette sales in supermarkets, which make up a significant share of the market, have declined by nearly 1% in 2013 [30] while volume sales for all smoking tobacco are forecasted to decline by 1% annually [31]. The only data that indicate plain packaging does not curb tobacco use are data compiled by the tobacco industry. A study funded by Philip Morris claims that the plain packaging law has not led to a decline in smoking among 14- to 17-year-old teens and that tobacco sales rose marginally in 2013 [32]. It may take years to see clear, indisputable outcomes from the plain packaging laws, but the early studies not funded by the industry show positive indicators.

India

India, the biggest movie producer in the world, enacted strict requirements in 2011 and 2012 around portraying tobacco use in movies or on TV. Any movie or TV programme showing tobacco use must display a fixed, noticeable anti-tobacco message during such scenes in addition to 30-second anti-tobacco ads at the beginning and in the middle of the show. New films and TV programmes must also include tobacco warnings at the beginning and in the middle in addition to justifying their portrayal of tobacco use. Brand names and product placement are prohibited, and any promotional materials for new films and TV programmes can-

not show tobacco use. Cinema owners and managers, and TV broadcasters are held responsible for the execution of these regulations and can be hit with penalties such as suspension or cancellation of licenses should they not comply [9].

Challenges from the Tobacco Industry

Despite – and partly due to – the tremendous gains in tobacco control legislation around the globe, there is one constant, ever-adapting challenge to progress: the tobacco industry. Particularly in countries where tobacco control is still beginning to develop, the industry fights, delays and evades legislation; uses their considerable monetary and political sway, and improves their image under the guise of Corporate Social Responsibility (CSR) [10].

Circumventing the Law
The tobacco industry spends its time and considerable resources working around the legislation countries put in place. For example, when a country enacts only a partial TAPS ban, the tobacco industry will then alter its focus to areas not covered in the legislation, such as point-of-sale advertising, discounts, coupons and product placement. Tobacco companies spent over USD 8 billion on these forms of marketing in the United States in just 1 year [14]. Even with comprehensive TAPS bans, tobacco companies can spend money on brand-stretching activities or new media, such as the Internet and social media, which have yet to be as heavily regulated.

Tobacco companies also attempt to circumvent TAPS bans by engaging in CSR, which is a form of advertising and promotion but is not always included in bans. Through CSR, tobacco companies are able to raise their profile and appear to positively contribute to society, even if their contribution to charity is marginal. They also run youth smoking prevention programmes that are not in fact intended to prevent youth from smoking [14].

Tobacco Control Interference
Over the past couple of decades, the tobacco industry has increasingly fought tobacco control. Tobacco companies spent over USD 16 million and employed 168 lobbyists in 2010 to pressure US political decisions [14]. In Europe, 9 tobacco companies, 22 lobbying groups, and 12 additional public relation and lobbying firms were active and spending over EUR 5.3 million in 2011 in Brussels, the capital of the European Union, according to the voluntary Transpar-

ency Register. However, because this Register is not mandatory, more organisations and funds are being used to influence European policy than are recorded [33] (for more details see chapter 3). Around the world, these companies are interfering with tobacco control legislation in countries through legal challenges, which threaten and delay implementation and are costly to defend. The tobacco industry currently focuses on packaging, labelling and TAPS, trying to weaken and defer enactment [34].

A prominent example is the plain packaging laws in Australia. After the legislation was passed, legal challenges to the law began within hours [35]. The High Court of Australia was presented with two cases of tobacco companies suing the Commonwealth of Australia, and in both cases the High Court ruled in favour of Australia. Philip Morris Asia brought a case against Australia over the *Agreement between the Government of Australia and the Government of Hong Kong for the Promotion and Protection of Investments*, which is still pending. The industry asserts that plain packaging infringes on their intellectual property rights and that Australia is impairing their investments in the country. They use scare tactics such as claiming that illicit trade and organised crime will increase [14]. Plain packaging scares the tobacco industry because it eliminates the power of branding, and they are doing everything in their power to resist the Australian legislation while the rest of the world – including countries considering enacting similar legislation – looks on.

Government Resistance
Article 5.3 of the WHO FCTC instructs countries that, 'In setting and implementing their public health policies with respect to tobacco control, Parties shall act to protect these policies from commercial and other vested interests of the tobacco industry in accordance with national law' [7]. However, given the sizeable resources available to the tobacco industry – the top six tobacco brands reported revenues over USD 346 billion in 2010 (for details see chapter 11) – countries must work particularly hard to resist their challenges [14]. A robust tobacco control programme is one of the best ways to resist interference, but governments must go further than the MPOWER measures in order to successfully defend against the tobacco industry.

There are different ways governments can resist industry interference. One pathway is setting up barriers between the industry and public officials to avoid conflicts of interest. A code of conduct can be established that outlines how members of the government may or may not deal with tobacco companies or those with vested interest in tobacco [9]. Legislation directly forbidding interference can be passed; for example, New South Wales in Australia passed legislation in 2010 banning political donations from tobacco companies. Political will is imperative in fighting the tobacco industry and protecting public health, and governments must rid themselves of interference in order to fight successfully.

Supply-Side Gap

Status of Supply-Side Interventions
The WHO FCTC lays out provisions to address demand- and supply-side tobacco control strategies. While demand-side interventions, such as warning labels, cessation assistance and TAPS bans, are frequently incorporated into tobacco control programmes, there is a gap regarding supply-side interventions. Most countries prohibit sales to minors, but do not go much further in looking at ways to curb the supply of tobacco from the general public. The WHO FCTC contains an Article ensuring the 'provision of support for economically viable alternative activities' for tobacco growers, but only 17 Parties reported establishing programmes that encourage viable alternatives [18]. There are a few reasons why demand-side interventions are far more commonplace than supply-side ones.

Supply-side strategies are popular in other public health strategies, but have not been as accepted by those working on tobacco control [36]. This is partly because while there is policy consensus on what works in reducing the demand for tobacco products, there is not the same agreement on supply-side measures. Some actors, such as the World Bank, believe that reducing supply is less promising than reducing demand because of the way economics works: when one supplier shuts down, other suppliers are then motivated to fill the gap in the market [37]. Furthermore, the research community which often provides the evidence base for tobacco control measures has chosen to focus more on smokers and cigarettes than on the supply of tobacco [34].

A large part of the problem is that governments put tobacco in the hands of companies and chose to allow them to supply cigarettes. Although some of these companies are owned or run by government, they are companies which aim for profit and not health. Governments establish how tobacco companies are governed and what legal rights they have; in high-income countries, this usually includes the right to maximise profits and be accountable only to shareholders [18]. If governments want to get serious about reducing the supply of tobacco items, they should reconsider the role they allow tobacco companies to have.

Chapter 13

Loddenkemper R, Kreuter M (eds): The Tobacco Epidemic, ed 2, rev. and ext.
Prog Respir Res. Basel, Karger, 2015, vol 42, pp 149–157 (DOI: 10.1159/000369441)

The WHO Framework Convention on Tobacco Control

Martina Pötschke-Langer[a] · Kerstin Schotte[b] · Tibor Szilagyi[c]

[a]German Cancer Research Center, Heidelberg, Germany; [b]World Health Organization and [c]Convention Secretariat,
WHO Framework Convention on Tobacco Control, Geneva, Switzerland

Tobacco is the biggest killer [1]
We need an international response
to an international problem [2]
Gro Harlem Brundtland
Former WHO Director-General

We must act now to reverse
the global tobacco epidemic
and save millions of lives [3]
Margaret Chan
WHO Director-General

Abstract

Tobacco is among the major preventable causes of death in the world today. The World Health Organization (WHO) estimates that tobacco kills about 6 million people yearly. The tobacco epidemic is devastating but preventable by strong political measures. This was the reason why in 1996 the World Health Assembly requested WHO to initiate the first treaty negotiated under the auspices of WHO in history: the WHO Framework Convention on Tobacco Control (WHO FCTC). In 2005, this Convention entered into force and changed the landscape of public health. Health was no longer the task of national health ministries, but also of the ministries of finance, economy, environment, consumer protection and many others. The WHO FCTC presents a blueprint for governments to reduce both the supply and the demand for tobacco. To support the Parties to the Convention to implement the WHO FCTC, guidelines on several articles have already been developed by the Parties and adopted by the Conference of the Parties, with others to follow. There is no doubt: the WHO FCTC is one of the most widely embraced treaties in the history of the United Nations, with 180 Parties involved (as of 15 January 2015), and many of them are implementing the WHO FCTC consistently. This success demonstrates sustained global political will to strengthen tobacco control and to reduce tobacco consumption.

© 2015 S. Karger AG, Basel

The World Health Organization Framework Convention on Tobacco Control (WHO FCTC) [4] is the first treaty negotiated under the auspices of WHO and a response to the globalization of the tobacco epidemic (see chapter 2). Since the establishment of WHO in 1948, its objective is 'the attainment by all peoples of the highest possible level of health' and Article 19 of its constitution gives the World Health Assembly (WHA), the WHO's governing body, the authority to adopt conventions with respect to any matter within the competence of WHO [5].

Two main reasons were responsible for using the instrument of a convention: First, the tobacco epidemic is a global public health threat with continuously increasing consumption of cigarettes and other tobacco products resulting in a raising avoidable tobacco-related death toll. The end of this epidemic is not yet in sight. Second, there was sufficient evidence that in most instances policy measures could stop this epidemic and could lead to a decline in tobacco use and related morbidity and mortality (see chapter 12). Only a convention was the appropriate means to establish mandatory measures for all member states, since previously developed and implemented recommendations and voluntary action plans were not effective enough.

The idea of using WHO's constitutional authority to develop an international regulatory mechanism for tobacco control first appeared in a report prepared by the WHO Expert Committee on Smoking Control in 1979 [6]. An article on the feasibility of such an international framework further explored this idea in 1989 [7]. A couple of years later, a successful process in setting up the agenda for the development of an international legal approach was conceptualized in the 1990s when US-based lawyers Ruth Roemer and Allyn Taylor [8] developed concrete proposals and worked together with the WHO Public Health Consultant Judith Mackay to eventually introduce a resolution during the 9th World Conference on Tobacco or Health held in Paris in 1994 'to achieve an International Convention on Tobacco Control adopted by the United Nations'.

Developing the Agenda of the WHO Framework Convention on Tobacco Control

It was an enormous effort of political will, creative work on policies and sustainable funding by many donors to finally establish an agenda for the convention [9]. Thanks to a careful conceptualization of an international legal approach and thanks to the Paris Resolution of the 9th World Conference on Tobacco or Health, the WHA requested the WHO Director-General in 1996 to initiate the preparation of the WHO FCTC. After her election as Director-General in 1998, Gro Harlem Brundtland made tobacco control one of her top priorities, created the WHO Tobacco Free Initiative (TFI) and started the preparations for the negotiations. In 1999, the WHA established an Intergovernmental Negotiating Body (INB) to draft and negotiate the convention and created a Technical Working Group open to all Member States to prepare for INB. Within only a few months, the Working Group presented a provisional text of potential parts of the WHO FCTC. The text elements were accepted by the WHA in 2000 to serve as a sound basis for initiating negotiations so that the first INB session could be realized in October 2000. During nearly 3 years, six sessions of negotiations were held in Geneva until the final WHO FCTC text was unanimously adopted by the WHA during its 56th Assembly on May 21, 2003. On June 16, the Convention was opened for signature and on the first day, 28 Member States and the European Union signed. By the end of the signing period 1 year later, 168 Member States had signed. The requirements for entry into force were met with the de-

posit of ratification, acceptance, approval, formal confirmation or accession by 40 Member States. And finally, 90 days after the deposition of the 40th instrument, the WHO FCTC entered into force on February 27, 2005 (fig. 1).

Pivotal Elements of the Successful Negotiations

The first pivotal element was a strong leadership of Gro Harlem Brundtland who launched the TFI with Derek Yach as first Director, who steered the process and was followed by Vera da Costa e Silva, Yumiko Mochizuki and Douglas Bettcher, who became the TFI Directors in the years to come. Brundtland's goals were clearly expressed: 'to build a "vibrant alliance" between WHO, UNICEF, the World Bank, and "Partnership with a purpose" with nongovernmental organizations, the private sector, academic/research institutions and donors' [1]. These alliances were extremely successful (fig. 2).

The second pivotal element was the World Bank Report in 1999 (Curbing the Epidemic: Governments and the Economics of Tobacco Control [10]). It concluded that successful tobacco control brings unprecedented health benefits without harming national economies. WHO used this report to provide the economic justification for the WHO FCTC and to counter economic arguments made by the tobacco industry (see also chapters 3 and 11). The controversy for the truth of science started before and during the negotiations and continues until today [11].

Third, the strong nongovernmental community including distinguished academics and researchers united under the umbrella of the Framework Convention Alliance (FCA) played a substantial role in pushing the negotiations forward and in countering permanent attempts by the tobacco industry to interfere with the WHO FCTC process. FCA was formed in 2000 when British-based Action on Smoking and Health mobilized tobacco control civil society around the world for the support of a strong WHO FCTC. During the negotiations in INBs, FCA produced a daily newsletter, The Alliance Bulletin, for Member State delegates, which provided them with basic information on the negotiated subject. The Alliance Bulletin became a main source of information for many delegates, especially in small delegations. It praised positive contributions and also used the tactic of shaming to influence country delegates and bluntly denounced the tobacco industry's efforts to influence delegates. FCA assigned two awards daily: the *Orchid Award* for recognizing leadership in the negotiations for a strong WHO FCTC and the *Dirty Ashtray Award* for attempts try-

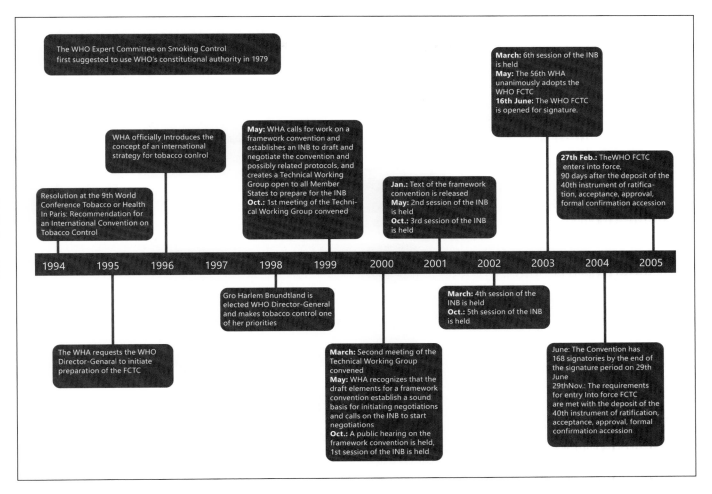

Fig. 1. The process of realization of the WHO FCTC.

ing to undermine it. Finally, FCA used a *death clock*, a large digital counter that displayed the number of worldwide tobacco-related deaths since the beginning of the negotiations, located at the entrance to the plenary sessions [12].

Continuing the Momentum: New International Instruments and Support to National Implementation

When the treaty had entered into force in 2005, the main task was beforehand: the Parties' complete implementation of all its requirements.

The translation from theory (articles of the WHO FCTC) into practice (full implementation) has been a challenge. As governing body for the Convention, the Conference of the Parties (COP) was formed. It provides guidance for the implementation and establishes the administrative and politi-

cal structures necessary for the Convention to achieve its goals. COP comprises all Parties to the WHO FCTC. Prepared by two sessions of an Intergovernmental Working Group in 2004 and 2005, the first COP session (COP1) took place in Geneva in 2006. Parties elected a Bureau of COP with six members, one representative from each WHO region. The Bureau elects its President from among its members. COP1 established a Convention Secretariat based at the WHO Headquarter in Geneva. The Secretariat supports the work of the Conference of the Parties and its subsidiary bodies, including the preparation of COP sessions, supports Parties in their implementation of WHO FCTC, coordinates the development of guidelines and elaborates global progress reports on the implementation of the Convention. COP1 adopted procedural and financial rules for COP and the Convention Secretariat. In summer 2007, Dr. Haik Nikogosian, former Health Minister of Armenia, was ap-

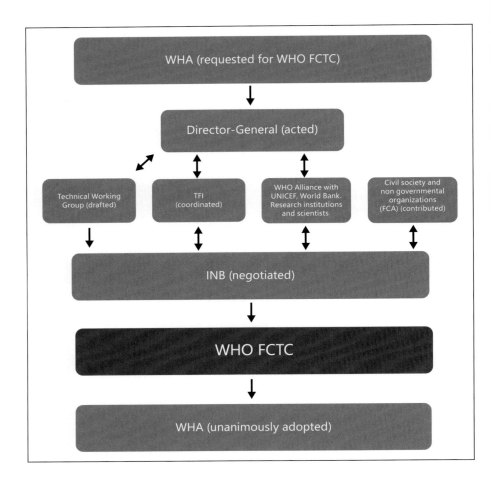

Fig. 2. The making of the WHO FCTC.

pointed as first head of the Convention Secretariat by the WHO Director-General [13].

During COP2 in Bangkok, Thailand, in 2007, Parties to the Convention decided to establish an INB to develop the first protocol to the convention, focusing on eliminating illicit trade in tobacco products. COP2 also adopted guidelines for the implementation of Article 8 (Protection from exposure to tobacco smoke) and decided to call for the elaboration of further guidelines in accordance with Article 7 of the treaty (Non-price measures to reduce the demand for tobacco).

COP3 took place in Durban, South Africa, in 2008, where Parties to the Convention adopted three other guidelines for implementation: on Article 5.3 (Protection of public health policies with respect to tobacco control from commercial and other vested interests of the tobacco industry), Article 11 (Packaging and labelling of tobacco products) and Article 13 (Tobacco advertising, promotion and sponsorship).

COP4 was conducted in Punta del Este, Uruguay, in 2010, where the Parties to the Convention adopted guidelines for the implementation of Article 12 (Education, communication, training and public awareness), Article 14 (Demand reduction measures concerning tobacco dependence and cessation) and partial guidelines for implementation of Articles 9 (Regulation of the contents of tobacco products) and 10 (Regulation of tobacco product disclosures).

COP5 took place in Seoul, Republic of Korea, in 2012, where the Parties to the Convention adopted the Protocol to Eliminate Illicit Trade in Tobacco Products, following the negotiations that took place in Geneva between 2008 and 2012. COP5 also adopted a set of guiding principles and recommendations to support the implementation of Article 6 on price and tax measures to reduce the demand for tobacco, and established an open-ended intercessional drafting group to finalize the full guidelines in this area for consideration at COP6. The Conference also amended the partial guidelines on Articles 9 and 10, requesting the Working Group to continue its work, and established a process for

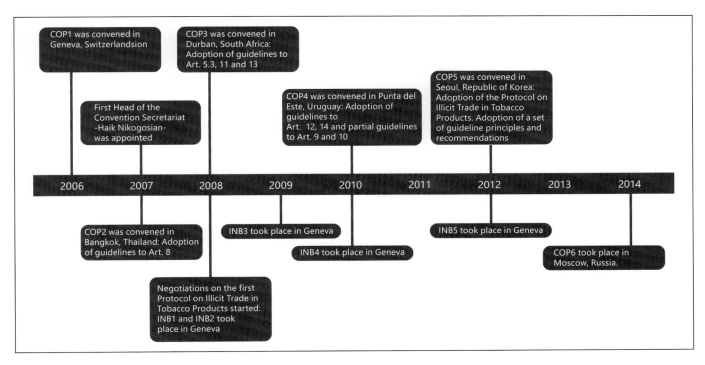

Fig. 3. Process of the implementation of the WHO FCTC.

further developing policy options and recommendations on Articles 17 and 18 regarding economically sustainable alternatives to tobacco growing for its next session.

COP6 took place in Moscow, Russia, in October 2014 (fig. 3). At this session, the Conference of the Parties adopted 29 decisions – the highest number of decisions at any session to date. These include several landmark decision on matters such as on Article 5.3 (to engage with international organizations on the matters of tobacco companies' influence); article 6 (to adopt guidelines on taxation of tobacco products); articles 17 and 18 (to adopt policy options and recommendations on economically sustainable alternatives to tobacco growing) and on electronic nicotine and non-nicotine delivery systems (ENDS), also known as electronic cigarettes. The latter acknowledges the need for regulations along the lines of policies concerning other tobacco products, including banning or restricting promotion, advertising and sponsorship of ENDS.

The WHO Framework Convention on Tobacco Control – A Milestone in International Public Health

The WHO FCTC contains 38 articles. The goal of the WHO FCTC is expressed in its objective: 'The objective of this Convention and its protocols is to protect present and fu-

ture generations from the devastating health, social, environmental and economic consequences of tobacco consumption and exposure to tobacco smoke by providing a framework for tobacco control measures to be implemented by the Parties at the national, regional and international levels in order to reduce continually and substantially the prevalence of tobacco use and exposure to tobacco smoke' [4].

The political will of the Parties is stated in the first preamble paragraph: 'Parties to this Convention (are) determined to give priority to their right to protect public health'.

The roadmap to fulfil this task is determined in Articles 6–17 requiring measures on both the demand and supply side of tobacco (fig. 4). In addition, three articles are to be implemented according to a specific timeline, set by Articles 11 and 13 of the Convention (packaging and labelling measures to be put in place within 3 years of entry into force of the Convention for the Party and measures to control advertising, promotion and sponsorship to be enacted within 5 years of entry into force of the treaty); in the case of Article 8 (Protection from exposure to tobacco smoke), the guidelines for implementation of this article adopted in 2008 recommend adoption of measures to ensure complete protection from exposure to tobacco smoke also within 5 years of entry into force of the Convention for the respective Party.

Measures reducing the demand for tobacco	Measures reducing the supply of tobacco	Further articles
Art. 6: Price and tax measures to reduce the demand for tobacco Art. 7: Non-price measures to reduce the demand for tobacco, namely Art. 8: Protection from exposure to tobacco smoke Art. 9: Regulation of the contents of tobacco products Art.10: Regulation of tobacco product disclosures Art. 11: Packaging and labelling of tobacco products Art. 12: Education, communication, training and public awareness Art. 13: Tobacco advertising, promotion and sponsorship Art. 14: Demand reduction measures concerning tobacco dependence and cessation	Art. 15: Illicit trade in tobacco products Art. 16: Sales to and by minors Art. 17: Provision of support for economically viable alternative activities	Art. 1–5: Terms, objectives, guiding principles and general obligations Art. 18: Protection of the environment and the health of persons Art. 19: Liability Art. 20–22: Scientific and technical cooperation and communication of information Art. 23–26: Institutional arrangements and financial resources Art. 27: Settlement of disputes Art. 28–29: Development of the Convention Art. 28–29: Final provisions

Fig. 4. WHO FCTC: core provisions.

Further articles address liability (Article 19), mechanisms for scientific and technical cooperation and exchange of information (Articles 20–22), institutional arrangements and financial resources (Articles 23–26), settlement of disputes (Article 27) and the further development of the Convention and final provisions (Articles 28–38).

Implementation of the Treaty in Member States

Each Party periodically submits reports on its implementation of the Convention to COP, as required by Article 21.1 of the WHO FCTC. These reports enable Parties to learn from each other's experience in implementing the WHO FCTC and are also the basis for reviews by COP on the progress of the international implementation of the Convention. The Secretariat of the WHO FCTC publishes global progress reports on the implementation on a regular basis.

The latest of these reports was published in 2014 [14] and summarized the submissions from 130 Parties (73% of all Parties that were due to report). The report showed that there are certain Articles with quite high implementation rates and articles with a relatively low reported implementation rate, with the remaining articles falling in between the above two groups (fig. 5).

Likewise, a substantial difference was reported in the progress Parties had made in implementing the respective Articles since their previous submission.

Parties report on their implementation of the WHO FCTC by using a standard questionnaire adopted and further refined by COP, but there is not yet a mechanism for the validation and assessment of compliance of the Parties with all requirements of the treaty in place. The Convention Secretariat reviews the reports for completeness and consistency, but no systematic 'correction' of the submitted reports takes place, for example on the basis of adopted tobacco control legislation, since this falls beyond the mandate of the Convention Secretariat. COP, using the experience of other international treaties, is currently considering the establishment of a mechanism to assist with the review of the reports submitted by the Parties, in accordance with Articles 23.5(d) and (f) of the Convention.

The reporting system of the Convention has evolved significantly over the years [15]. It currently comprises not only standardized instruments to assist Parties to provide information on their implementation efforts, but also promotes, among the Parties, the use of specific WHO FCTC indicators and terms/definitions to allow for better comparability of reported data in the future. This will ensure that

Articles with relatively high implementation rates more than 65% average implementation rate across 130 reporting Parties	Articles with relatively low implementation rates less than 40% average implementation rate across 130 reporting Parties	Articles with relatively high change in implementation rates overall change in all substantive articles was plus 7 percentage points (from 52% between 2007 and 2010 to 59% in 2014)
Art. 8: Protection from exposure to tobacco smoke	**Art. 17:** Provision of support for economically viable alternative activities	**Art. 8:** Protection from exposure to tobacco smoke: +18 percentage points
Art. 11: Packaging and labelling of tobacco products	**Art. 18:** Protection of the environment and the health of persons	**Art. 12:** Education, communication, training and public awareness: +11 percentage points
Art. 12: Education, communication, training and public awareness	**Art. 19:** Liability	**Art. 13:** Tobacco advertising, promotion and sponsorship: +14 percentage points (for comprehensive advertising ban)
Art. 16: Sales to and by minors	**Art. 22:** Cooperation in the scientific, technical, and legal fields and provision of related expertise	**Art. 16:** Sales to and by minors: +13 percentage points

Fig. 5. Implementation of WHO FCTC.

the reporting system of the WHO FCTC is suited to track progress within a Party, but will also contribute to better comparability of data across the Parties.

Effects and Lives Saved by the WHO Framework Convention on Tobacco Control

As the implementation of the WHO FCTC progresses globally, the need has emerged to conduct an impact assessment of the WHO FCTC. At its 5th session, COP initiated the establishment of such process [16]. In some areas, and groups of interventions, literature is already available to indicate the significant impact the Convention has on shaping countries' tobacco control policies, as well as on tobacco use and its health, and economic, social and environmental consequences, as foreseen in Article 3 of the Convention.

One significant comprehensive work was published in July 2013 [17]. The paper examined the effect of selected tobacco control demand reduction measures on lives saved since the WHO FCTC went into force in 2005. The authors of the study projected that 7.4 million premature deaths will be averted by 2050 through the implementation of one or more of the 'MPOWER measures' (see chapters 2 and 12) (the MPOWER measures correspond to one or more of the demand reduction provisions included in the WHO FCTC [18]). The study focused on the 41 countries (2 of which are not Parties to the WHO FCTC) that had implemented the MPOWER measures at 'the highest level of achievement', that is at a level proven to attain the greatest impact. These countries represented nearly 1 billion people or one seventh of the world's population of 6.9 billion in 2008. Of the 41 countries, 33 had put in place one MPOWER measure and the remaining 8 had implemented more than one. Given that 1 in every 2 smokers dies prematurely from smoking-related diseases, the authors calculated that the MPOWER measures put in place in the 41 countries would prevent the premature deaths of half of the 14.8 million smokers who quit – that is 7.4 million people – by 2050. The study showed that almost half of the averted deaths would be attributable to increased cigarette taxes (3.5 million).

Outlook

The WHO FCTC is one of the most widely embraced treaties in the history of the United Nations (UN), with 180 Parties participating (as of 15 January 2015) and covering more than 88% of the world population. This success demonstrates sustained global political will to strengthen tobacco control and save lives. The last couple of years have brought about an increased awareness of the importance and harm caused by tobacco specifically and by noncommunicable diseases (NCDs) in general: not only in high-income countries but also globally. This has been reflected by a high-level meeting of the UN General Assembly on the prevention and control of NCDs that took place in New York City in September 2011 [19]. This high-level meeting was the second health-related high-level meeting in the history of the UN and addressed the prevention and control of NCDs worldwide, with a particular focus on developmental and other challenges, and social and economic impacts, particularly for developing countries.

World leaders agreed in this meeting that the global burden and threat of NCDs constitutes one of the major challenges for development in the 21st century and that business as usual was no longer an option. Countries committed to take action by setting national targets, developing national plans and implementing proven interventions to prevent, control and monitor NCDs. To support the development of national targets, in May 2013, the WHA adopted the WHO global action plan for the prevention and control of NCDs 2013–2020 [20], in which reducing tobacco use is identified as one of the critical elements of effective NCD control. The global action plan comprises a set of actions which – when performed collectively by Member States, WHO and international partners – will set the world on a new course to achieve nine globally agreed targets for NCDs; these include a reduction in premature mortality from NCDs by 25% in 2025 and a 30% relative reduction in prevalence of current tobacco use in persons aged 15 years and older. It is proposed that WHO Member States undertake the following actions to achieve this target:

- Accelerate full implementation of the WHO FCTC; Member States that have not yet become a Party should consider action to accede to the treaty at the earliest opportunity
- Protect tobacco control policies from commercial and other vested interests of the tobacco industry
- Putting in place a set of tobacco control measures, including the MPOWER measures
- Regulate the contents and emissions of tobacco products, and manufacturers and importers of tobacco products are required to disclose information about their contents and emissions to governmental authorities

Similarly to this global action plan, the UN Economic and Social Council adopted a resolution to support UN system-wide coherence on tobacco control. The resolution calls upon UN agencies to contribute and assist countries in meeting their obligations under the WHO FCTC.

Examples from countries that have put in place strong tobacco control measures in line with the WHO FCTC show that premature tobacco-related death can be prevented. Turkey or Uruguay are examples of countries that have had a long tradition of tobacco use and high smoking prevalence. However, after implementing a set of tobacco control measures at the highest level of achievement, smoking prevalence has been declining at unprecedented rates. Turkey, for example, has seen a relative decline in smoking of 13.4% in just 4 years [21, 22]. The successes demonstrated by many countries in using demand reduction measures to build capacity to implement the WHO FCTC show that it is possible to effectively address the tobacco epidemic and save lives, regardless of size or income. However, efforts to incorporate all provisions of the WHO FCTC into national tobacco control programs must be accelerated in all countries to save even more lives.

To make this a reality, WHO FCTC knowledge hubs are being established in several WHO regions. Three hubs either have been or are in the process of being established (Australia: McCabe Center for Cancer Control, focusing on trade and tobacco matters; Finland: National Institute for Public Health, focusing on surveillance, and Uruguay: Center for International Cooperation in Tobacco Control), with other hubs to follow.

Key Points

- The WHO FCTC is the first international treaty negotiated under the auspices of WHO.
- The WHO FCTC was developed in response to the globalization of the tobacco epidemic and is an evidence-based treaty that reaffirms the right of all people to the highest standard of health.
- Adopted by the World Health Assembly in 2003 and entered into force in 2005, the WHO FCTC has since become one of the most rapidly and widely embraced treaties in United Nations history.
- The Convention represents a milestone for the promotion of public health and provides new legal dimensions for international health cooperation.
- Substantial progress has been made in implementing the WHO FCTC. However, efforts to incorporate all provisions of the WHO FCTC into national tobacco control programmes must be accelerated in all countries to save even more lives.

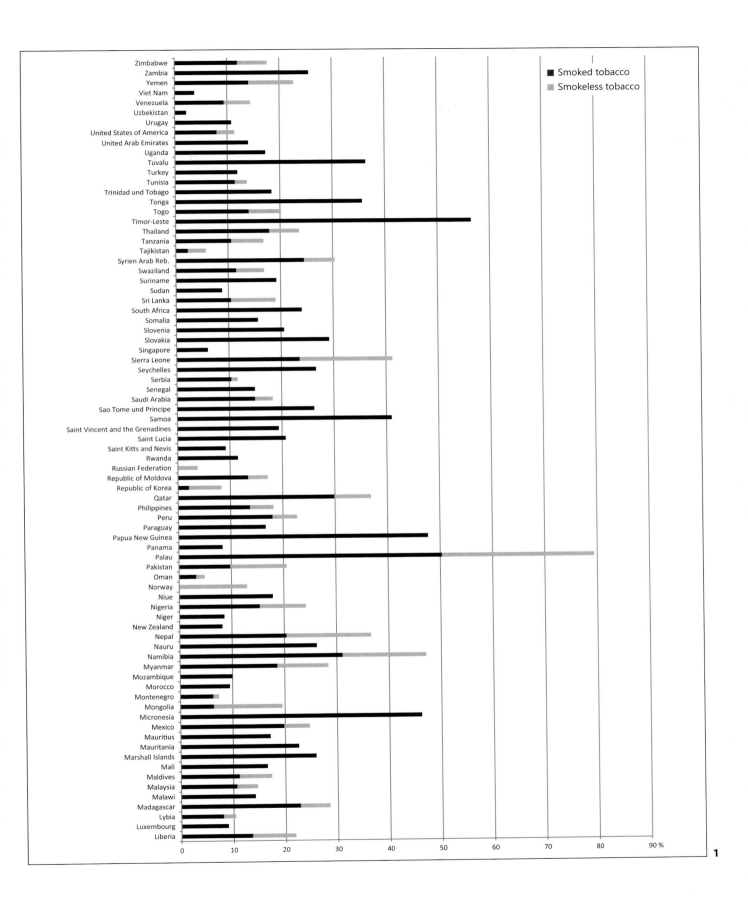

cigarettes (e-cigarettes) [13]. For some years, a decline in the prevalence of cigarette smoking among adolescents has been observed in developed countries, whereas a reversal has occurred in several low- and middle-income countries [8]. Among other things, this is due to the widespread availability of smuggled cigarettes, which make international brands more affordable to the low-income consumers and the youth, thus stimulating consumption [14]. Even if the prevalence of cigarette smoking is still significantly higher than that of other tobacco usage in the regions of America, Europe and Western Pacific, it is significantly lower than that of other tobacco formulations used in Eastern Mediterranean regions and Southeast Asia regions, while it is nearly equally distributed in the African regions [15, 16]. Cigarette volume sales have still increased at higher rates in the Asia-Pacific region, the Middle East and Africa than in the rest of the world.

The use of smokeless tobacco products has remained unchanged in several developed and developing regions of the world, but the types of smokeless tobacco products vary widely. In the Western World, low-nitrosamine products, such as Swedish-style snus, have continued to increase in popularity, whereas most smokeless tobacco users of certain European countries commonly use the conventional or the traditional products with a relatively high level of toxins, including oral and nasal snuff [8] (see also chapter 21).

Over the past 5 years, more and more young people tended to smoke some kind of waterpipe, even in countries where smoking a waterpipe is not part of the traditional lifestyle [17] (see also chapter 22). 'According to the World Health Organization, it is quickly becoming the largest epidemic or public health epidemic in the world because of how many people are doing it' [18]. Its popularity is due to its easy availability, attractive designs and flavored aromatic tobacco [19]. Young people enjoy the socializing, mingling with friends and the relaxing moments associated with this type of tobacco consumption, but they are not aware of the harmful effects of nicotine, chemicals and charcoal carcinogens. They assume waterpipe smoking is healthier and has less addictive effects than cigarette smoking, and they do not realize the added risk of transmissible and communicable diseases associated with this type of tobacco usage.

It appears that the usage of e-cigarettes is increasing rapidly among young people over the last years [20, 21, 22] (see also chapter 23). Between 2011 and 2013, in the USA, the number of never-smoking young people who used e-cigarettes increased from 79,000 to over 263,000, and the intention to smoke conventional cigarettes was 43.9% among ever e-cigarette users and 21.5% among never e-cigarette us-

ers. This finding suggests that e-cigarette use is aggravating rather than ameliorating the tobacco epidemic among youths [22, 23]. E-cigarettes used by adolescents are a unique concern, as the extent of the adverse health effects are unknown and the reasons for their use are still under further investigation. Whereas the use of e-cigarettes among adults is often associated with the attempt to stop smoking, different reasons apply to adolescents. The increasing desire to experiment with e-cigarettes is more a consequence of seeking new and different sensations and experiences, combined with the willingness to accept the added risks to achieve them. Adolescents trying out cigarettes are also more inclined to try out e-cigarettes and vice versa. This is especially troubling, as the majority of young adults do consider e-cigarettes to be safer than cigarettes, and, therefore, it is unclear if the use of e-cigarettes may reduce inhibition thresholds towards tobacco and other harmful substances. It is conceivable that e-cigarettes may help to make cigarettes more acceptable again and act as a potential gateway for increased tobacco usage [20].

Recognition of Adolescents' Behavior

A person's path to daily smoking and nicotine dependency can be described in five stages: susceptibility to smoking (having never smoked before); initiation (trying the first cigarette); experimentation (repeatedly trying, may show signs of addiction); established smoking (regular smoking, likely to show signs of addiction), and finally nicotine dependency. Adolescents are especially susceptible to initiate smoking and willing to experiment. From the early experiments leading to addiction, it can take up to 2 years, although some children and adolescents progress much more rapidly towards a state of nicotine dependence [24]. The duration of smoking and the number of cigarettes required to establish nicotine addiction are lower for adolescents than for adults [25]. Furthermore, people who start smoking at younger ages – and about two-thirds of adults who had ever smoked daily began smoking daily already by 18 years of age (fig. 2) – are more likely to develop high levels of nicotine dependence than those who start later, leading to more difficulty quitting [26].

Therefore, it is of critical importance to prevent (or at least to delay) the start of tobacco use in early adolescence [27]. Tobacco usage is also associated with other aspects of risk behavior with negative effects on the health of adolescents. Therefore, it can be considered to be part of a broader unhealthy behavior pattern frequently shown in adolescence [25].

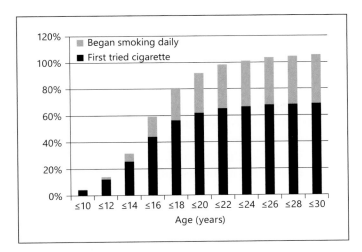

Fig. 2. Cumulative percentages of recalled age at which a respondent first tried a cigarette and when they began smoking daily, by smoking status among subjects 30–39 years old [30].

It is known that the strongest determinants (see also chapter 16) regarding health are structural factors such as national wealth, inequality of income and access to education. Furthermore, safe and supportive families, safe and supportive schools and positive and supportive peers are crucial in helping young people to attain the best level of health during the transition to adulthood [28]. Therefore, it is not astonishing that there are some characteristics which increase the likelihood that an adolescent will smoke.

Factors Influencing the Onset of Tobacco Use

In order to reduce the health and social impact of tobacco use worldwide, it is important to understand factors that contribute to the onset and perpetuation of tobacco use among young people. Adolescence is a critical period with a high risk to develop a lifelong smoking habit [29]. There are many different factors reported on why young people start to smoke, including the disintegration of the urban community, poverty as well as personal factors associated with emotional and psychosocial problems, little involvement at school, academic failure/dropping out of the education system altogether, antisocial behavior, early pregnancy/young parenthood, dissociation within the family, homelessness, stress, feeling a lack of belonging, little supervision, and familial (mis)use of cigarettes, alcohol and other drugs. Furthermore, curiosity, peer pressure and the feeling of maturity have been shown to be the key factors among youths for starting to smoke [11]. Besides these social and environ-

mental aspects leading to tobacco use, additional genetic susceptibilities are being discussed. Maternal smoking during pregnancy has been associated with increased risks for the offspring of ever smoking, regular (or current) smoking, and dependence on tobacco as preadolescent, adolescent and young adult [30].

The Role of the Family
The parent-child relationship during adolescence may introduce additional challenges into the family structure. There is some evidence that adolescents with a perception that their parents give them opportunities for their own decision making may be less inclined to seek unhealthy ways to express themselves. Furthermore, it was shown that adolescents developing a more independent relationship towards their parents, whilst remaining positively connected to them, have an added factor of protection against taking up smoking [31]. In addition, smoking behavior of adolescents is influenced by the role model the parents adopt, in other words, adolescents are likely to follow parental smoking habits. Interestingly, a stronger link concerning current smoking habits seems to be based on maternal smoking rather than paternal smoking [32].

The Role of Peers
Peer influence is a consistent predictor of smoking onset among adolescents [33, 34]. Smoking may be deemed to be one of the ways to gain acceptance from other peers and this is one of the most important aspects during adolescence. To be accepted, the adolescent takes on the attitudes and behaviors of the group. Yet, some young people report that the general peer pressure is not a factor for their smoking, but sometimes it is the experience of being pressurized by an individual to smoke in the presence of other adolescents, who are also smoking [35]. Unlike this socialization, in which an individual conforms to group norms, peer selection of a person does also play an important role. When some members of a peer group begin smoking or experimenting with other substances, other members of this group can respond by dropping out of the group (de-selection), conforming to the new norms of the group (socialization), risking disapproval of the group or by living with the dissonance between their own norms and those of the group.

The Role of School Education
It seems that adolescent smoking behavior is strongly linked to their own educational level. The percentage of smokers among adolescents with a lower education is higher than

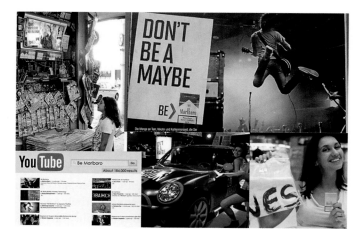

Fig. 3. Tobacco advertising using different media [37].

among adolescents with a higher education [36]. An international European study revealed that vocational secondary school students are more likely to smoke than academic students. This might represent effects of differential peer clusters and school-related factors, such as achievement motivation and school performance [10]. Furthermore, educational upward mobility seems to protect adolescents from becoming smokers; on the other hand, educational downward mobility seems to stimulate tobacco smoking, at least among boys.

The Role of the Tobacco Industry
The tobacco industry still engages in ways to attract the youth. While tobacco companies claim publicly that they do not market to young people or design marketing campaigns that target the youth, volumes of internal industry documents and decades of peer-reviewed research show that tobacco companies target children as young as 13 years of age, and such marketing increases youth smoking rates [37] (see also chapter 3). They advertise in magazines, promote their products in convenience stores, market their brands through direct mail, Internet Web sites and social media networks (fig. 3). Adolescents and young adults are uniquely susceptible to social and environmental influences when it comes to using tobacco products, and tobacco companies continue to spend billions of dollars on cigarette and smokeless tobacco marketing. The evidence is sufficient to conclude that there is a causal relationship between advertising and promotional efforts of the tobacco companies and the initiation to and the progression of tobacco usage among young people (see also chapter 15). Evidence is also suggesting that tobacco companies have changed the

packaging and design of their products in ways that have increased the appeal of these products to adolescents and young adults [31].

The Genetic Impact
Why do some adolescents use tobacco while others avoid substance misuse? Not all adolescents who attend a school with a large number of smokers, or who have parents who smoke, do smoke themselves. Certain characteristics may render adolescents more susceptible to these social influences than others. A systematic review of gene studies found some evidence to support the hypothesis that people with certain genetic variants are more likely to experiment and persist in smoking [38] (see also chapter 5). The effects of genetic risks seem to be limited to people who start smoking as teens. This suggests that there may exist some genetic background on tobacco addiction. Genetic risk scores seem to be unrelated to smoking initiation, but there are increased risks to convert to daily smoking as teenagers, to progress more rapidly from smoking initiation to heavy smoking, to persist longer in smoking heavily, to develop nicotine dependence more frequently, to be more reliant on smoking to cope with stress and to be more likely to fail in cessation attempts [39].

Strategies to Prevent Youths from Smoking

Many strategies are developed, many initiatives are undertaken and many programs are implemented to prevent young people from using tobacco. These smoking prevention efforts occur within large community environments (mass media campaigns or tobacco control programs at state level), small social environments (families, health care settings or schools), or through regulatory or legislative approaches (taxation and pricing, or regulations on youth access) [40]. However, all these strategies can only be successful if they really reach the young and are appreciated by them.

School-Based Educational Interventions
The school environment has been a particular focus for substance use prevention programs for nearly 4 decades, since the school environment offers the ability to reach almost all children, and a focus on education fits naturally with the daily activities of schools. All prevention strategies should be sensitive to represent a student population that is multicultural, multiethnic and socioeconomically diverse [41]. To be most effective, school-based prevention programs

must target children and adolescents prior to the onset of tobacco use or their dropping out of school [41, 42]. There are five types of school-based educational interventions, which are commonly used, each based on a different theoretical approach [43].

The first type assumes that information alone will lead to behavioral changes; therefore, this attempt provides only information on the harmfulness and the actual rate of tobacco usage, as well as on the inaccurate beliefs on the social acceptability of smoking. Most often information is provided to arouse concern or fear. However, findings from school-based prevention research revealed that providing information alone may be able to help to change knowledge and attitudes, but it is not sufficient to effect a change in behavior [44].

A second type of intervention aims to improve the adolescents' general social competence. Social competence plays a primary and fundamental role in promoting the initiation of substance use among adolescents. Therefore, social learning processes or life skills, such as problem solving, decision making, resisting interpersonal or media influences, increased self-control and self-esteem, as well as strategies for stress management and general assertive and social skills, can decrease the susceptibility to tobacco use [43]. The Life Skills Training program, for example, teaches these skills using a combination of proven cognitive-behavioral skill training methods that include instruction and demonstration, behavioral rehearsal (in-class practice), feedback and reinforcement and extended (out-of-class) practice through behavioral homework assignments [45].

Prevention programs of the third type focus on social resistance skills and want to increase the adolescents' awareness of the various social influences that support substance use. These influences come from different sources, including peers, family and mass media [44]. The aim of these prevention programs is to teach adolescents how to best deal with peer pressure and other high-risk situations, and how to handle these situations when they become unavoidable. These programs can also make students aware of the techniques used by advertisers to promote tobacco products. Findings indicate that social resistance skill interventions can considerably reduce the number of young people beginning to consume tobacco products [44].

A fourth type of prevention program uses combined social competence and social influence approaches.

Finally, the fifth type involves multimodal programs combining curricular approaches with wider initiatives within and beyond the school, including programs for parents, schools or communities, and initiatives to change school policies about tobacco use [43]. These programs include, among other topics, the following strategies: to develop and enforce a school policy on tobacco use, provide instructions about the negative physiologic and social consequences of tobacco use, social influences on tobacco use, peer norms regarding tobacco use and refusal skills, provide tobacco use prevention education from nursery to class 12, provide program-specific training for teachers, involve parents or families in support of school-based tobacco prevention programs, support cessation efforts among students and all school staff who use tobacco, and assess the effectiveness of the tobacco use prevention program at regular intervals [46].

The effectiveness of such school-based intervention programs is controversially discussed. Evaluations of different specific programs and a recent Cochrane meta-analysis of tobacco prevention programs in school settings strongly suggest that programs that use a social competence approach and those that combine a social competence with a social influence approach are more effective than other programs [43]. However, it is important that these programs are implemented in a setting with broad policy support [4].

Community Interventions
Since the decisions to smoke are often influenced by environmental, social and cultural conditions, emphasis is often placed on interventions that include comprehensive, community-based approaches. Such an approach comprises the involvement of families, schools, community organizations, churches, businesses, the media, social service and health agencies, government bodies and law enforcement agencies. These intervention strategies generally focus on making changes in both the environment and the individuals' behavior. The essence of the community approach aiming to influence smoking behavior, in particular the prevention of smoking, lies in its multidimensionality, in the coordination of different activities to maximize the chance of reaching all members, and in the ongoing and widespread support for the upkeep of nonsmoking behavior. Although some evidence is available to suggest that multicomponent community interventions are effective in influencing smoking behavior and preventing the uptake of smoking in young people [47], broad-based community interventions alone seem not to be sufficient to bring about a substantial and sustained decline in smoking in the young. However, the effectiveness of school-based programs appears to be enhanced when they are included in broad-based community efforts in which parents, mass media and community organizations are involved and in

which the social policy or social environment, as well as individual knowledge, attitudes and behavior are targeted for change [4].

Mass Media/Public Education

Media-based health promotion efforts have the potential to reach and modify the knowledge, attitudes and behavior of large segments of the population, especially those who are less educated [4] (see also chapter 15). Media channels commonly used for tobacco control advertising include television, radio, print and billboards. By the age of 18 years, a young person will have spent more time being entertained by the media than doing any other activity except sleeping [48]. In particular, YouTube, a free video-sharing service, is currently one of the fastest growing Web sites in the United States and the fourth most-accessed site on the Internet. Among the visitors of the Web site, youths aged 12–17 years comprise a greater portion than any other demographic. Due to this popularity among youth and the potential to influence their behavior, YouTube has already been noticed by the business world as an ideal platform for advertising and marketing [49]. Due to this great interest in these media, it has been suggested that the mass media are particularly appropriate for delivering antismoking messages to young people [48]. Themes that are used in this advertising include the health consequences of smoking, tobacco industry manipulation, dangers of secondhand smoking and the declining social acceptability of smoking. The latest antismoking campaign of the FDA focuses on cosmetic consequences such as tooth loss and skin damage, as well the loss of control nicotine addiction creates. The development of a strong negative emotion is more likely to be associated with changes in youth attitudes about tobacco (social norms) and lower smoking initiation compared to other advertising messages [50]. However, the effectiveness of smoking-focused mass media interventions is also determined by the target audiences, as well as by the duration and the intensity of the exposure. There is good evidence that media campaigns can be effective, but they may be more effective in combination with other approaches, such as school and/or community-based programs, than on their own [51].

Tobacco Advertising Restrictions

Adolescents are vulnerable targets for the tobacco industry, being easily influenced by television, cinema and advertisements [7] (see chapter 15). Therefore, tobacco advertising and marketing – including the distribution of promotional products such as clothing, sporting equipment and gear for outdoor activities – is causally associated with tobacco usage, particularly by the young [4, 51]. Since adolescents are in the process of forming their own identity, they are very susceptible to distinct lifestyle images. Tobacco companies have therefore created distinct lifestyle images, e.g. masculinity (for boys), thinness (for girls), independence, extroversion, coolness, temerity and sex appeal [52], and associated them with different cigarette brands. On that basis, young people associate smoking with certain characteristics and images which they are trying to assimilate [52]. It appears that cigarette advertising increases adolescents' awareness of smoking at a generic level and encourages them to take up the behavior. Thus, a significant number of youth experimenting with smoking can be attributed to tobacco promotional activities [4]. Therefore, the WHO Framework Convention on Tobacco Control (FCTC) recognized 'that a comprehensive ban on advertising, promotion and sponsorship would reduce the consumption of tobacco products' [52]. Several countries all over the world (e.g. Finland, Italy and New Zealand) have already implemented strong tobacco-marketing regulations. Other countries (including the United States and Germany) have, however, implemented considerably weaker tobacco-marketing policies. Germany, for example, has banned tobacco advertisements in television, radio, newspapers and magazines, but tobacco marketing is still allowed at point of sale, on billboards and in cinema commercials prior to movies which are shown after 6.00 p.m. It could be shown that exposure to antismoking media messages on television, radio, billboards, posters, newspaper, magazines and movies are associated with adapting a nonsmoking attitude. Especially antismoking messages on television proved to be very effective in hindering smoking among adolescents [53].

Youth Access Restrictions

Programs that effectively disrupt tobacco sales to minors have been shown to reduce smoking among youth. In the last years, comprehensive tobacco control strategies were created, recommending legislation and enforcement to restrict tobacco sales to minors [54]. These strategies include prohibition of the sale and distribution of tobacco products to people under the age of 18 years [4], reduced availability of cigarette vending machines and the need of an identity card to use it, as well as a ban on providing free samples of cigarettes and smokeless tobacco. Furthermore, training programs for tobacco vendors are necessary for them to understand the health effects of tobacco use and the importance of preventing youth from initiating its use and to gain the skills to deal with smoking adolescents. Although com-

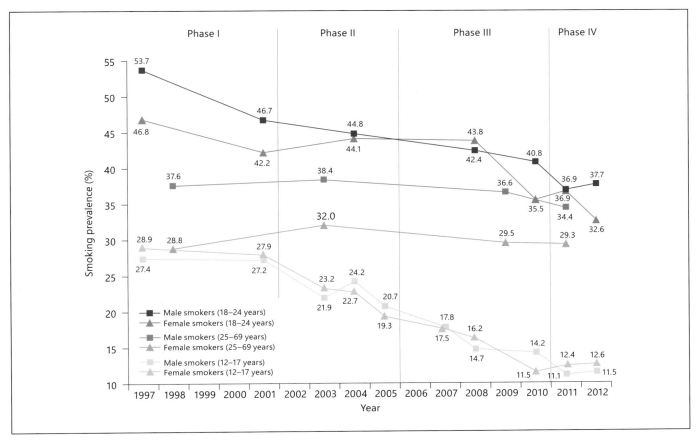

Fig. 4. Development of smoking habits in the different German age groups during the four phases of tax increase. Phase I (1997–2001) = Largely constant tobacco tax; phase II (2002–2005) = considerable and continuing rise in the tobacco tax; phase III (2006–2010) = largely constant tobacco tax; phase IV (2011–2012) = moderate rise in the tobacco tax [modified from ref. 61].

mercial supply does become more important as nicotine addiction develops and smoking frequency increases, adolescents' friends, peers and even families remain the key supply routes adolescents use to procure tobacco [55]. Therefore, policy makers need to generally reduce the easiness on how people buy and supply tobacco products (see chapter 12).

Tobacco Excise Taxes
Theoretically, increasing the price of cigarettes through taxation could reduce adolescent cigarette consumption through three mechanisms: Quitting smoking, reducing the rate of smoking and preventing to start smoking. The extent to which higher cigarette taxes will achieve these objectives depends upon how responsive smokers and potential smokers are to price increases [4] (see also chapters 11 and 12). The addictive nature of cigarette consumption suggests that youths should be more responsive to changes in cigarette prices than adults (fig. 4).

They spend a larger share of their income on cigarettes, and the larger the share of disposable income spent on a product becomes, the more responsive the individual will be to price changes [3]. However, higher cigarette prices are also found to have an impact on cigarette purchasing patterns. As a response to the increase in tobacco prices, people change the type of tobacco they consume to cheaper brands, smokeless tobacco and hand-rolled cigarettes [56]. The evidence on the degree to which teenagers are responsive to changes in cigarette prices is diverse, but the general consensus is that higher prices are an effective tobacco control policy not only in reducing the rate of smoking but also in preventing adolescents from smoking altogether [57]. However, as long as cigarette prices differ arbitrarily from region to region on a worldwide basis, increasing the price of cigarettes will not be as effective as it otherwise could be, since cigarettes can be bought cheaper elsewhere, or even tax free, e.g. when travelling by air.

Recent Innovations in Youth Smoking Prevention and Cessation

Despite multiple strategies which have contributed to reductions in youth smoking during the past 2 decades, the impact of once effective strategies may diminish over time [34, 50]. These trends suggest the need for novel, not yet widely tested or evaluated intervention strategies to prevent the onset of tobacco use and support cessation strategies for adolescents. These strategies take advantage of the possibilities of new media (e.g. Internet and smartphones), because their use is widespread among adolescents. An example of such a new way could be the Internet-delivered intervention, which seems to have the potential to be effective in promoting a healthy lifestyle behavior among adolescents. Prior studies have shown that frequent use of an Internet-delivered intervention resulted in higher smoking cessation rates among adults and adolescents. To stimulate reuse of an Internet-delivered intervention, periodic prompts may be a valuable tool, because the provision of prompts can have a positive effect on reuse of an intervention Web site [58]. Furthermore, SMS (short message service) programs, which deliver text support that is highly tailored to a smoker (e.g. iQuit system) seem to be effective in long-term abstinence and could be supportive in smoking cessation [59].

A further major trend is establishing peer education programs, in which older students are trained to become positive role models for their younger classmates [4, 34]. Furthermore, a new, youth-oriented generation of antitobacco advertising, which is high energy, aggressive, fast paced and in turn angry, sarcastic and irreverent, has been developed, even partially designed by young people [4]. Other initiatives focus on fining juveniles for smoking in public or possessing tobacco products, actions against retail vendors who sell tobacco products, further restrictions on the sale and marketing of tobacco products, recently developed school smoking policies, adolescent risk taking in general and/or problem behavior and on direct restrictions on smoking in public facilities, restaurants, bars and hotels, and on trains and airline flights, for example.

Conclusions and Recommendations

In the past 2 decades, many efforts and measures were taken to combat the tobacco epidemic worldwide. The most important step in this respect was the WHO FCTC (see chapter 13), which came into force on February 27, 2005. It had been signed by 168 countries and is legally binding in 178 ratifying countries. This convention includes rules that govern the production, sale, distribution, advertisement and taxation of tobacco. However, FCTC standards represent only the minimum requirements, and much more stringent measures have to be implemented to prevent the onset of tobacco use.

Since all over the world young people grow to adulthood within a complex web of family, peer, community, and social and cultural influences, the common factors that help protect young people from harm are similar across high-, middle- and low-income countries. However, this complex web is designed differently in different nations and cultures. Therefore, intervention programs to prevent young people from the onset of tobacco consumption have to include several components targeting diverse mediating mechanisms and may not focus on just one [57].

It is important to note that preventing the onset of tobacco use not only implies 'preventing the onset of cigarette smoking'. Many other tobacco products, which are also very harmful, play an increasingly important role all over the world (see chapter 22). Therefore, preventing the onset of tobacco implies to act on many fronts. A lot has already been done up to now, but much still remains to be done to reach our goal of 'preventing the onset of tobacco use'!

Key Points

- Adolescence is the most decisive phase to prevent the onset of tobacco consumption.
- A worrying increase in e-cigarette use among young people is observed over the last years.
- Smoking behavior of young people is influenced by the family environment, smoking behavior of peers, peer attitudes and norms, own intentions, attitudes and beliefs, educational environment, accessibility to and availability of tobacco products, affordability, tobacco advertising and promotion, and the creation of new tobacco products.
- Due to the diversity of key factors for smoking uptake, effective youth smoking prevention requires a comprehensive multifaceted approach, involving a range of well-researched, coordinated and complementary strategies that reinforce each other.
- For continued progress in youth smoking prevention, the importance of preventive programs must be positioned in the minds of parents, professionals, communities and policy makers.
- Since the determinants of tobacco use amongst young people are diverse, future research must aim at differentiating use patterns to improve existing tobacco prevention.

References

1 McNeill A: Preventing the onset of tobacco use; in Bolliger CT, Fagerström KO (eds): The Tobacco Epidemic. Prog Respir Res. Basel, Karger, 1997, vol 28, pp 213–229.

2 Phanikumar SP: Advancing Global Tobacco Control: Exploring Worldwide Youth Attitudes and Behaviors toward Tobacco Use and Control; thesis, East Tennessee State University, 2012, http://dc.etsu.edu/etd/1223.

3 Nikaj S, Chaloupka FJ: The effect of prices on cigarette use among youths in the global youth tobacco survey. Nicotine Tob Res 2014; 16(suppl 1):S16–S23.

4 Lantz PM, Jacobson PD, Warner KE, Wasserman JV, Pollack HA, Berson J, Ahlstrom A: Investing in youth tobacco control: a review of smoking prevention and control strategies. Tob Control 2000;9:47–63.

5 Catalano RF, Fagan AA, Gavin LE, Greenberg MT, Irwin CE Jr, Ross DA, Shek DTL: Worldwide application of prevention science in adolescent health. Lancet 2012;379:1653–1664.

6 Johnston V, Liberato S, Thomas D: Incentives for preventing smoking in children and adolescents. Cochrane Database Syst Rev 2012; 10:CD008645.

7 Mukherjee A, Sinha A, Taraphdar P, Basu G, Chakrabarty D: Tobacco abuse among school going adolescents in a rural area of West Bengal, India. Indian J Public Health 2012;56: 286–289.

8 Agaku IT, Ayo-Yusuf OA, Vardavas CI, Connolly G: Predictors and patterns of cigarette and smokeless tobacco use among adolescents in 32 countries, 2007–2011. J Adolesc Health 2014;54:47–53.

9 WHO: Tobacco Free Initiative (TFI) – Tobacco control country profiles. 2013, http://www.who.int/tobacco/surveillance/policy/country_profile/en/.

10 de Looze M, ter Bogt T, Hublet A, Kuntsche E, Richter M, Zsiros E, Godeau E, Vollebergh W: Trends in educational differences in adolescent daily smoking across Europe, 2002–10. Eur J Public Health 2013;23:846–852.

11 Al-Sadat N, Misau AY, Zarihah Z, Maznah D, Tin Su T: Adolescent tobacco use and health in Southeast Asia. Asia Pac J Public Health 2010;22:175S–180S.

12 SAMHSA: Prevention of Substance Abuse and Mental Illness. http://www.samhsa.gov/prevention/.

13 Office of Adolescent Health: Trends in Adolescent Tobacco Use. http://www.hhs.gov/ash/oah/adolescent-health-topics/substance-abuse/tobacco/trends.html.

14 Ali AY, Safwat T, Onyemelukwe G, Otaibi MA, Amir AA, Nawas YN, Aouina H, Afif MH, Bolliger CT: Smoking prevention and cessation in the Africa and Middle East region: a consensus draft guideline for healthcare providers – executive summary. Respiration 2012;83:423–432.

15 Centers for Disease Control and Prevention (CDC): Use of cigarettes and other tobacco products among students aged 13–15 years – worldwide, 1999–2005. MMWR Morb Mortal Wkly Rep 2006;55:553–556.

16 Warren CW, Jones NR, Peruga A, Chauvin J, Baptiste JP, Costa de Silva V, el Awa F, Tsouros A, Rahman K, Fishburn B, Bettcher DW, Asma S; Centers for Disease Control and Prevention (CDC): Global youth tobacco surveillance, 2000–2007. MMWR Surveill Summ 2008;57:1–28.

17 Revelesa CC, Segrib NJ, Botelhoc C: Factors associated with hookah use initiation among adolescents. J Pediatr (Rio J) 2013;89:583–587.

18 Winconek S: Hookah Smoking Is on the Rise among Teens. 2013, http://www.metroparent.com/Blogs/Views-on-the-News/September-2013/Hookah-Smoking-is-on-the-Rise-Among-Teens/.

19 Anjum Q, Ahmed F, Ashfaq T: Knowledge, attitude and perception of water pipe smoking (shisha) among adolescents aged 14–19 years. J Pak Med Assoc 2008;58:312–317.

20 Chapman SLC, Wu LT: E-cigarette prevalence and correlates of use among adolescents versus adults: a review and comparison. J Psychiatr Res 2014;54:43–54.

21 Sutfina E, McCoyb T, Morrell H, Hoeppnere B, Wolfsona M: Electronic cigarette use by college students. Drug Alcohol Depend 2013; 131:214–221.

22 Dutra LM, Glantz SA: Electronic cigarettes and conventional cigarette use among U.S. adolescents – a cross-sectional study. JAMA Pediatr 2014;168:610–617.

23 Bunnell RE, Agaku IT, Arrazola RA, Apelberg BJ, Caraballo RS, Corey CG, Coleman BN, Dube SR, King BA: Intentions to smoke cigarettes among never-smoking U.S. middle and high school electronic cigarette users, National Youth Tobacco Survey, 2011–2013. Nicotine Tobacco Res 2014, Epub ahead of print.

24 Moyer VA, U.S. Preventive Services Task Force: Primary care interventions to prevent tobacco use in children and adolescents: U.S. Preventive Services Task Force recommendation statement. Ann Intern Med 2013;159: 552–557.

25 WHO Regional Office for Europe: Tobacco: Why Pay Attention to This Issue during Adolescence? Copenhagen, WHO Regional Office for Europe, 2012.

26 Mermelstein R: Teen smoking cessation. Tob Control 2003;12:i25–i34.

27 Skara S, Sussman S: A review of 25 long-term adolescent tobacco and other drug use prevention program evaluations. Prev Med 2003; 37:451–474.

28 Viner RM, Ozer EM, Denny S, Marmot M, Resnick M, Fatusi A, Currie C: Adolescence and the social determinants of health. Lancet 2012;379:1641–1652.

29 Gilman SE, Rende R, Boergers J, Abrams DB, Buka SL, Clark MA, Colby SM, Hitsman B, Kazura AN, Lipsitt LP, Lloyd-Richardson EE, Rogers ML, Stanton CA, Stroud LR, Niaura RS: Parental smoking and adolescent smoking initiation: an intergenerational perspective on tobacco control. Pediatrics 2009;123:274–282.

30 US Department of Health and Human Services: Preventing Tobacco Use among Youth and Young Adults: A Report of the Surgeon General. Atlanta, US Department of Health and Human Services, Centers for Disease Control and Prevention, National Center for Chronic Disease Prevention and Health Promotion, Office on Smoking and Health, 2012.

31 Gutman LM, Eccles JS, Peck S, Malanchuk O: The influence of family relations on trajectories of cigarette and alcohol use from early to late adolescence. J Adolesc 2011;34:119–128.

32 Mak KK, Ho SY, Day JR: Smoking of parents and best friend – independent and combined effects on adolescent smoking and intention to initiate and quit smoking. Nicotine Tob Res 2012;14:1057–1064.

33 Villanti A, Boulay M, Juon HS: Peer, parent and media influences on adolescent smoking by developmental stage. Addict Behav 2011; 36:133–136.

34 Kreuter M, Bauer CM, Ehmann M, Kappes J, Drings P, Herth FJF: Wirksamkeit und Nachhaltigkeit eines Raucherpräventionsprogramm für Schüler – 'ohnekippe'. Dtsch Med Wochenschr 02014;1390:1–7.

35 Simons-Morton B, Farhat T: Recent findings on peer group influences on adolescent smoking. J Prim Prev 2010;31:191–208.

36 Crone MR, Reijneveld SA, Willemsen MC, van Leerdam FJM, Spruijt RD, Hira Sing RA: Prevention of smoking in adolescents with lower education: a school based intervention study. J Epidemiol Community Health 2003; 57:675–680.

37 Alliance for the Control of Tobacco Use (ACT Brazil), Campaign for Tobacco-Free Kids, Tobacco Control Alliance, Corporate Accountability International, Framework Convention Alliance, InterAmerican Heart Foundation, Southeast Asia Tobacco Control Alliance: You Are the Target. 2014, http://global.tobaccofreekids.org/en/.

38 Sandford A: Trends in smoking among adolescents and young adults in the United Kingdom – implications for health education. Health Educ 2008;108:223–236.

39 Belsky DW, Moffitt TE, Baker TB, Biddle AK, Evans JP, Harrington HL, Houts R, Meier M, Sugden K, Williams B, Poulton R, Caspi A: Polygenic risk and the developmental progression to heavy, persistent smoking and nicotine dependence: evidence from a 4-decade longitudinal study. JAMA Psychiatry 2013;70: 534–542.

40 Patnode CD, O'Connor E, Whitlock EP, Perdue LA, Soh C, Hollis J: Primary care-relevant interventions for tobacco use prevention and cessation in children and adolescents: a systematic evidence review for the U.S. Preventive Services Task Force. Ann Intern Med 2013;158:253–260.

41 Guidelines for school health programs to prevent tobacco use and addiction. Centers for Disease Control and Prevention. MMWR Recomm Rep1994;43(RR-2):1–18.

42 Inman DD, van Bakergem KM, LaRosa AC, Garr DR: Evidence-based health promotion programs for schools and communities. Am J Prev Med 2011;40:207–219.

43 Thomas RE, McLellan J, Perera R: School-based programmes for preventing smoking. Cochrane Database Syst Rev 2013;4: CD001293.

44 Botvin GJ, Griffin KW: School-based programmes to prevent alcohol, tobacco and other drug use. Int Rev Psychiatry 2007;19:607–615.

45 Botvin GJ: Preventing drug abuse in schools: social and competence enhancement approaches targeting individual-level etiologic factors. Addict Behav 2000;25:887–897.

46 Montana State Office of Public Instruction: Curriculum Planning Guidelines for Tobacco Use Prevention and Education. Helena, Montana State Office of Public Instruction, 2000.

47 Carson KV, Brinn MP, Labiszewski NA, Esterman AJ, Chang AB, Smith BJ: Community interventions for preventing smoking in young people. Cochrane Database Syst Rev 2011;7:CD001291.

48 Brinn MP, Carson KV, Esterman AJ, Chang AB, Smith BJ: Mass media interventions for preventing smoking in young people (review). Cochrane Database Syst Rev 2010;11: CD001006.

49 Paek HJ, Kim K, Hove T: Content analysis of antismoking videos on YouTube: message sensation value, message appeals, and their relationships with viewer responses. Health Educ Res 2010;25:1085–1099.

50 Pierce JP, White VM, Emery SL: What public health strategies are needed to reduce smoking initiation? Tob Control 2012;21:258–264.

51 Jackson CA, Henderson M, Frank JW, Haw SJ: An overview of prevention of multiple risk behaviour in adolescence and young adulthood. J Public Health (Oxf) 2012;34:i31–i40.

52 Hanewinkel R, Isensee B, Sargent JD, Morgenstern M: Cigarette advertising and teen smoking initiation. Pediatrics 2011;127:271–279.

53 Rao S, Aslam SK, Zaheer S, Shafique K: Antismoking initiatives and current smoking among 19,643 adolescents in South Asia: findings from the Global Youth Tobacco Survey. Harm Reduc J 2014;11:8.

54 Diemert L, Dubray J, Babayan A, Schwartz R: Strategies Affecting Tobacco Vendor Compliance with Youth Access Laws – A Review of the Literature. Toronto, Ontario Tobacco Research Unit, 2013.

55 Gendall Ph, Hoek J, Marsh L, Edwards R, Healey B: Youth tobacco access: trends and policy implications. BMJ Open 2014;4:e004631.

56 Kim HC, Kwon SM, Cho KS, Lim JY: The effect of the increase in tobacco price on adolescent smoking in Korea: smoking reduction and brand switching. Health Soc Welfare Rev 2012;32:429–460.

57 White VM, Warne CD, Spittal MJ, Durkin S, Purcell K, Wakefield MA: What impact have tobacco control policies, cigarette price and tobacco control program funding had on Australian adolescents' smoking? Findings over a 15-year period. Addiction 2011;106:1493–1502.

58 Cremers HP, Mercken L, Crutzen R, Willems P, de Vries H, Oenema A: Do email and mobile phone prompts stimulate primary school children to reuse an Internet-delivered smoking prevention intervention? J Med Internet Res 2014;16:e86.

59 Naughton F, Jamison J, Boase S, Sloan M, Gilbert H, Prevost AT, Mason D, Smith S, Brimicombe J, Evans R, Sutton S: Randomized controlled trial to assess the short-term effectiveness of tailored web- and text-based facilitation of smoking cessation in primary care (iQuit in practice). Addiction 2014;109: 1184–1193.

60 United States Department of Health and Human Services, Substance Abuse and Mental Health Services Administration, Center for Behavioral Health Statistics and Quality: National Survey on Drug Use and Health, 2010 (ICPSR 32722). https://nsduhweb.rti. org/respweb/homepage.cfm.

61 Deutsches Krebsforschungszentrum in der Helmholtz-Gemeinschaft: Tabaksteuererhöhungen und Rauchverhalten in Deutschland. Aus der Wissenschaft – für die Politik. 2014, http://www.dkfz.de/de/tabakkontrolle/ download/Publikationen/AdWfP/AdWfdP_ Tabaksteuererhoehungen_und_Rauchverhalten_in_Deutschland.pdf.

Claudia Bauer
Department of Pneumology and Respiratory Critical Care Medicine
Smoking Prevention Unit, Thoraxklinik, University of Heidelberg, Amalienstrasse 5
DE–69126 Heidelberg (Germany)
E-Mail claudia.bauer@med.uni-heidelberg.de

Sargent et al. [16] used this method to determine exposure to movie smoking in a representative sample of young US adolescents. The authors surveyed 6,522 nationally representative US adolescents aged 10–14 years and performed content analysis of 534 contemporary box-office hits for movie smoking. Each movie was assigned to a random subsample of adolescents (mean: 613) who were asked whether they had seen the movie. Forty-one percent of the 534 movies was rated PG-13 (parents are urged to be cautious as the motion picture contains some material that parents might consider inappropriate for children under 13 years). Another 40% was rated R (people under 17 years may only be admitted if accompanied by a parent or guardian). Overall, 74% of the movies contained smoking (3,830 total smoking occurrences). On average, each movie was seen by 25% of the adolescents surveyed. Viewership was higher with increased age and lower for R-rated movies. Overall, at the date of the survey in 2003, these movies delivered 13.9 billion gross smoking impressions, an average of 665 to each US adolescent aged 10–14 years. US media companies (Hollywood studios) produce and/or distribute 80–90% of all box-office hits that are viewed in many countries. Using similar methodology, Hanewinkel and Sargent [17] surveyed adolescents in Germany and found that popular US movies deliver billions of smoking images and character smoking depictions to young US adolescents and to adolescents worldwide.

Relationship between Exposure to On-Screen Smoking and Youth Smoking

Experimental Studies
Quasi-experimental and randomized study designs allow a better control for risk factors and influences that eventually could confound the effect of on-screen smoking on smoking-related attitudes and behaviors. A 2008 National Cancer Institute review summarized the results from eight experimental studies on viewers' beliefs about smoking and their reactions to movie smoking [5]. A further recent nine experimental studies have been summarized by a 2012 Surgeon General review [18]. The paragraphs below summarize the findings.

Functional magnetic resonance imaging responses to smoking scenes in movies in smokers and nonsmokers naïve to the focus on smoking were studied by Wagner et al. [19]. Brain responses to movie smoking segments were compared to responses to segments without smoking. This study suggests that smokers may have larger responses in reward cir-

cuits and also larger responses in motor planning areas for the right hand, suggesting that the smoking scenes may prompt motor planning for smoking. The study provides a biological basis for the idea that cues could prompt autonomous smoking events – when smokers find themselves lighting up without remembering doing it, or when they find themselves having lit two cigarettes at the same time.

Few studies have assessed the association between exposure to movie smoking and urge to smoke under real-world conditions. Sargent et al. [20] conducted exit interviews with 2,817 adult movie patrons of whom 536 were smokers. Subjects had exited 26 movies, of which 12 contained smoking. After controlling for movie rating, age, sex, Heaviness of Smoking Index and time since last cigarette smoked, attendance of a movie with smoking was associated with a significant increase in the urge to smoke. The effect size was consistent with responses seen in cue reactivity experiments.

A strong design was realized by Shmueli et al. [21]. Young adult smokers were randomly assigned to watch an 8-min film consisting of clips that either did or did not contain smoking. After watching the film, participants were asked to leave the room for 10 min. Smokers who were exposed to the film with smoking scenes were more likely to smoke during the break than those who watched the smoke-free film. Furthermore, young adult smokers who saw the film with smoking were more likely to smoke a cigarette within 20 min after completion of the experiment compared to those who watched the smoke-free film.

To sum up, experimental studies offer evidence for an effect of the exposure to on-screen smoking on behavior and biological evidence for cue-based craving related to movie images and automaticity, as well as some evidence to support the idea that movie smoking prompts immediate smoking.

Cross-Sectional Observational Studies
Several cross-sectional studies using a variety of approaches to assess exposure to movie smoking have been conducted to examine the association between past exposure to movie smoking and current youth smoking status. A random-effect meta-analysis of four cross-sectional studies using the Beach method to estimate the exposure to movie smoking included more than 20,000 early adolescents from the United States, Germany and Mexico, and produced a pooled adjusted odds ratio of 2.32 (95% CI: 1.98–2.73) for adolescents smoking in the highest quartile of movie smoking exposure compared with the lowest quartile of exposure [18].

Similarly, a recent cross-sectional survey of more than 16,000 pupils recruited from six European countries (Iceland, Italy, Germany, the Netherlands, Poland and

Scotland), all with substantial differences regarding tobacco control policies, indicated a robust association between movie smoking exposure and youth smoking regardless of what country the adolescents lived in [22]. The sample quartile (Q) exposure was significantly associated with the prevalence of ever smoking: 14% of adolescents in Q1 had tried smoking, 21% in Q2, 29% in Q3 and 36% in Q4. The association remained after controlling for a number of covariates, including age, gender, family affluence, school performance, television screen time, number of movies seen, sensation seeking and rebelliousness and smoking within the social environment (peers, parents and siblings).

Longitudinal Observational Studies
Compared to cross-sectional studies, longitudinal studies have the methodological advantage of enabling the investigation of the incidence of behavioral transitions (smoking onset vs. becoming an established smoker) and in establishing temporality, placing the exposure (movie smoking) prior to these transitions.

A random-effect meta-analysis of six longitudinal studies, conducted in the United States, Germany and Mexico, included more than 20,000 early adolescents who had never smoked at baseline [18]; exposure to movie smoking was estimated by the Beach method. Outcome was the rate of smoking initiation during the observational period. A pooled covariate-adjusted relative risk of 1.76 (95% CI: 1.31–2.37) was found for adolescents in the highest quartile of movie smoking exposure compared with the lowest quartile of exposure.

A first cross-cultural comparison of the movie smoking effect was conducted with a German and a Northern New England cohort [17]. A very similar dose-response curve for the relation between a continuous measure of exposure to movies smoking and smoking initiation was found for the two cohorts, which is illustrated in figure 4, but with smoking incidence shifted higher in Germany, where tobacco faces fewer governmental controls compared to the US, and where youth smoking is consequently higher.

A second longitudinal cross-cultural comparison of the movie effect was carried out in six European countries – Iceland, Italy, Germany, the Netherlands, Poland and Scotland [23]. After 1 year, 17% of the 9,987 baseline never smokers initiated smoking. The crude relationship between movie smoking exposure and smoking initiation was significant in all countries. After controlling for a wide range of covariates, including age, gender, family affluence, school performance, TV screen time, personality characteristics, and smoking status of peers, parents and siblings, the

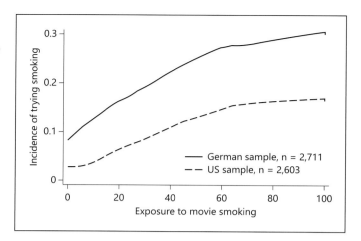

Fig. 4. Shape of the crude dose-response between exposure to movie smoking and adolescent smoking initiation, comparing the response curves for a German and a US adolescent sample. Of note, for the German sample, exposure was to 398 internationally distributed box-office hits in the German market; for the US sample, exposure was to 601 box-office hits in the North American market. Because the sample of movies for the US study was larger, those individuals had higher average levels of exposure to movie smoking. To compare the dose-response curves, we standardized movie smoking exposure for each study so that the lowest value was 0 and the highest was 100, with both distributions trimmed at the 95th percentile. For the German sample, the median (interquartile range) was 23 (7–48), and for the US sample it was 32 (18–56) (source Hanewinkel and Sargent [17]; reprinted with permission from the American Academy of Pediatrics, © 2008).

relationship remained significant in Germany, Iceland, the Netherlands, Poland and Scotland, but not Italy.

The study with the longest follow-up was conducted by Primack et al. [24]. A sample of 2,049 nonsmoking students was first surveyed at the age of 10–14 years and was followed up 7 years later. Results indicated that early exposure to movie smoking was significantly related to established smoking, defined as having smoked >100 cigarettes in their lives at follow-up when they were young adults.

Association between On-Screen Smoking and Population Trends in Smoking
Sargent and Heatherton [25] compared trends of smoking in the top 25 box-office hits each year from 1990 to 2007 with trends in adolescents smoking. Figure 5 illustrates a parallel downward trend for movie smoking and smoking among eighth graders from the Monitoring the Future surveys.

Jamieson and Romer [26] performed a content analysis of 15 movies randomly selected from the top 30 box-office hits each year from 1950 through 2006 (n = 825 movies). They

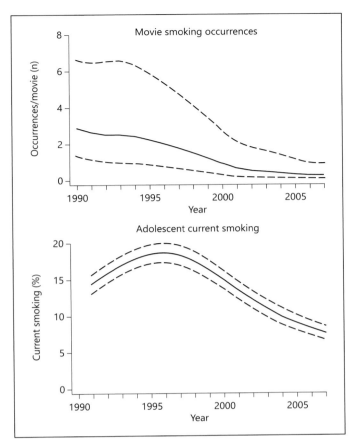

Fig. 5. Smoking occurrences in highest-grossing movies and adolescent smoking in the United States. Trends for the geometric mean for the number of smoking occurrences in the 25 movies with the highest US box-office gross revenues released each year between 1990 and 2007 and current (past 30-day) smoking among eighth graders from the Monitoring the Future study for each year between 1991 and 2007. Dashed lines indicate 95% confidence intervals (source Sargent and Heatherton [25]; reprinted with permission from the American Medical Association, © 2009).

Do Scientists Agree That the Movie Smoking-Youth Smoking Association Is Causal?

There is widespread agreement that smoking in movies is a key determinant of youth smoking. In 2012, the US Surgeon General determined that: 'The evidence is sufficient to conclude that there is a causal relationship between depictions of smoking in the movies and the initiation of smoking among young people' [18]. Longitudinal observational studies indicate a dose-response effect: the more smoking youth see, the more likely they are to smoke, with heavily exposed youth about two times as likely to begin smoking as lightly exposed youth. These initial results from the United States have been confirmed both qualitatively and quantitatively in other countries with different regulatory environments surrounding smoking and tobacco marketing (Germany, Iceland, Italy, Mexico, the Netherlands, New Zealand, Poland and Scotland). Because of the dose-response relationship, the World Health Organization (WHO) [27] has called for reductions in youth exposure to on-screen smoking by modernizing rating systems to give films with smoking a 'mature content' rating (e.g. 'R' in the United States, '18' in the United Kingdom and 'FSK-18' in Germany) to reduce youth exposure and the attendant smoking. The WHO Framework Convention on Tobacco Control recommended this measure as part of the implementation process of the convention in the countries. This policy has also been endorsed by the US Centers for Disease Control and Prevention, the New York State and Los Angeles County Health Departments, leading US national health and medical organizations as well as organizations outside the USA, such as the German alliance for tobacco control [ABNR (Aktionsbündnis Nichtrauchen)].

What to Do about Smoking in Movies

Movies are considered artistic expression in the United States. Therefore, their content is subject to first amendment protections of free speech, with government censorship of such content not allowable. Other countries do not allow movies such broad protections; however, most countries, regardless of how they regard censorship, control youth access to movies through their rating systems and would not allow overt censorship of movie content. There are two exceptions to this rule. Thailand requires pixilation of the cigarette image in movies, a process that electronically covers the image of the cigarette. India requires a subtext to be displayed during any scene with movie smoking.

compared the trend of tobacco use in movies and the per capita cigarette consumption among US adults. A downward trend for both outcomes, beginning in 1964–1965, could be found. Tobacco content declined considerably since 1950. Total tobacco-related content peaked around 1961, while the decline in portrayal of main character use was already underway in 1950. Cigarette consumption peaked around 1966 with a trend that closely paralleled total tobacco content and that coincided with major tobacco control events. The authors concluded that despite the inability to draw causal conclusions, tobacco portrayal in movies may serve as a barometer of societal support for the habit and thus efforts should continue to limit exposure to such content.

In the USA, the movie rating system is a voluntary system operated by the USA Motion Picture Association of America (MPAA) and the National Association of Theatre Owners. The ratings are intended to provide parents with advanced information so they can decide for themselves which films are appropriate for viewing by their children. Movie ratings in European countries also use age categories to classify films, but the rating systems differ substantially, not only from the MPAA system, but also within Europe. For example, there is high variance in the number of age categories used, ranging from only two categories in Belgium to 10 categories in Switzerland.

In a recent study, smoking content was present in over two thirds of a large sample of the most commercially successful movies (n = 464) shown in cinemas of six European countries and the United States between 2004 and 2009 [28]. Consistent with previous research, it was found that 'mature'-rated movies more often contain smoking episodes. Study results indicate that a substantially higher number of movies portraying smoking can be legally viewed by European youth than by US youth: 85% of the movies that portrayed smoking were 'youth' rated in Europe compared with only 59% in the USA.

Concerns over the effects of smoking in the movies on youth smoking initiation has led the WHO to call for reductions in youth exposure to movies that portray smoking in the implementation guidelines of Article 13 of the WHO Framework Convention on Tobacco Control [27]. Given that an outright ban on portrayal of smoking in movies is not a realistic option in most countries, most tobacco control policy makers are calling for a 'mature' rating for new movies including smoking. The WHO has taken up this suggestion and recommends reducing on-screen smoking as one key in the implementation guidelines of Article 13 of the Framework Convention on Tobacco Control. Addressing smoking through the rating system allows movie makers to still include smoking in the event they see it as integral to the artistic value of their film if they are willing to accept a mature rating. This policy option plays the artistic value of the film against the revenue that is lost when a film cannot be marketed to the adolescent market (contrary to the popular belief that youths flock to movies that are rated for adults, the adolescent viewership rate of most mature-rated movies is much lower than for youth-rated movies). Because most production companies would be unwilling to give up the adolescent market, it is thought that a mature rating for smoking would cause movie producers to eliminate smoking scenes from movies aimed at youth, just as they routinely eliminate scenes of violence of such movies now. The mature rating would represent only a partial solution to the health problems created by smoking in movies because, while less likely to see mature content-rated films than youth-rated films, youth still see some of these films and, thus, are exposed to their pro-tobacco influence. Despite widespread agreement that movie smoking is one cause of adolescent smoking, no country to date has integrated movie smoking into their movie ratings or movie censorship rules.

Many governments around the world go even further than tolerating rating systems that certify movies with tobacco use as appropriate for children and adolescents by funding the promotion of smoking to youth through generous subsidies to the movie industries. Government support ('state aid') for movie production currently makes no distinction between projects whose tobacco content plays an important role in recruiting adolescents to smoke and those that do not. It has been estimated that public subsidies for top-grossing movies with tobacco was more than EUR 1 billion between 2008 and 2011 in the USA, Canada, Australia, New Zealand and several European countries. Given the growing evidence of a causal link between exposure to tobacco imagery in movies and smoking initiation among youth, health experts have called governments to end their subsidies for movies with tobacco imagery [29].

To try to 'immunize' youth against the movie smoking exposure, the WHO and other organizations have recommended showing an antismoking advertisement before any film showing smoking. Hanewinkel et al. [30] assessed the effect of an antismoking advertisement under real-world conditions. A quasi-experimental study design in a multiplex cinema in Kiel, Germany, was realized. In the intervention condition (weeks 1 and 3), a 30-second antismoking advertisement accentuating long-term health consequences of smoking and promoting cessation was shown prior to all movies; in the control condition (weeks 2 and 4), no such spot was shown. A total of 4,073 patrons were surveyed after having viewed a movie. After controlling for gender differences, patrons exposed to the antismoking advertisement had (i) higher awareness of smoking in the movies, (ii) lower levels of approval of smoking in the movies, and (iii) a more negative attitude towards smoking in general compared with those not exposed. While these effects occurred at all ages, they were bigger in youth than in adults. In line with earlier experimental studies on youth in the United States and real-world observational studies in theaters in Australia, study results suggest the benefits of antismoking advertisements before smoking films is not heavily dependent upon the cultural context.

How Well Has the Movie Industry Done to Limit Smoking in Movies?

According to a recent report by Polansky et al. [8], up to now the major Hollywood studios or their parent companies have responded to the problem of on-screen smoking but in relatively modest ways:

(1) At their own expense, all MPAA member companies now add State of California-produced antitobacco spots to their youth-rated DVDs with smoking, which are distributed in the United States; movies distributed at theaters or aired on television are not preceded by antitobacco spots.

(2) Between 2005 and 2007, three MPAA member companies – Disney, Warner Bros. and Universal – published corporate policies related to tobacco depictions. In 2012 and 2013, the three other MPAA member companies – Fox, Sony and Paramount – followed.

(3) Most of these policies prohibit tobacco product placement deals with the companies themselves; none extend that stipulation to, or require certification of no payoffs from, the production companies contracted to make the films that the studios develop, finance, promote and distribute.

(4) Subjective language allows any youth-rated film to justify inclusion of tobacco imagery. None prohibits tobacco brand display in films they produce or distribute.

(5) Since 2007, the MPAA has added small-print 'smoking' labels to 12% of all youth-rated films with smoking.

Conclusion

There is ample theoretical reason to believe that actors smoking in movies would serve as models to adolescents, who are in the midst of determining their identity and are highly observant of the behaviors of others in their environment. There is also extensive empirical evidence to support the notion that exposure to movie smoking is one cause of adolescent smoking, along with functional magnetic reso-nance imaging to support the biological plausibility of this association. Several reviews conducted by bodies of behavioral scientists and reviewed by independent panels of scientists have concluded that movie smoking is one cause of adolescent smoking. Hollywood studios have decreased smoking depictions in their movies by integrating some oversight of smoking into the production process. Furthermore, it is known that more than half of current youth exposure to smoking in movies derives from youth-rated movies; therefore, a mature rating for smoking would limit about half of new exposure. Yet no country has adopted a mature rating for smoking into their movie censorship laws; this represents a serious failure of western governments to protect children from a key determinant of ill health.

Key Points

- Entertainment media, especially popular US movies, deliver billions of smoking images and character smoking depictions to young US adolescents and to adolescents worldwide. In addition, tobacco content is common in popular television programs in many countries.
- The US Surgeon General and the US National Cancer Institute concluded that the evidence from cross-sectional, longitudinal and experimental studies indicates a causal relationship between exposure to movie smoking depictions and youth smoking initiation.
- Concerns over the effects of smoking in the movies on youth smoking uptake has led the WHO to call for reductions in youth exposure to movies that portray smoking in the implementation guidelines of Article 13 of the WHO Framework Convention on Tobacco Control.
- Given that an outright ban on portrayal of smoking in movies is not a realistic option in most countries, most tobacco control policy makers are calling for a 'mature' rating for new movies including smoking.
- Showing an antismoking advertisement before any film showing smoking is another key prevention measure.

References

1 Strasburger VC: Pediatricians, schools, and media. Pediatrics 2012;129:1161–1163.
2 Bandura A: Social Foundations of Thought and Action: A Social Cognitive Theory. Englewood Cliffs, Prentice-Hall, 1986.
3 St Romain T, Hawley SR, Ablah E, Kabler BS, Molgaard CA: Tobacco use in silent film: precedents of modern-day substance use portrayals. J Community Health 2007;32:413–418.
4 Lum KL, Polansky JR, Jackler RK, Glantz SA: Signed, sealed and delivered: 'Big Tobacco' in Hollywood, 1927–1951. Tob Control 2008;17:313–323.
5 National Cancer Institute: The Role of Media in Promoting and Reducing Tobacco Use. Tobacco Control Monograph No. 19. Bethesda, US Department of Health and Human Services, National Institutes of Health, National Cancer Institute, 2008, NIH Publ No 07-6242.
6 Arora M, Mathur N, Gupta VK, Nazar GP, Reddy KS, Sargent JD: Tobacco use in Bollywood movies, tobacco promotional activities and their association with tobacco use among Indian adolescents. Tob Control 2012;21:482–487.
7 Bergamini E, Demidenko E, Sargent JD: Trends in tobacco and alcohol brand placements in popular US movies, 1996 through 2009. JAMA Pediatr 2013;167:634–639.

8 Polansky JR, Titus K, Lanning N, Glantz SA: Smoking in Top-Grossing US Movies. San Francisco, Center for Tobacco Control Research & Education, University of California, 2014.

9 Glantz SA, Iaccopucci A, Titus K, Polansky JR: Smoking in top-grossing US movies, 2011. Prev Chronic Dis 2012;9:120170.

10 Worth KA, Dal Cin S, Sargent JD: Prevalence of smoking among major movie characters: 1996–2004. Tob Control 2006;15:442–446.

11 Lyons A, McNeill A, Britton J: Tobacco imagery on prime time UK television. Tob Control 2014; 23:257–263.

12 Cullen J, Sokol NA, Slawek D, Allen JA, Vallone D, Healton C: Depictions of tobacco use in 2007 broadcast television programming popular among US youth. Arch Pediatr Adolesc Med 2011;165: 147–151.

13 McGee R, Ketchel J: Tobacco imagery on New Zealand television 2002–2004. Tob Control 2006; 15:412–414.

14 Hanewinkel R, Wiborg G: Smoking in contemporary German television programming. Int J Public Health 2007;52:308–312.

15 Sargent JD, Worth KA, Beach M, Gerrard M, Heatherton TF: Population-based assessment of exposure to risk behaviors in motion pictures. Commun Methods Meas 2008;2:134–151.

16 Sargent JD, Tanski SE, Gibson J: Exposure to movie smoking among US adolescents aged 10 to 14 years: a population estimate. Pediatrics 2007; 119:e1167–e1176.

17 Hanewinkel R, Sargent JD: Exposure to smoking in internationally distributed American movies and youth smoking in Germany: a cross-cultural cohort study. Pediatrics 2008;121:e108–e117.

18 US Department of Health and Human Services: Preventing Tobacco Use among Youth and Young Adults: A Report of the Surgeon General. Atlanta, US Department of Health and Human Services, Centers for Disease Control and Prevention, National Center for Chronic Disease Prevention and Health Promotion, Office on Smoking and Health, 2012.

19 Wagner DD, Dal Cin S, Sargent JD, Kelley WM, Heatherton TF: Spontaneous action representation in smokers when watching movie characters smoke. J Neurosci 2011;31:894–898.

20 Sargent JD, Morgenstern M, Isensee B, Hanewinkel R: Movie smoking and urge to smoke among adult smokers. Nicotine Tob Res 2009;11:1042–1046.

21 Shmueli D, Prochaska JJ, Glantz SA: Effect of smoking scenes in films on immediate smoking: a randomized controlled study. Am J Prev Med 2010;38:351–358.

22 Morgenstern M, Poelen EAP, Scholte RH, Karlsdottir S, Jonsson SH, Mathis F, Faggiano F, Florek E, Sweeting H, Hunt K, Sargent JD, Hanewinkel R: Smoking in movies and adolescent smoking: cross-cultural study in six European countries. Thorax 2011;66:875–883.

23 Morgenstern M, Sargent JD, Engels RC, Scholte RH, Florek E, Hunt K, Sweeting H, Mathis F, Faggiano F, Hanewinkel R: Smoking in movies and adolescent smoking initiation: longitudinal study in six European countries. Am J Prev Med 2013; 44:339–344.

24 Primack BA, Longacre MR, Beach ML, Adachi-Mejia AM, Titus LJ, Dalton MA: Association of established smoking among adolescents with timing of exposure to smoking depicted in movies. J Natl Cancer Inst 2012;104:549–555.

25 Sargent JD, Heatherton TF: Comparison of trends for adolescent smoking and smoking in movies, 1990–2007. JAMA 2009;301:2211–2213.

26 Jamieson PE, Romer D: Trends in US movie tobacco portrayal since 1950: a historical analysis. Tob Control 2010;19:179–184.

27 World Health Organization: Smoke-Free Movies: From Evidence to Action, ed 2. Geneva, WHO, 2011.

28 Hanewinkel R, Sargent JD, Karlsdottir S, Jonsson SH, Mathis F, Faggiano F, Poelen EA, Scholte R, Florek E, Sweeting H, Hunt K, Morgenstern M: High youth access to movies that contain smoking in Europe compared with the USA. Tob Control 2013;22:241–244.

29 Millett C, Hanewinkel R, Britton J, Florek E, Faggiano F, Ness A, McKee M, Polansky JR, Glantz SA: European governments should stop subsidizing films with tobacco imagery. Eur J Public Health 2012;22:167–168.

30 Hanewinkel R, Isensee B, Sargent JD, Morgenstern M: Effect of an antismoking advertisement on cinema patrons' perception of smoking and intention to smoke: a quasi-experimental study. Addiction 2010;105:1269–1277.

Prof. Reiner Hanewinkel, PhD
Institute for Therapy and Health Research, IFT-Nord
Harmsstrasse 2
DE–24114 Kiel (Germany)
E-Mail hanewinkel@ift-nord.de

Chapter 16

Loddenkemper R, Kreuter M (eds): The Tobacco Epidemic, ed 2, rev. and ext.
Prog Respir Res. Basel, Karger, 2015, vol 42, pp 181–198 (DOI: 10.1159/000369508)

Social Determinants of Cigarette Smoking

Dona Upson

New Mexico Veterans Affairs Health Care Services, and University of New Mexico, Albuquerque, N. Mex., USA

Abstract

As the tobacco epidemic has evolved, within countries and between them, tobacco dependence has become more stratified, increasingly affecting those less advantaged. Rates of illness and premature death are considerably higher for those in lower socioeconomic strata in most countries; much of that disparity is due to higher rates of smoking cigarettes. Disadvantage appears to be cumulative, with smoking rates over 60% for some groups with multiple attributes of risk. Those risks include mental illness, lower economic status and educational level, homelessness, disability, incarceration, military experience and some racial, ethnic and sexual minority identities. Some individuals are more susceptible to the harmful effects of tobacco because of genetic or environmental risk factors and/or comorbid conditions. It is highly likely that the changing face of the epidemic, from one affecting the population as a whole to one that affects specific segments, is a major contributor to health inequalities worldwide. Aggressive marketing by the tobacco industry has largely driven the high rates of tobacco dependence by people who lack advantage. Limited coping mechanisms to deal with high levels of stress and variations in the social acceptability of smoking contribute to the disparities. Marginalized groups have been disenfranchised from clinical research, as well as from society. Further study is needed, especially in methods to treat tobacco dependence. Action is of the utmost importance. There is good evidence that public health strategies work. Broad implementation of the tenets of the World Health Organization Framework Convention on Tobacco Control is needed to decrease the scourge of tobacco dependence worldwide.

© 2015 S. Karger AG, Basel

'The World Health Organization (WHO) has defined tobacco use as a marker of social inequity, because the health consequences of smoking are disproportionately borne by the most disadvantaged groups in society' [1, 2].

Some of the social determinants of health that influence tobacco use are common to many vulnerable populations. Low socioeconomic status (SES), unemployment and lack of access to health care cross racial, ethnic and geographic lines, but are more common among some minority populations. The minority stress model posits that the negative experiences endured by individuals because of their minority status culminate in a unique type and level of stress [3]. The importance of stigma – the 'co-occurrence of labeling, stereotyping, separation, status loss and discrimination in a context in which power is exercised' – is increasingly recognized [4]. It is pervasive and often insidious, negatively impacting social relationships and coping mechanisms, and has been associated with increased rates of smoking [4, 5]. Stigma is often compound, in that an individual may have several different attributes to which stigma is attached, thus further increasing their marginalization [5].

The tobacco industry has a very long history of aggressively marketing to youth and disenfranchised groups (see also chapters 1 and 14) [6]. As highlighted in the US Surgeon General's Report in 2000, 'Many public health and smoking prevention groups are concerned about the tobacco industry's practice of targeting cultural and ethnic minorities through product development, packaging, pricing, advertising and promotional activities' [7]. Targeted marketing provides acknowledgment and validation to some marginalized individuals and communities [8].

Point-of-sale advertising, cigarette displays and promotions by retailers are less tightly regulated than other types of marketing, and hence emphasized by the tobacco industry [9–11]. Henriksen [11] found that young adults (age 18–24 years) are twice as likely as older adults to make unplanned cigarette purchases in response to point-of-sale advertising (see also chapter 14) [12]. There is a higher density of point-of-sale advertising in stores located in areas of lower SES and in places where youth shop frequently, including close to schools [10, 12–14]. Lovato et al. [15] found that across five provinces in Canada, stores near schools with high smoking prevalence had significantly lower cigarette prices, more in-store promotions and fewer government-sponsored health warnings compared to those near schools with low smoking prevalence.

Socioeconomic Status

Low SES, based on a person's position in society due to social and economic factors, places people at risk for tobacco use [6, 2]. Tobacco use, in turn, contributes to poverty, with the poorest segments of society, in some of the poorest countries, spending more on tobacco than on food, housing or education [2, 16]. The burden from tobacco-related illness and premature death is having devastating health and economic consequences for low- and middle-income countries (LMIC) [17, 18]. The gap in prevalence rates of tobacco use between individuals at either end of the socioeconomic spectrum increases as countries move along the four stages of the tobacco epidemic (see also chapter 2). In the first stage, tobacco dependence begins primarily among men, with prevalence increasing rapidly during the next stage, concomitant with rising use among women. In the third stage, smoking begins to decline, especially among men. During the fourth, use continues to decrease, but SES inequalities become more obvious [19, 20]. With appropriate interventions, the as yet undefined next stage may represent progressive decreases in tobacco dependence among all segments of society.

Rates of illness and death are considerably higher for those in lower SES in most countries. Much of the disparity is due to different rates of tobacco use [19, 21]. Individuals between 35 and 69 years of age in disadvantaged groups are much more likely to die from tobacco-related illness than their higher SES counterparts, accounting for a third to a half of the difference in mortality rates [19, 21]. In England, 25% of manual workers smoke compared to 16% of other workers. Almost 50% of pregnant women in lower-level occupations in the UK have been found to be current smokers [19]. In the US, 16% of the population, 48.8 million people, lived below the federal poverty level in 2012 [22]; 27.9% of those adults were current smokers, compared with 23.6% of near-poor adults (100 to <200% poverty threshold] and 14.9% of the rest [23].

Smoking prevalence varies greatly by educational level. In the US, 41.9% of individuals with a general educational development certificate smoke cigarettes, compared with 24.5% of those with less than a high school diploma, 23.1% for high school graduates (without further education), 9.1% with an undergraduate degree and 5.9% with a graduate degree [24]. The general educational development test is available for people over 16 years of age who are not enrolled in school; passing the test certifies high school equivalency skills for the US and Canada. High smoking prevalence rates for those with a general educational development diploma have been consistent over time. The reasons are unknown. Although most of the data collected and research on SES and tobacco use have been done in high-income countries, the socioeconomic inequities are also widening in most LMIC [19].

Distinct from the usual objective measures of SES, subjective social status refers to an individual's perception of their place in society and is typically perceived in relationship to others [25]. While closely related to educational level, occupational status and material wealth, subjective social status encompasses quality of education, job-related control, workplace prestige, satisfaction with financial resources, experience with social inequities (e.g. discrimination or stigmatization), social trust, acculturation and beliefs about future opportunities and security [25]. Subjective social status is a strong independent and incremental predictor of self-related health, as well as for health indicators and behaviors. Even after adjusting for objective SES measures and demographic variables, people with higher subjective social status have better success quitting smoking. Reitzel et al. [25] also found that they are more likely to be nondaily smokers (p = 0.17), a trait mediated, at least in part, by greater life satisfaction (p = 0.003). Lower subjective social status is associated with lower positive affect, higher negative affect, less social support and more depressive symptoms, all of which can impact tobacco use [19, 25].

Although not as easily measured in youth, SES is also an important determinant of initiation of smoking cigarettes and continued use for them (see also chapter 14). The reasons include: greater likelihood of having parents, siblings and peers who smoke; targeted marketing, including higher density of tobacco retail outlets, advertising and promotions by the tobacco industry in disadvantaged locales, including near schools; less understanding of adverse health effects, and, possibly, more stressful lives with limited means of coping [19]. Having a greater number of people who smoke in one's environment impacts modeling behavior, access to cigarettes, ability to resist peer pressure and social norms, with the belief that more people smoke than actually do [19, 26].

The Global Youth Tobacco Survey (GYTS) does not measure SES; however, an increasing number of local and regional studies are documenting higher smoking rates and earlier initiation among less advantaged youth using proxy measures [26–30]. The Health Behavior in School-Aged Children survey uses 'family affluence' to estimate youth SES in 39 countries, mostly in Europe, Russia, Canada and the US [19]. The 2005/2006 survey found that adolescent girls from low-income families in countries in stage 4 of the tobacco epidemic (northern and western Europe, Canada and the USA) were more likely to smoke than those from higher-income families, an association that was not seen in stage 3 countries (Ukraine, Estonia and Russia). In northern Europe, 15-year-old girls from low-income families were also more likely to have started smoking before age 14 [19]. Data from the UK and the US have shown that disparities in tobacco use widen when other aspects of social disadvantage, such as some racial, ethnic and sexual minority identities, are included. Youth who leave school before graduating have among the highest rates of tobacco dependence [19, 24].

In India, the second most populous country in the world, 35% of people over age 15 years use tobacco; about 40% of them in its combustible forms [31]. GYTS data indicate that initiation rates appear to have stabilized since 2003, but India is experiencing the most rapid rise in tobacco-attributable deaths worldwide [28]. They are projected to increase from 1% in recent years to over 13% by 2020. Using the type of school attended (private or government, in urban settings) as a proxy for SES in 2004, Mathur et al. [28] initially found low SES youth 1.5 times more likely to be current tobacco users than those with higher SES. When that cross-sectional survey was continued longitudinally, however, it showed increasing trends toward tobacco use, which were especially pronounced in the higher SES students. By 2006, there was no longer a significant difference in prevalence rates; this shift was thought to have been mediated by increased 'Westernization' of high SES students [28].

As in wealthier countries, high levels of receptivity to advertising, greater numbers of family members and friends who use tobacco, normative beliefs and expectations, low levels of refusal skill efficacy and lack of awareness of the specific adverse health effects of tobacco use and benefits of cessation are all significantly associated with current tobacco use among India's youth [28, 32]. If India follows the 4-stage model of the tobacco epidemic, so that increasing

numbers of low SES youth will initiate and continue using tobacco and have more difficulty quitting than those of higher SES, the tobacco epidemic will rapidly accelerate, since 60–80% of children and adolescents live in low-resource settings [32].

In Chinese cities, middle and high school students in schools that have a low academic rank smoke at higher rates than those in better-ranked schools [19]. In China, 67% of adult men smoke and 3% of women [29]. Ding et al. [29] found that men with involuntary unemployment were more than six times more likely to smoke than those who were employed or retired.

Using 2007 GYTS data for Argentina, Linetzky et al. [26] found that 13- to 15-year-old students who attended schools receiving social assistance were more likely to smoke [adjusted odds ratio (AOR) 1.35, confidence interval (CI) 1.02–1.80] and/or buy single cigarettes (AOR 1.66, CI 1.08–2.54) than those attending schools that did not receive aid. Students who attended schools located in poor neighborhoods, but which were not necessarily receiving social assistance, were more likely to be exposed to secondhand smoke (AOR 1.27, CI 1.04–1.58). The overall prevalence of smoking was 31.1% for girls and 25.6% for boys [26].

There is a paucity of data on tobacco use from LMIC in sub-Saharan Africa. Youth (aged 13–18 years) with some measures of low SES in Ghana have been found to have higher levels of having ever used tobacco than their higher SES counterparts, although rates were relatively low overall [30]. In a cross-sectional study by Doku et al. [30], students' plans for postgraduation – continue schooling, learn a trade, look for a job, not sure – but not their school performance – were associated with tobacco use. A lower level of familial material affluence was associated with having ever used tawa, the local smokeless tobacco, but not with smoking cigarettes. Both smoking and tawa use were associated with a lower educational level of fathers, but not with parental occupation or maternal education. Death of one or, especially, both parents was strongly linked to both forms of tobacco use [30].

People with low SES are not only more likely to initiate smoking, they are less successful at cessation, although the desire to quit and number of attempts are similar [19, 33–35] (see chapters 16 and 18). The reasons are numerous and interrelated (fig. 1). Data from the English Smoking Toolkit have depicted similar numbers of quit attempts in the past year, with success rates of 11% in the lowest social grade compared with 20% in higher grades [35]. Similar findings have been replicated in many countries, especially those in the later stages of the tobacco epidemic [2]. In addition to cost barriers, people with low SES have concerns about the

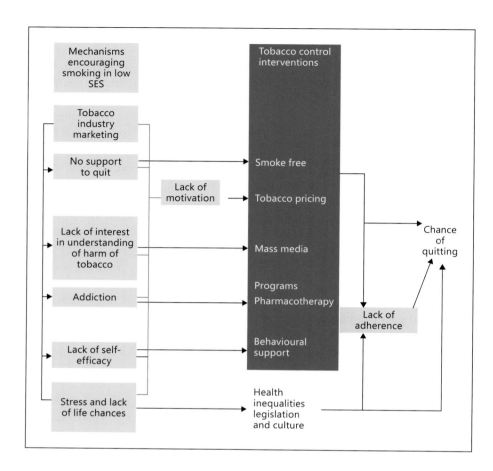

Fig. 1. Model of relationships among mechanisms encouraging smoking in low SES, tobacco control interventions and chances of quitting smoking [19].

safety of nicotine replacement therapy [19, 36]. They are more likely to discontinue pharmacotherapy prematurely and are less likely to complete counseling and support programs. It is unknown whether their lack of adherence causes relapse or vice versa. Health care providers in the US are less likely to address tobacco dependence in people with lower SES, and resources are not as available as for those with higher SES [19].

Persistent, nondirective social support for addressing tobacco dependence improves cessation rates, especially in the short term, and possibly has greater impact than health concerns [19]. Although having 'buddies' in tobacco dependence programs has not proven fruitful, work in China that focused on providing tobacco-related health information to nonsmoking mothers increased cessation among their partners [37]. People with low SES are more likely to be around people who smoke, which is known to hinder long-term success. Many people with low SES believe that smoking rates are higher than they are, and this may contribute to a lack of social pressure to quit [19]. The International Tobacco Control Survey found higher rates of nicotine addic-

tion among those with low SES, making social support and adequate treatment, including pharmacotherapy, more crucial [38]. Often by necessity, people with low SES are more likely to have a present-day orientation; the challenges of daily survival often supersede prospects of future negative health effects of tobacco or benefits of cessation [36].

As highlighted by the Centers for Disease Control and Prevention in 2013, 'addressing the social determinants of health (e.g. socioeconomic status, cultural characteristics, acculturation, stress, targeted advertising, price of tobacco products, and varying capacities of communities to mount effective tobacco-control initiatives) will be necessary to disrupt the cycle of smoking among low-socioeconomic status populations' [39].

Gender, Race and Ethnicity

Men continue to have significantly higher prevalence rates of current smoking than women in most countries: 20.5 compared to 15.8% in the US in 2012, respectively (see also

Table 1. Percentage of persons aged ≥18 years who were current cigarette smokers[1] – National Health Interview Survey, United States, 2012

Race/ethnicity[2]	Men, % (95% CI)	Women, % (95% CI)	Total, % (95% CI)
White	21.1 (19.9–22.2)	18.4 (17.4–19.3)	19.7 (18.9–20.4)
Black	22.1 (19.9–24.4)	14.8 (13.2–16.3)	18.1 (16.7–19.4)
Hispanic	17.2 (15.2–19.2)	7.8 (6.6–8.9)	12.5 (11.3–13.7)
American Indian/Alaska Native	25.5 (15.5–35.6)	18.7 (9.3–28.0)	21.8 (15.0–28.6)
Asian[3]	16.7 (13.7–19.8)	5.5 (4.0–7.0)	10.7 (9.1–12.3)
Multiple race	28.6 (21.0–36.3)	23.9 (17.6–30.2)	26.1 (21.3–31.0)

Adapted from Agaku et al. [40] (all material in the *MMWR* Series is in the public domain and may be used and reprinted without permission) .
[1] Persons who reported smoking ≥100 cigarettes in their lifetime and who were smoking every day or some days at the time of the interview.
[2] Unless otherwise indicated, all racial/ethnic groups are non-Hispanic; Hispanics can be of any race.
[3] Does not include Native Hawaiians or other Pacific Islanders.

chapter 2) [40]. Also in the US, by race and ethnicity, adults who reported being of multiple races had the highest prevalence of smoking, 26.1% (28.6% of men and 23.9% of women), and those of Asian descent had the lowest, 10.7% (16.7% of men and 5.5% of women; table 1) [40]. Within each of the broad categories used for racial/ethnic identity in the US, there are subgroups that represent more accurate identities and may better depict disparities in tobacco use. There is a tremendous cultural diversity among Asian Americans; smoking rates between 2002 and 2005 varied from 8.8% for Chinese Americans to 26.6% for Korean Americans [41]. Smoking prevalence in women ranged from 3.5% among Asian Indians to 20.1% among Koreans, and in men from 13.9% among Chinese to 37.4% among Koreans. Among Hispanic populations, Puerto Ricans had much higher rates of smoking than people of Central or South American origin; Mexicans and Cubans were in between [41].

Targeted marketing by the tobacco industry and variation in the social acceptability of smoking, in addition to differences in SES and education levels, account for much of the disparity between racial/ethnic groups as well as genders [40]. The tobacco industry has targeted American Indians and Alaska Natives by funding cultural events (powwows/rodeos) and using iconic symbols and designs in their cigarette packaging and advertising [42]. Counter advertising is complicated because tobacco is sacred for many American Indians, and its ceremonial use is important [42]. Many tribes profit from commercial sales of tobacco that are exempt from state taxes; lower prices offset the impact of that key element of tobacco control. Groups that garner a large proportion of their revenue from casinos may be hesitant to pass comprehensive smoke-free laws, in part due to concern that while people are outside smoking they are not inside gambling. Indigenous people in other high-income coun-

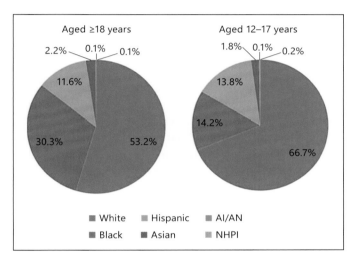

Fig. 2. Percent of menthol cigarette use among past-month cigarette smokers aged 12 years and older by race and ethnicity: 2004–2008, National Survey on Drug Use and Health (by courtesy of the Tobacco Products Scientific Advisory Committee [120]). AI/AN = Asian Indian/Alaska Native; NHPI = Native Hawaiian and Pacific Islander.

tries (Australia, New Zealand and Canada) also have rates of tobacco use that are much higher than the corresponding national populations [43, 44].

Some people are more susceptible to the harmful effects of tobacco because of genetic or environmental risk factors and/or comorbid conditions. In the US, among those who smoke less than 10 or between 11 and 30 cigarettes/day, African Americans and Native Hawaiians are more likely to develop lung cancer than are Whites, Latinos or Japanese Americans [45]. Targeted advertising of African Americans in the US has been identified in tobacco industry documents, especially for menthol brands, which are preferentially used by African Americans and women (fig. 2, 3) [46,

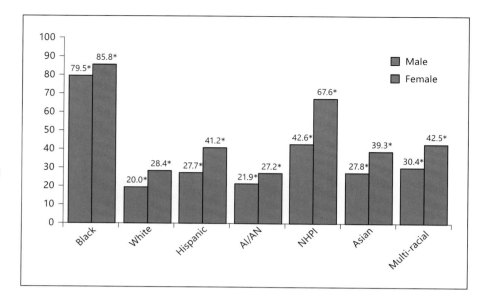

Fig. 3. Percent of menthol cigarette use among past-month cigarette smokers aged 12 years and older by race, ethnicity and gender: 2004–2008, National Survey on Drug Use and Health (by courtesy of the Tobacco Products Scientific Advisory Committee [120]). AI/AN = Asian Indian/ Alaska Native; NHPI = Native Hawaiian and Pacific Islander. Statistically significant differences are marked with an asterisk.

47]. There is disproportionate exposure to cigarette advertisements, on billboards and at point of sale, in neighborhoods with more African American residents [10, 14, 48]. Dauphinee et al. [48] found that African American students aged 11–15 years were three times more likely than other students to recognize the Newport brand and less likely to recognize Marlboro. Regardless of race, recognition of Newport cigarette advertising at baseline was associated with higher rates of smoking initiation within the next 12 months.

Tobacco imagery in film plays an important and well-established role in smoking initiation and continuation (see chapter 15) [6, 49–53]. Acknowledging substantial evidence from cross-sectional, longitudinal and experimental studies, the US Surgeon General's 2012 report stated that 'The evidence is sufficient to conclude that there is a causal relationship between depictions of smoking in movies and the initiation of smoking among young people' [49]. An estimated 37% of adolescent smoking initiation is attributed to exposure to smoking in movies [51, 52, 54].

Personal relevance may moderate the impact of depictions of tobacco use on smoking initiation [55]. African American youth in the US see more tobacco use in mainstream media than do White youth, but are less responsive to it, unless it is connected with African-American-oriented themes or characters [56, 57]. Among Mexican-born youth living in the US, exposure to smoking imagery in movies is a strong independent predictor of initiation, more so than for US-born Mexican American youth, possibly as part of the acculturation process [58]. Popular media are more influential among adolescents who are at low to moderate risk

for smoking, rather than those at either extreme [57]. Perhaps of greatest impact, the vast majority of popular films that are viewed in many countries are produced and/or distributed by US companies; 80% of them show images of smoking tobacco, almost always depicting lifestyle behavior to which youth aspire [59].

Individuals with lower education and/or income are more likely than others to smoke daily (vs. nondaily) in the US. However, race and ethnicity may be protective, with nondaily use among 24% of African American and 36% of Latino smokers, compared with 17% of non-Latino White smokers [25]. The prevalence of nondaily smoking has increased to 21.6% of all adult smokers [40]. Although some health risks are lower with less consumption, cardiovascular effects are not as easily mitigated (see also chapter 8). Health care providers may not offer the same degree of tobacco dependence counseling and treatment for those with intermittent use, and therapeutic modalities may need to be modified [25].

Homelessness

In high-income countries, people who experience homelessness have extremely high rates of tobacco use: more than 60% in the US and Canada. The numbers are even higher for White men (84%), those currently using alcohol (88%) or illicit drugs (81%), or those who have mental illness (79%) [60–62]. Two to 3.5 million people in the US experience homelessness every year [25, 63]. One million are served in federally supported emergency, or transitional

66 Centers for Disease Control and Prevention: Homelessness is a Risk Factor for TB. Atlanta, Centers for Disease Control and Prevention, 2012, http://www.cdc.gov/Features/dsTB2011Data/.

67 Haddad MB, Wilson TW, Ijaz K, Marks SM, Moore M: Tuberculosis and homelessness in the United States, 1994–2003. JAMA 2005; 293:2762–2766.

68 Centers for Disease Control and Prevention: TB in the Homeless Population. Atlanta, Centers for Disease Control and Prevention, 2013, http://www.cdc.gov/tb/topic/populations/Homelessness/default.htm.

69 Lindsay RP, Shin SS, Garfein RS, Rusch ML, Novotny TE: The association between active and passive smoking and latent tuberculosis infection in adults and children in the United States: results from NHANES. PLoS One 2014;9:e93137.

70 Bates MN, Khalakdina A, Pai M, Chang L, Lessa F, et al: Risk of tuberculosis from exposure to tobacco smoke: a systematic review and meta-analysis. Arch Intern Med 2007;167: 335–342.

71 US Department of Housing and Urban Development: HUD's 2013 Continuum of Care Homeless Assistance Programs: Homeless Populations and Subpopulations. 2013, https://www.hudexchange.info/reports/CoC_PopSub_NatlTerrDC_2013.pdf.

72 Gaetz S, Donaldson J, Richter T, Gulliver T: The State of Homelessness in Canada. Toronto, Canadian Homelessness Research Network Press, 2013, http://www.wellesleyinstitute.com/wp-content/uploads/2013/06/SOHC2103.pdf.

73 Apollonio DE, Malone RE: Marketing to the marginalised: tobacco industry targeting of the homeless and mentally ill. Tob Control 2005;14:409–415.

74 Baggett TP, Tobey ML, Rigotti NA: Tobacco use among homeless people – addressing the neglected addiction. N Engl J Med 2013;369: 201–204.

75 RJ Reynolds Tobacco: Project SCUM. 1995, bates No. 518021121/1129, http://legacy.library.ucsf.edu/tid/mum76d00.

76 Ling PM, Glantz SA: Using tobacco-industry marketing research to design more effective tobacco-control campaigns. JAMA 2002;287: 2983–2989.

77 Baggett TP, Anderson RH, Freyder PJ, et al: Addressing tobacco use in homeless populations: a survey of health care professionals. J Health Care Poor Underserved 2012;23:1650–1659.

78 Arnsten JH, Reid K, Bierer M, Rigotti N: Smoking behavior and interest in quitting among homeless smokers. Addict Behav 2004; 29:1155–1161.

79 Businelle MS, Cuate EL, Kesh A, Poonawalla IB, Kendzor DE: Comparing homeless smokers to economically disadvantaged domiciled smokers. Am J Public Health 2013; 103(suppl 2):S218–S220.

80 Okuyemi KS, Goldade K, Whembolua GL, Thomas JL, Eischen S, Guo H, et al: Smoking characteristics and comorbidities in the power to quit randomized clinical trial for homeless smokers. Nicotine Tob Res 2013;15:22–28.

81 Connor SE, Cook RL, Herbert MI, Neal SM, Williams JT: Smoking cessation in a homeless population: there is a will, but is there a way? J Gen Intern Med 2002;17:369–372.

82 Businelle MS, Kendzor DE, Kesh A, Cuate EL, Poonawalla IB, Reitzel LR, Oluyemi KS, Wetter DW: Small financial incentives increase smoking cessation in homeless smokers: a pilot study. Addict Behav 2014;39:717–720.

83 Jun H-J, Rich-Edwards JW, Boynton-Jarrett R, Wright RJ: Intimate partner violence and cigarette smoking: association between smoking risk and psychological abuse with and without co-occurrence of physical and sexual abuse. Am J Public Health 2008;98: 527–535.

84 Blosnich JR, Farmer GW, Lee JGL, Silenzio VMB, Bowen DJ: Health inequalities among sexual minority adults: evidence from ten U.S. states, 2010. Am J Prev Med 2014;46:337–349.

85 Corliss HL, Wadler BM, Jun H, Rosario M, Wypij D, Frazier AL, Austin SB: Sexual-orientation disparities in cigarette smoking in a longitudinal cohort study of adolescents. Nicotine Tob Res 2013;15:213–222.

86 Cochran SD, Bandiera FC, Mays VM: Sexual orientation-related differences in tobacco use and secondhand smoke exposure among US adults aged 20 to 59 years: 2003-2010 National Health and Nutrition Examination Surveys. Am J Public Health 2013;103:1837-1844.

87 Centers for Disease Control and Prevention: Tobacco product use among adults – United States, 2012–2013. MMWR Morb Mortal Wkly Rep 2014;63:542–547.

88 Kann L, Olsen EO, McManus T, et al; Centers for Disease Control and Prevention (CDC): Sexual identity, sex of sexual contacts, and health-risk behaviors among students in grades 9–12 – youth risk behavior surveillance, selected sites, United States, 2001–2009. MMWR Surveill Summ 2011;60:1–133.

89 Shelton J: National LGBT Health Education Center. Boston, Fenway Institute, 2014.

90 Blosnich JR, Horn K: Associations of discrimination and violence with smoking among emerging adults: differences by gender and sexual orientation. Nicotine Tob Res 2011;13: 1284–1295.

91 Stevens P, Carlson LM, Hinman JM: An analysis of tobacco industry marketing to lesbian, gay, bisexual, and transgender (LGBT) populations: strategies for mainstream tobacco control and prevention. Health Promot Pract 2004;5:129S–134S.

92 Smith EA, Offen N, Malone RE: What makes an ad a cigarette ad? Commercial tobacco imagery in the lesbian, gay, and bisexual press. J Epidemiol Community Health 2005;59:1086–1091.

93 Padilla J: New Mexico's Progress in Collecting Lesbian, Gay, Bisexual, and Transgender Health Data and Its Implications for Addressing Health Disparities. Albuquerque, New Mexico Department of Health, unpubl data.

94 US Department of Health and Human Services: Healthy People 2020. Topics and Objectives. Lesbian, Gay, Bisexual and Transgender Health. http://healthypeople.gov/2020/topicsobjectives2020/overview.aspx?topicid=25.

95 VanKim NA, Padilla JL, Lee JG, Goldstein AO: Adding sexual orientation questions to statewide public health surveillance: New Mexico's experience. Am J Public Health 2010;100:2392–2396.

96 Institute of Medicine: The Health of Lesbian, Gay, Bisexual, and Transgender People: Building a Foundation for Better Understanding. Washington, The National Academies, 2011.

97 Jones G, Sinclair L: Multiple health disparities among minority adults with mobility limitations: an application of the ICF framework and codes. Disabil Rehabil 2008;30: 901–915.

98 Courtney-Long E, Stevens A, Caraballo R, Ramon I, Armour BS: Disparities in current cigarette smoking prevalence by type of disability, 2009–2011. Public Health Rep 2014; 129:252–260.

99 Borrelli B, Busch AM, Trotter DRM: Methods used to quit smoking by people with physical disabilities. Rehabil Psychol 2013; 58:117–123.

100 Plummer SB, Findley PA: Women with disabilities' experience with physical and sexual abuse: review of the literature and implications for the field. Trauma Violence Abuse 2012;13:15–29.

101 Centers for Disease Control and Prevention (CDC): Racial/ethnic disparities in self-rated health status among adults with and without disabilities – United States, 2004–2006. MMWR Morb Mortal Wkly Rep 2008;57: 1069–1073.

102 Rutkow L, Vernick, JS, Tung GJ, Cohen JE: Creating smoke-free places through the UN Convention on the Rights of Persons with Disabilities. Am J Public Health 2013;103: 1748–1753.

103 Wagner P, Sakala L: Mass Incarceration: The Whole Pie – A Prison Policy Initiative Briefing. Northampton, Prison Policy Initiative, 2014, http://www.prisonpolicy.org/reports/pie.html.

104 Cropsey KL, Jones-Whaley S, Jackson DO, Hale GJ: Smoking characteristics of community corrections clients. Nicotine Tob Res 2010;12:53–58.

105 Cropsey K, Eldridge G, Weaver M, et al: Smoking cessation intervention for female prisoners: addressing an urgent public health need. Am J Public Health 2008;98:1894–1901.

106 Torchalla I, Strehlau V, Okoli CTC, Li K, Schuetz C, Krausz M: Smoking and predictors of nicotine dependence in a homeless population. Nicotine Tob Res 2011;13:934–942.

107 Centers for Disease Control and Prevention: Quick Stats: Current smoking among men aged 25 to 64 years, by age group and veteran status – National Health Interview Survey (NHIS), United States, 2007 to 2010. MMWR 2012;61:929, http://www.cdc.gov/tobacco/campaign/tips/resources/data/cigarette-smoking-in-united-states.html#asterisk.

108 Institute of Medicine: Combating Tobacco Use in Military and Veteran Populations. Washington, The National Academies, 2009.

109 Talcott GW, Cigrang J, Sherrill-Mittleman D, Snyder DK, Baker M, Tatum JL, Cassidy D, Sonnek S, Balderrama-Durbin C, Klesges RC, Ebbert JO, Slep AM Heyman RE: Tobacco use during military deployment. Nicotine Tob Res 2013;15:1348–1354.

110 Smith B, Ryan MAK, Wingard DL, Patterson TL, Slymen DJ, Macera CA; Millennium Cohort Study Team: Cigarette smoking and military deployment: a prospective evaluation. Am J Prev Med 2008;35:539–546.

111 CDC 2014. Military Service Members and Veterans. http://www.cdc.gov/tobacco/campaign/tips/resources/data/cigarette-smoking-in-united-states.html#asterisk.

112 Centers for Disease Control and Prevention: Best Practices for Comprehensive Tobacco Control Programs – 2007. Atlanta, US Department of Health and Human Services, Centers for Disease Control and Prevention, National Center for Chronic Disease and Health Promotion, Office on Smoking and Health, 2007.

113 Chaloupka FJ, Yurekli A, Fong GT: Tobacco taxes as a tobacco control strategy. Tob Control 2012;21:172–180.

114 Vijayaraghavan M, Messer K, White MM, Pierce JP: The effectiveness of cigarette price and smoke-free homes on low-income smokers in the United States. Am J Public Health 2013;103:2276–2283.

115 Farrelly MC, Nonnemaker JM, Watson KA: The consequences of high cigarette excise taxes for low-income smokers. PLoS One 2012;7:e43838.

116 Siahpush M, Thrasher JF, Yong HH, Cummings KM, Fong GT, Miera BS, Borland R: Cigarette prices, cigarette expenditure and smoking-induced deprivation: findings from the International Tobacco Control Mexico survey. Tob Control 2013;22:223–226.

117 Siahpush M, Borland R, Yong H: Sociodemographic and psychosocial correlates of smoking-induced deprivation and its effect on quitting: findings from the International Tobacco Control Policy Evaluation Survey. Tob Control 2007;16:e2.

118 Kostova D, Andes L, Erguder T, et al; Office on Smoking and Health, National Center for Chronic Disease Prevention and Health Promotion, CDC: Cigarette prices and smoking prevalence after a tobacco tax increase – Turkey, 2008 and 2012. MMWR Morb Mortal Wkly Rep 2014;63:457–461.

119 Zhou H, Tsoh JY, Grigg-Saito D, Tucker P, Liao Y: Decreased smoking disparities among Vietnamese and Cambodian communities – Racial and Ethnic Approaches to Community Health (REACH) Project, 2002–2006. MMWR Surveill Summ 2014; 63(suppl 1):37–45.

120 Tobacco Products Scientific Advisory Committee: Menthol cigarettes and public health: review of the scientific evidence and recommendations, submitted to FDA, 2011, http://www.fda.gov/downloads/AdvisoryCommittees/CommitteesMeetingMaterials/TobaccoProductsScientificAdvisoryCommittee/UCM269697.pdf.

Dona Upson, MD
New Mexico Veterans Affairs Health Care Services
Pulmonary, Critical Care & Sleep Medicine
111A-Pulm
1501 San Pedro SE
Albuquerque, NM 87108 (USA)
E-Mail djupson@aol.com

apy (CBT) approaches, individual and group counselling and health care provider interventions, with length of treatment associated with outcome [7]. CBT approaches typically target cognitions that may be acting as a barrier to quitting or encourage continued smoking (e.g. 'I can't cope with this, I need a smoke') by bringing these thoughts to the person's awareness and encouraging their replacement with more helpful thoughts. CBT will also target the reduction in behaviours associated with smoking that may help to maintain the addiction, and initiation of new behaviours that support smoking cessation/reduction and maintain cessation and avoid relapse (e.g. having a shower rather than a cigarette on first rising or avoiding going to the pub for a period of time). CBT has been used effectively for depression, anxiety and the positive symptoms of psychotic illness [61], and can be used to address both smoking and mental health symptoms concurrently [62]. CBT may also be enhanced by the addition of motivational interviewing to help the client build readiness to change by exploring and resolving ambivalence about change [63].

As mentioned previously, pharmacological interventions with evidence supporting use in people with mental health conditions include NRT, varenicline, nortriptyline, bupropion and clonidine (table 1; see also chapter 20) [7]. Emerging treatments that have not yet been evaluated in people with mental health conditions, but have some support in general population studies as smoking cessation aids, also hold promise. These include cytisine, extracted from the seed of *Cytisus laburnum* L. (Golden Rain acacia) and the substance from which varenicline is derived. Cytisine has been used as a smoking cessation aid for over 40 years in former Soviet economy countries [64]. Also, preliminary smoking cessation studies have been carried out on N-acetyl cysteine (NAC), the acetylated precursor to cysteine, which replenishes the antioxidant glutathione and modulates glutamatergic and inflammatory pathways (table 1). Glutathione is thought to have a role in the neurobiology of addiction, and some clinical trials also suggest potential utility of NAC for the treatment of cannabis and cocaine addiction [65]. Evidence is also emerging that NAC may be used for the symptomatic treatment of mental health conditions, including bipolar disorder, depression and schizophrenia [66].

Hitsman et al. [7] identified NRT, bupropion and varenicline as first-line medications for smoking cessation, with nortriptyline and clonidine as second-line medications, although their use was cautioned due to side effect profiles (table 1). It was also recommended that pharmacological and counselling interventions be combined to optimise outcomes. The evidence supporting these pharmacological and psychological interventions for smoking cessation in people with psychotic illness, major depression (MD), post-traumatic stress disorder (PTSD) and substance use disorders is described in the following.

People Diagnosed with Psychotic Disorders
Banham and Gilbody [6] have reviewed randomised controlled trials of smoking cessation interventions among people with severe mental illnesses, including schizophrenia, and schizo-affective, bipolar or delusional disorders. The primary outcome was smoking cessation, with secondary outcomes also reported (smoking reduction, change in weight, change in psychiatric symptoms and adverse events). Eight randomly controlled trials combining psychological interventions with either NRT or bupropion were reported to show moderately positive results, with point prevalence abstinence rates ranging from 4 to 22% at the final follow-up, which was compared with 4–43% in the general population and interpreted as approximately equally effective. Some studies reported reductions in smoking at some time points but not others. No studies reported a worsening of psychiatric symptomatology in the intervention versus control groups except for one study on day 2 (Abnormal Involuntary Movement Scale). Only one study reported data on changes in participants' weight. There were few adverse events. Banham and Gilbody [6] concluded that combined pharmaceutical and behavioural interventions are effective among people with severe mental illness, and recommended that general practitioners and secondary care services develop collaborative and tailored interventions to enhance acceptability and effectiveness.

Varenicline has also been evaluated among smokers with severe mental illness [67]. Recently, findings were reported from a randomised, double-blind, placebo-controlled, parallel-group, clinical trial on relapse prevention conducted among 247 smokers with schizophrenia or bipolar illness who received 12-week open-label varenicline and CBT [68]. Those who had 2 weeks or more of continuous abstinence at week 12 (n = 87) entered the relapse prevention intervention and were randomly assigned to receive CBT and double-blind varenicline (1 mg, 2 per day) or placebo up to week 52. Participants then discontinued study treatment and were followed up to week 76. At week 52, point prevalence abstinence rates were significantly different, 60% in the varenicline group (24 of 40) versus 19% (9 of 47) in the placebo group. From weeks 12 through 76, 30% (12 of 40) in the varenicline group versus 11% (5 of 47) in the placebo group reported continuous abstinence. As in the studies reviewed above, there were no significant treatment effects on psychiatric symptom ratings or psychiatric adverse events.

People Diagnosed with Major Depressive Disorder

Hitsman et al. [69] have recently conducted a systematic review and meta-analysis of 42 studies as to whether past MD is associated with smoking cessation. Most studies involved a combination of CBT and pharmacotherapy (n = 34) and CBT face to face only, and another four involved CBT self-help only. Overall, past MD was associated with a significant decrease in abstinence rates. Interestingly, among trials permitting recent MD episodes, those with depression performed better than those without depression when treated with CBT self-help. For those with past MD, buproprion, nortriptyline and NRT were recommended as effective. Only one trial had evaluated varenicline. The authors noted the possible antidepressant effects of these medications. They also recommended the addition of CBT for mood management in addition to CBT for smoking cessation with the aim of improving abstinence rates for smokers with past MD.

Weinberger et al. [70] examined the gender and racial composition in smoking cessation treatment studies published in the 2 decades between 1990 and 2010. They noted important gaps in the treatment literature, including (i) that the majority of the literature focuses on samples with lifetime MD rather than current MD, dysthymia and minor depression; (ii) lack of clarity regarding how smokers taking antidepressants respond to behavioural or pharmaceutical smoking cessation treatments; (iii) the need to identify treatments and treatment-related variables that can best assist woman smokers regarding the greater negative impact of depression on their smoking cessation outcomes; (iv) the lack of data on racial differences in the relationship of depression and smoking cessation outcomes; (v) the focus on depression rather than on smoking-related differences such as withdrawal symptoms, cue reactivity and smoking reward between those with and without depression, and (vi) the absence of information regarding the concurrent or sequential delivery of treatment.

Post-Traumatic Stress Disorder

The results of a multisite randomised controlled trial have recently been reported among 943 smokers with military-related PTSD who were recruited from outpatient PTSD clinics and followed up for 18–48 weeks. Smoking cessation treatment was either integrated within mental health care for PTSD delivered by mental health clinicians (integrated)

or delivered following referral to Veterans Affairs smoking cessation clinics. Integrated care delivered CBT for smoking cessation and pharmacological treatment (NRT, bupropion or varenicline) if desired by the participant. Integrated care was significantly better than smoking cessation clinics on prolonged abstinence (8.9 vs. 4.5%) with differences largest at 6 months for 7-day point prevalence abstinence. Participants in the integrated condition attended significantly more sessions and took medication for a longer time period. Number of counselling sessions received and days of cessation medication used explained 39.1% of the treatment effect. Between baseline and 18 months, psychiatric status did not differ between treatment conditions. PTSD symptoms improved for the sample as a whole, with non-quitters worsening slightly on the Patient Health Questionnaire relative to quitters. The authors recommended integration of smoking cessation treatment into mental health care.

People with Alcohol and Other Drug Disorders

Smoking rates among drug treatment populations range from 74 to 100% [71–75]. Smokers with alcohol and drug disorders are more likely to die from tobacco-related causes [76], such as cardiovascular disease, cancer, stroke and chronic lung disease, than from causes related to the use of any other drug. Prochaska et al. [8] conducted a meta-analysis of smoking cessation interventions with individuals in substance use treatment or recovery, reporting on 18 randomised controlled trials. Post-treatment abstinence rates collapsing across treatment studies were 12% in the intervention condition and 3% in the comparison condition (non-significant). In a subgroup analysis, more recently published treatment studies that provided NRT indicated significant effects. For participants in recovery, there was a significant 77% increase in the likelihood of smoking abstinence among intervention versus control participants. At the long-term follow-up, there was no difference in abstinence rates between conditions. Smoking cessation interventions were associated with a significant 25% increased likelihood of long-term abstinence from alcohol and other drugs. The authors thus concluded that, contrary to widely held views, smoking cessation interventions during substance use treatment enhance substance use outcomes.

A review of smoking cessation interventions among individuals in methadone maintenance treatment reported on the results of five randomised controlled trials and three pre-test post-test non-equivalent group designs [9]. Approaches included pharmacotherapy incentives (increases in methadone dose), CBT and counselling usually in conjunction with NRT. Smoking cessation interventions were associated with a significant reduction in smoking and expired carbon monoxide but not abstinence. No study reported any worsening in substance abuse. The authors suggested either increased intensity of treatment or new strategies are required with this population. They further suggested that maintenance treatment may be required for smoking cessation, alongside methadone maintenance. Furthermore, the authors noted that none of the intervention components addressed specific mental health issues faced by participants and that integration of treatment for mental health issues such as depression may be important.

some subgroups such as methadone maintenance patients. Certainly, integration of smoking cessation treatment into mental health or substance use treatment seems indicated, with provision of pharmacotherapy of adequate dosage and duration. The development of pharmacotherapies which address multiple symptoms, such as nicotine withdrawal and symptoms of anxiety and depression, enhancing cognition and motivation (with a negligible side effect profile) are a priority. Staff and management of treatment facilities should work further to develop policies conducive to smoking cessation to allow dissemination of evidence-based treatment into practice as new treatments emerge.

Conclusions

In a previous review of the smoking cessation literature [77], it was noted that further reductions in the prevalence of smoking are unlikely to be achieved unless specific attention and interventions are directed to high-prevalence subgroups. We recommend that while the high rates of smoking are associated with low socio-economic status, limited education and other factors, there are specific and potentially correctable factors associated with smoking that need to be considered for each sub-population. Although Banham and Gilbody [6] have noted that similar abstinence rates can be achieved among people with mental health problems in the general community, abstinence rates are variable, diminished in the longer term and abstinence is elusive among

Key Points

- Dysregulated balance between brain reward and brain aversion systems may promote addiction to nicotine.
- Improved pharmacological treatments for nicotine addiction may include specific modulators of hypothalamic receptor systems, metabotropic glutamate receptors and specific nicotinic acetylcholine receptor subunits.
- Unique interactions between nicotine and the pathophysiology of an illness may necessitate different approaches to smoking interventions.
- Smoking cessation interventions consisting of behavioural and pharmacological approaches should be available within mental health and substance use treatment settings.
- Smoking cessation does not worsen mental health symptoms or alcohol and other drug use.

References

1 Lasser K, Boyd J, Woolhandler S, Himmelstein DU, McCormick D, Bor DH: Smoking and mental illness: a population-based prevalence study. JAMA 2000;284:2606–2610.

2 Williams JM, Ziedonis D: Addressing tobacco among individuals with a mental illness or an addiction. Addict Behav 2004;29:1067–1083.

3 Degenhardt L, Hall W: The Relationship between Tobacco Use, Substance Use Disorders and Mental Disorders: Results from the National Survey of Mental Health and Well-Being. Sydney, National Drug & Alcohol Research Centre, UNSW, 1999.

4 Cook B, Wayne G, Kafali E, Liu Z, Shu C, Flores M: Trends in smoking among adults with mental illness and association between mental health treatment and smoking cessation. JAMA 2014; 311:172–182.

5 Siru R, Hulse GK, Tait RJ: Assessing motivation to quit smoking in people with mental illness: a review. Addiction 2009;104:719–733.

6 Banham L, Gilbody S: Smoking cessation in severe mental illness: what works? Addiction 2010;105: 1176–1189.

7 Hitsman B, Moss TG, Montoya ID, George TP: Treatment of tobacco dependence in mental health and addictive disorders. Can J Psychiatry 2009;54:368–378.

8 Prochaska JJ, Delucchi K, Hall SM: A meta-analysis of smoking cessation interventions with individuals in substance abuse treatment or recovery. J Consult Clin Psychol 2004;72:1144–1156.

9 Okoli CTC, Khara M, Procyshyn RM, Johnson JL, Barr AM, Greaves L: Smoking cessation interventions among individuals in methadone maintenance: a brief review. J Subst Abuse Treat 2010;38: 191–199.

10 Castagnoli K, Steyn S, Magnin G, Van Der Schyf C, Fourie I, Khalil A, et al: Studies on the interactions of tobacco leaf and tobacco smoke constituents and monoamine oxidase. Neurotox Res 2002; 4:151–160.

11 Corrigall W, Coen K: Nicotine maintains robust self-administration in rats on a limited-access schedule. Psychopharmacology 1989;99:473–478.

12 Koob GF, Le Moal M: Neurobiological mechanisms for opponent motivational processes in addiction. Philos Trans R Soc Lond B Biol Sci 2008;363:3113–3123.

13 Caille S, Clemens K, Stinus L, Cador M: Modeling nicotine addiction in rats. Methods Mol Biol 2012; 829:243–256.

14 Edwards S, Koob GF: Escalation of drug self-administration as a hallmark of persistent addiction liability. Behav Pharmacol 2013;24:356–362.

15 Ahmed SH, Kenny PJ, Koob GF, Markou A: Neurobiological evidence for hedonic allostasis associated with escalating cocaine use. Nat Neurosci 2002;5:625–626.

16 Changeux J-P: Nicotine addiction and nicotinic receptors: lessons from genetically modified mice. Nat Rev Neurosci 2010;11:389–401.

17 Bossert J, Marchant N, Calu D, Shaham Y: The reinstatement model of drug relapse: recent neurobiological findings, emerging research topics, and translational research. Psychopharmacology 2013;229:453–476.

18 Clemens K, Caillé S, Cador M: The effects of response operandum and prior food training on intravenous nicotine self-administration in rats. Psychopharmacology 2010;211:43–54.

19 Koob GF: A role for brain stress systems in addiction. Neuron 2008;59:11–34.

20 Picciotto MR, Mineur YS: Molecules and circuits involved in nicotine addiction: the many faces of smoking. Neuropharmacology 2014;76(pt B):545–553.

21 Exley R, Maubourguet N, David V, Eddine R, Evrard A, Pons S, et al: Distinct contributions of nicotinic acetylcholine receptor subunit α4 and subunit α6 to the reinforcing effects of nicotine. Proc Natl Acad Sci 2011;108:7577–7582.

22 Orejarena MJ, Herrera-Solís A, Pons S, Maskos U, Maldonado R, Robledo P: Selective re-expression of β2 nicotinic acetylcholine receptor subunits in the ventral tegmental area of the mouse restores intravenous nicotine self-administration. Neuropharmacology 2012;63:235–241.

23 Fowler CD, Lu Q, Johnson PM, Marks MJ, Kenny PJ: Habenular α5 nicotinic receptor subunit signalling controls nicotine intake. Nature 2011;471:597–601.

24 Pons S, Fattore L, Cossu G, Tolu S, Porcu E, McIntosh J, et al: Crucial role of α4 and α6 nicotinic acetylcholine receptor subunits from ventral tegmental area in systemic nicotine self-administration. J Neurosci 2008;28:12318–12327.

25 Caillé S, Guillem K, Cador M, Manzoni O, Georges F: Voluntary nicotine consumption triggers in vivo potentiation of cortical excitatory drives to midbrain dopaminergic neurons. J Neurosci 2009;29:10410–10415.

26 Reisiger A-R, Kaufling J, Manzoni O, Cador M, Georges F, Caillé S: Nicotine self-administration induces CB1-dependent LTP in the bed nucleus of the stria terminalis. J Neurosci 2014;34:4285–4292.

27 Hikosaka O: The habenula: from stress evasion to value-based decision-making. Nat Rev Neurosci 2010;11:503–513.

28 McCallum SE, Cowe MA, Lewis SW, Glick SD: α3β4 nicotinic acetylcholine receptors in the medial habenula modulate the mesolimbic dopaminergic response to acute nicotine in vivo. Neuropharmacology 2012;63:434–440.

29 Frahm S, Ślimak MA, Ferrarese L, Santos-Torres J, Antolin-Fontes B, Auer S, et al: Aversion to nicotine is regulated by the balanced activity of β4 and α5 receptor subunits in the medial habenula. Neuron 2011;70:522–535.

30 Görlich A, Antolin-Fontes B, Ables JL, Frahm S, Ślimak MA, Dougherty JD, et al: Reexposure to nicotine during withdrawal increases the pacemaking activity of cholinergic habenular neurons. Proc Natl Acad Sci U S A 2013;110:17077–17082.

31 Bierut L, Stitzel J, Wang J, Hinrichs A, Grucza R, Xuei X, et al: Variants in nicotinic receptors and risk for nicotine dependence. Am J Psychiatry 2008;165:1163–1171.

32 Hung RJ, McKay JD, Gaborieau V, Boffetta P, Hashibe M, Zaridze D, et al: A susceptibility locus for lung cancer maps to nicotinic acetylcholine receptor subunit genes on 15q25. Nature 2008;452:633–637.

33 Saccone NL, Schwantes-An TH, Wang JC, Grucza RA, Breslau N, Hatsukami D, et al: Multiple cholinergic nicotinic receptor genes affect nicotine dependence risk in African and European Americans. Genes Brain Behav 2010;9:741–750.

34 Thorgeirsson TE, Geller F, Sulem P, Rafnar T, Wiste A, Magnusson KP, et al: A variant associated with nicotine dependence, lung cancer and peripheral arterial disease. Nature 2008;452:638–642.

35 Boutrel B, Kenny PJ, Specio SE, Martin-Fardon R, Markou A, Koob GF, et al: Role for hypocretin in mediating stress-induced reinstatement of cocaine-seeking behavior. Proc Natl Acad Sci U S A 2005;102:19168–19173.

36 Harris GC, Wimmer M, Aston-Jones G: A role for lateral hypothalamic orexin neurons in reward seeking. Nature 2005;437:556–559.

37 Hollander JA, Lu Q, Cameron MD, Kamenecka TM, Kenny PJ: Insular hypocretin transmission regulates nicotine reward. Proc Natl Acad Sci U S A 2008;105:19480–19485.

38 Corrigall WA: Hypocretin mechanisms in nicotine addiction: evidence and speculation. Psychopharmacology 2009;206:23–37.

39 Yeoh JW, Campbell EJ, James MH, Graham BA, Dayas CV: Orexin antagonists for neuropsychiatric disease: progress and potential pitfalls. Front Neurosci 2014;8:36.

40 Plaza-Zabala A, Martín-García E, de Lecea L, Maldonado R, Berrendero F: Hypocretins regulate the anxiogenic-like effects of nicotine and induce reinstatement of nicotine-seeking behavior. J Neurosci 2010;30:2300–2310.

41 James MH, Charnley JL, Levi EM, Jones E, Yeoh JW, Smith DW, et al: Orexin-1 receptor signalling within the ventral tegmental area, but not the paraventricular thalamus, is critical to regulating cue-induced reinstatement of cocaine-seeking. Int J Neuropsychopharmacol 2011;14:684–690.

42 Lerman C, LeSage MG, Perkins KA, O'Malley SS, Siegel SJ, Benowitz NL, et al: Translational research in medication development for nicotine dependence. Nat Rev Drug Discov 2007;6:746–762.

43 Simonnet A, Cador M, Caille S: Nicotine reinforcement is reduced by cannabinoid CB1 receptor blockade in the ventral tegmental area. Addict Biol 2013;18:930–936.

44 Markou A: Metabotropic glutamate receptor antagonists: novel therapeutics for nicotine dependence and depression? Biol Psychiatry 2007;61:17–22.

45 Carlsson A, Carlsson ML: A dopaminergic deficit hypothesis of schizophrenia: the path to discovery. Dialogues Clin Neurosci 2006;8:137–142.

46 Kumari V, Postma P: Nicotine use in schizophrenia: the self medication hypotheses. Neurosci Biobehav Rev 2005;29:1021–1034.

47 Chambers RA: A nicotine challenge to the self-medication hypothesis in a neurodevelopmental animal model of schizophrenia. J Dual Diagn 2009;5:139–148.

48 Smith GN, Wong H, MacEwan GW, Kopala LC, Ehmann TS, Thornton AE, et al: Predictors of starting to smoke cigarettes in patients with first episode psychosis. Schizophr Res 2009;108:258–264.

49 Velligan DI, Mahurin RK, Diamond PL, Hazleton BC, Eckert SL, Miller AL: The functional significance of symptomatology and cognitive function in schizophrenia. Schizophr Res 1997;25:21–31.

50 Hong LE, Schroeder M, Ross TJ, Buchholz B, Salmeron BJ, Wonodi I, et al: Nicotine enhances but does not normalize visual sustained attention and the associated brain network in schizophrenia. Schizophr Bull 2011;37:416–425.

51 Sacco KA, Termine A, Seyal A, et al: Effects of cigarette smoking on spatial working memory and attentional deficits in schizophrenia: involvement of nicotinic receptor mechanisms. Arch Gen Psychiatry 2005;62:649–659.

52 Smith RC, Singh A, Infante M, Khandat A, Kloos A: Effects of cigarette smoking and nicotine nasal spray on psychiatric symptoms and cognition in schizophrenia. Neuropsychopharmacology 2002;27:479–497.

53 Barr RS, Culhane MA, Jubelt LE, Mufti RS, Dyer MA, Weiss AP, et al: The effects of transdermal nicotine on cognition in nonsmokers with schizophrenia and nonpsychiatric controls. Neuropsychopharmacology 2007;33:480–490.

54 Depatie L, O'Driscoll GA, Holahan A-LV, Atkinson V, Thavundayil JX, Kin NNY, et al: Nicotine and behavioral markers of risk for schizophrenia: a double-blind, placebo-controlled, cross-over study. Neuropsychopharmacology 2002;27:1056–1070.

55 George TP, Vessicchio JC, Termine A, Sahady DM, Head CA, Pepper WT, et al: Effects of smoking abstinence on visuospatial working memory function in schizophrenia. Neuropsychopharmacology 2002;26:75–85.

56 Adler LE, Hoffer LD, Wiser A, Freedman R: Normalization of auditory physiology by cigarette smoking in schizophrenic patients. Am J Psychiatry 1993;150:1856–1861.

57 Turetsky B, Dent G, Jaeger J, Zukin S: P50 amplitude reduction: a nicotinic receptor-mediated deficit in first-degree relatives of schizophrenia patients. Psychopharmacology 2012;221:39–52.

58 Hong LE, Wonodi I, Lewis J, Thaker GK: Nicotine effect on prepulse inhibition and prepulse facilitation in schizophrenia patients. Neuropsychopharmacology 2007;33:2167–2174.

59 George TP, Termine A, Sacco KA, Allen TM, Reutenauer E, Vessicchio JC, et al: A preliminary study of the effects of cigarette smoking on prepulse inhibition in schizophrenia: involvement of nicotinic receptor mechanisms. Schizophr Res 2006;87:307–315.

Similar results derived from the National Health Interview Survey showed that smokers who attained a college degree (compared to those who did not finish high school) were up to 83% more likely to achieve abstinence lasting greater than 7 months [27]. Indeed, US prevalence data indicate that, each year, approximately 11% of smokers who have attained a college degree are able to quit smoking for at least 6 months, compared to only 3.4% among smokers with less than 12 years of education, despite much less discrepancy in quitting attempts [12] (fig. 1). Due to observed discrepancies in the prevalence of tobacco smoking and successful quitting across SES stratifications, researchers have concluded that low SES smokers experience multiple disadvantages (e.g. greater perceived stress, and lower social support, self-efficacy for quitting and treatment access/adherence) that may have an additive effect on cessation outcomes [25].

Smoking-Related Factors That Have Been Shown to Influence Cessation

Nicotine/Tobacco Dependence and Smoking Behavior before Cessation

Nicotine/tobacco dependence may be characterized by a range of factors, including tolerance (e.g. needing more of the substance to produce desired effects), withdrawal effects (e.g. craving, irritability, depression, anxiety, insomnia and increased appetite) and indices of smoking heaviness (e.g. frequency and quantity of tobacco smoking). Widely used measures of this construct include the Fagerström Test for Nicotine Dependence (FTND) [28] (see chapter 5) and the Heaviness of Smoking Index (HSI) [29], which is comprised of two FTND items that assess the number of cigarettes smoked per day and the time to the first cigarette after waking. In general, individuals who smoke more and/or score higher on measures of nicotine/tobacco dependence tend to be *less likely to attempt* smoking cessation and *more likely to relapse* following a quit attempt [30]. Whereas FTND scores have been shown to predict smoking cessation, converging data, including the results of population-based studies in the UK, US, Canada and Australia, indicate that the two HSI items tend to be the strongest predictors of abstinence outcomes [31]. Furthermore, it appears that a single item on the FTND and HSI (i.e. the latency to the first cigarette in the morning) may predict relapse to smoking as well, if not better than longer multidimensional measures [32]. The latency to the first cigarette has been described as an item that taps a pattern of heavy, uninterrupted and au-

tomatic smoking [32], and quit rates appear to be highest among those who report smoking their first cigarette after 60 min or later after waking (36%), and lowest among those who report smoking within 5 min of waking (8%) [11]. Finally, there is some evidence that the predictive utility of these measures may be most robust during the early period (i.e. 1 week to 1 month) of a quit attempt [33] and decline precipitously following approximately 3 months of smoking abstinence [14].

Nicotine/Tobacco Withdrawal Symptoms

The nicotine/tobacco withdrawal syndrome has been described as an aversive state characterized by a constellation of cognitive-affective, behavioral and physiological symptoms, including craving to smoke, anxiety, depression, irritability, difficulty concentrating, sleep disturbance, restlessness, decreased heart rate and increased appetite [34] (see also chapter 5). Withdrawal symptoms begin to emerge within 30 min of smoking abstinence [34], typically peak within the first 3 days of quitting and last for up to 4 weeks following smoking cessation [35], though there is substantial heterogeneity across individuals with respect to the duration and pattern of nicotine withdrawal [36]. Although nicotine withdrawal has long been considered an important antecedent of relapse to smoking, variability in the timing and measurement of specific withdrawal symptoms has contributed to somewhat inconsistent findings across studies [37]. Despite these limitations, recent research has highlighted the predictive utility of self-reported craving to smoke, but only when measured over the first few days following a quit attempt [38]. Withdrawal-induced negative affect (e.g. anxiety or depression) has also been shown to predict cessation outcomes [14, 35], with some evidence that anxiety may evince the most robust pattern of relations [39]. Other withdrawal symptoms found to predict relapse include sleep disturbance [14] and concentration difficulties [39]. Finally, converging evidence from studies that utilized ecological momentary assessment and/or daily diaries indicates that spikes in nicotine/tobacco withdrawal symptoms tend to immediately precede relapse to smoking [40]. There is also some evidence that smokers who perceive themselves as having greater control over their withdrawal symptoms may be less likely to relapse [41].

Motivation and Self-Efficacy for Quitting

Motivational factors associated with smoking cessation include expressed desire and readiness or intention to engage a serious quit attempt [14, 42]. Overall, the extant empirical literature indicates that although motivational factors consistently predict *attempts* to quit smoking [14], such factors have less utility in the prediction of *smoking abstinence*. A recent systematic review of prospective general population studies found that, whereas measures of motivation to stop smoking were highly predictive of future quit attempts, only measures of nicotine/tobacco dependence were consistently predictive of success in those attempts [30]. Similar data gleaned from the ITC (the International Tobacco Control) Four Country Project suggested that although motivation is necessary to prompt a quit attempt, such motivation is not sufficient to predict the maintenance of cessation [42]. However, it is also important to note that some researchers have conceptualized motivation as more of a dynamic process that peaks during the early stages of a quit attempt and diminishes with the passage of time [43]. Indeed, the few studies that have measured motivation at multiple time points following a quit attempt have demonstrated sharp declines in abstinence motivation prior to relapse [43].

In contrast to motivation for smoking cessation, there is converging evidence that greater self-efficacy or confidence in one's ability to abstain from smoking is predictive of both future quit attempts *and* successful quitting [30]. For example, among self-quitters (i.e. those not seeking treatment for tobacco addiction), greater levels of confidence/self-efficacy are consistently associated with more successful quitting and abstinence from smoking for greater than 6 months [44]. In addition, the results of a recent prospective study revealed that smokers who reported greater self-efficacy for smoking cessation during the first few weeks following a quit attempt were less likely to relapse [41]. Finally, a meta-analysis revealed differences in the predictive utility of self-efficacy/confidence for quitting depending on the timing of assessment, such that relations between self-efficacy and future smoking were observed to be fairly modest when assessed before quitting and stronger when assessed after quitting [45]. These authors concluded that many studies may overestimate the magnitude of self-efficacy-abstinence relations due to a failure to appropriately control for smoking behavior at the point of assessment.

Other Individual Differences Associated with Smoking Cessation

Comorbid Depression and Anxiety
Symptoms of anxiety and depression are more prevalent among smokers than nonsmokers [46], and there is reason

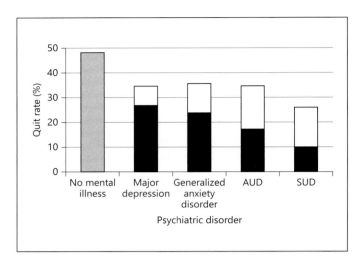

Fig. 2. Quit rate for individuals with no lifetime history of mental illness (leftmost column) versus history of select psychiatric diagnoses during the past year (solid bar) and any point in their life (full bar) in the United States. Data were derived from the National Epidemiologic Survey on Alcohol and Related Conditions, 2001–2002 [50]. Quit rate was defined as the proportion of lifetime smokers who were not current smokers (i.e. had not smoked in the past year) at the time of the survey.

to suspect that relations between smoking and symptoms of anxiety/depression may be bidirectional in nature [47] (see also chapter 17). There is also evidence that smokers with comorbid anxiety/depression may be more dependent on nicotine and have a harder time quitting. For example, the findings of two nationally representative US health surveys indicated that individuals with anxious/depressive disorders tended to be heavier smokers who evinced greater physiological dependence on tobacco [48] and experienced more severe withdrawal when attempting to quit [49]. Consistent with these findings, results derived from the 2001–2002 US National Epidemiologic Survey on Alcohol and Related Conditions revealed that a greater percentage of ever smokers with no history of psychiatric disorders reported having successfully quit smoking (48%), compared to those with a history of major depression during the past year (27%) or at any point in their life (35%), and those with a history of generalized anxiety disorder during the past year (24%) or at any point in their life (35%) [50] (fig. 2). There is also converging prospective evidence that smokers who meet diagnostic criteria for either anxiety [51] or depressive disorders [52] prior to quitting may be less likely to engage a quit attempt and more likely to relapse. Finally, there is some empirical evidence to support the notion that tailored cog-

Table 1. Clinical manifestations of disordered motivation systems in the brain [33]

- Excessive engagement in addictive behaviors, often at higher frequencies/quantities than intended
- Persistent desire for, and unsuccessful attempts at, behavioral control
- Adverse impact on social function or interpersonal relationships
- Continued use despite persistent or recurrent physical or psychological consequences
- A narrowing of the behavioral repertoire related to environmental cues and emotional triggers
- Ambivalence about ameliorative action despite recognition of problems with continued use
- Increased sensitivity to stressors and recruitment of brain stress systems, such that 'things seem more stressful' as a result

fers to the activities or decisions made in the course of caring for patients with tobacco dependence. In contrast, organizational responsibilities extend beyond the boundary of self to incorporate the systems and processes expected to influence the probability of abstinence among a patient population [23, 24]. The third perspective, less frequently considered, is the institutional responsibility. In the sociological context of the word, institution refers not to a specific building, but the well-established and structured patterns of behavior that are accepted as a fundamental part of the health care culture. Our institutional responsibilities refer to the long-established customs that frame assumptions and resource dedication, as we pursue solutions to this monumental threat to health.

The Professional's Individual Role
The evidence that the advice and support given to smokers by health care professionals can achieve abstinence rates of 5–10% with minimal interventions, and 15–30% with more intense interventions, is well established [25] and has been available for several decades [26, 27]. Given that nearly 80% of adults have contact with the primary care setting each year, the potential population health impact of integrating sophisticated tobacco use treatment into the primary care context is enormous [28, 29]. Providers will identify tobacco use status and will frequently make directive recommendations that the patient works toward abstinence, particularly when tobacco use is related to the reason for acute presentation [30, 31]. However, clinicians are much less likely to engage in the 'next steps' consistent with sophisticated management of chronic illness [32].

Clinical interventions can be quite effective in altering the course of nicotine addiction. Close monitoring of the patient's behaviors and aggressive pharmacologic management over prolonged periods of time contribute dramatically to positive clinical outcomes [25]. Clinicians should seek not to simply change behavior but also to assess control of the underlying compulsion to smoke (table 1) [33] (see also chapters 5 and 6). Excessive focus on 'quit rates' ob-

scures other equally important markers of clinical impact, including sustained periods of remission, decreased frequency and intensity of relapse, and optimized control over smoking-related illnesses during periods of remission [14].

Pharmacologic support is an effective mechanism for minimizing emotional barriers to cessation (see also chapter 20). By reducing withdrawal symptoms, improving control over the compulsion to smoke and offering a mechanism for the smoker to be actively engaged in addiction treatment, pharmacotherapy represents an extremely powerful tool for minimizing the impact of compulsion and the associated ambivalence about abstinence. Generally speaking, as the intensity of tobacco use treatment increases, outcomes improve. A number of treatment strategies have been recommended by the US Public Health Service as both cost and clinically effective (table 2) [25] (for details see chapter 20). Excellent toolkits are also available that help guide clinicians in the implementation of these strategies within a practice setting [34, 35].

Nearly 20% of people seek complementary and alternative treatments prior to seeking conventional medical care [36]. In addition to pharmacologic support, providers should be prepared to address questions about the utility of alternative methods of cessation, such as hypnotherapy, acupuncture, acupressure and auricular therapy. Although proposed to act by weakening the desire to smoke and strengthening the will to stop, and widely promoted as methods to aid smoking cessation, the effects described in uncontrolled studies have been notoriously difficult to confirm in randomized controlled trials [37]. Recent rigorous evidence-based reviews suggest there is no clear evidence of a benefit for either acupuncture or hypnotherapy [38, 39]. Acupuncture was less effective than nicotine replacement therapy, and hypnotherapy did not have a greater effect than any other intervention or no therapy. When a patient indicates an interest in either of these methods, rather than be dismissive, the health care professional recognizes the opportunity to engage the patient in a discussion about why

Table 2. Effectiveness and abstinence rates for various medications and medication combinations compared to placebo 6 months after quitting (n = 83 studies)

Medication	Arms, n	Estimated odds ratio (95% CI)	Estimated abstinence rate (95% CI)
Placebo	80	1.0	13.8
Monotherapies			
Varenicline, 2 mg/day	5	3.1 (2.5–3.8)	33.2 (28.9–37.8)
Nicotine nasal spray	4	2.3 (1.7–3.0)	26.7 (21.5–32.7)
High-dose nicotine patch (>25 mg; standard or long-term duration)	4	2.3 (1.7–3.0)	26.5 (21.3–32.5)
Long-term nicotine gum (>14 weeks)	6	2.2 (1.5–3.2)	26.1 (19.7–33.6)
Varenicline, 1 mg/day	3	2.1 (1.5–3.0)	25.4 (19.6–32.2)
Nicotine inhaler	6	2.1 (1.5–2.9)	24.8 (19.1–31.6)
Clonidine	3	2.1 (1.2–3.7)	25.0 (15.7–37.3)
Bupropion SR	26	2.0 (1.8–2.2)	24.2 (22.2–26.4)
Nicotine patch (6–14 weeks)	32	1.9 (1.7–2.2)	23.4 (21.3–25.8)
Long-term nicotine patch (>14 weeks)	10	1.9 (1.7–2.3)	23.7 (21.0–26.6)
Nortriptyline	5	1.8 (1.3–2.6)	22.5 (16.8–29.4)
Nicotine gum (6–14 weeks)	15	1.5 (1.2–1.7)	19.0 (16.5–21.9)
Combination therapies			
Patch (long term; >14 weeks) + ad libitum NRT (gum or spray)	3	3.6 (2.5–5.2)	36.5 (28.6–45.3)
Patch + bupropion SR	3	2.5 (1.9–3.4)	28.9 (23.5–35.1)
Patch + nortriptyline	2	2.3 (1.3–4.2)	27.3 (17.2–40.4)
Patch + inhaler	2	2.2 (1.3– 3.6)	25.8 (17.4–36.5)
Patch + second generation antidepressants (paroxetine/venlafaxine)	3	2.0 (1.2–3.4)	24.3 (16.1–35.0)

NRT = Nicotine replacement therapy (adapted from Fiore et al. [25]).

those methods are appealing. Understanding the request as either (1) an expression of underlying ambivalence, (2) a response to prevalent myths about pharmacotherapy or (3) an expression of self-reliance allows both parties to work together to develop a trusting and respectful tobacco treatment plan.

Fundamental to exploring counseling methods as part of the health care professional's individual role is the realization that no single approach or message is sufficient to meet the myriad needs of dependent patients. The professional caring for tobacco-dependent patients will find it useful to begin by first considering the question 'What can I do to help *this* patient with *this* problem at *this* time?' In this manner, success is individually defined, and overemphasis on unrealistic goals is avoided. Understanding tobacco dependence as the behavioral manifestation of a chronic illness of the brain, *defined* by the patient's lack of readiness to abstain, shifts the clinical imperative 'forward' – toward intervening with all tobacco users, not only the small minority of tobacco users who might affirm readiness while at the office [40, 41] (see also chapters 5 and 6). Familiarity with proven approaches for dealing with ambivalence can help clinicians

be more effective and can help uneasy patients find the resolve necessary to take the fateful next steps (fig. 1). Motivational interviewing is the technique by which providers can enhance motivation to change by focusing on the obstacles to cessation and resolving ambivalence [42]. Through reflective listening and addressing disincentives without judgment or confrontation, this approach allows providers to engage in a meaningful conversation with their patients. The goal is for the patient to seek his/her own reasons for change, or not to change, recognizing that pushing against resistance only amplifies it. 'Reluctance' is not unique to smoking. Physicians face reluctance in their daily practice in a myriad of ways. Perhaps it is reluctance to begin a new inhaler or to get the annual flu vaccine. Or maybe it is an unwillingness to wear oxygen or engage in physical therapy. We accept reluctance as part of our routine interactions with patients, and we accept the responsibility of managing reluctance so that our patients enjoy the best possible outcomes.

Addressing tobacco dependence within the established paradigm of chronic illness management includes ensuring the patient's integral need for long-term follow-up is met. Health care professionals can more completely affect their

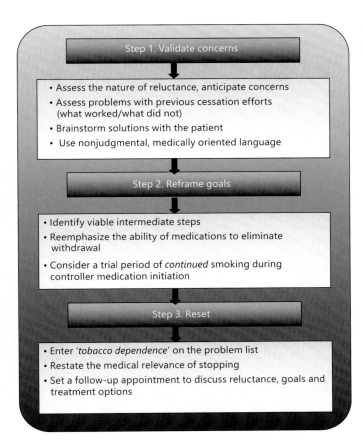

Step 1. Validate concerns

- Assess the nature of reluctance, anticipate concerns
- Assess problems with previous cessation efforts (what worked/what did not)
- Brainstorm solutions with the patient
- Use nonjudgmental, medically oriented language

Step 2. Reframe goals

- Identify viable intermediate steps
- Reemphasize the ability of medications to eliminate withdrawal
- Consider a trial period of *continued* smoking during controller medication initiation

Step 3. Reset

- Enter *'tobacco dependence'* on the problem list
- Restate the medical relevance of stopping
- Set a follow-up appointment to discuss reluctance, goals and treatment options

Fig. 1. A simple 3-step plan for successfully working through patient reluctance [35].

individual role responsibilities by ensuring follow-up visits are arranged, in order to assess the patient's response to interventions, manage factors that place the patient at risk for relapse and to reassert control at the earliest stages of illness exacerbation [25, 32, 34]. The chronic disease paradigm shifts attribution of culpability away from the patient (i.e. continued smoking as a failure of motivation) [43] and more appropriately onto the biology of addiction (i.e. continued smoking is an uncontrolled compulsion) in a manner consistent with our own long-standing, research-based position on addictions [44].

While brief tobacco cessation interventions are effective, more intensive longitudinal interventions are more effective and most cost-effective [45]. Evidence-based guideline recommendations for treating tobacco use as a chronic medical condition through sophisticated and longitudinal pharmacologic approaches are available for free, and can help clinicians feel empowered to intervene, even on the most addicted of their patients [25, 34]. Unfortunately, the degree to which individual clinicians have adopted these recommen-

dations has remained less than ideal [46–49]. Clinicians have reported prohibitive time requirements, treatment ineffectiveness, disinterest among patients, lack of reimbursement and lack of self-efficacy as rationales for lacking engagement in tobacco treatment [50, 51]. However, these explanations are inconsistent with both the observed patterns of evidence uptake in other difficult chronic illnesses and the widespread availability of reimbursement for professional services [34, 52–55]. Beliefs regarding illness causation, and inferences about responsibility in the matter, profoundly influence the willingness to invest effort in help giving [56]. Even medical students distinguish between onset-controllable and onset-uncontrollable problems, and are more willing to prescribe drugs for the latter, even though disease severities and distress are equal [57]. Awareness of our visceral reactions to stigmatized individuals and the potential implications of this emotional response is a crucial component of the health care professional's individual responsibility for minimizing the observed disparities in diagnosis rates and treatment outcomes among dependent patients [58].

The Professional's Organizational Role

A large number of organizational health care changes have been proposed to help reduce the prevalence of tobacco use among patients served. Direct organizational interventions, such as the creation of smoke-free hospital environments, provision of telephone- or text-based counseling, or implementation of systematic health risk assessments, for example, are intended to primarily influence patient behaviors. Conversely, indirect organizational interventions, such as integration of computerized decision support tools into electronic health record systems, health care financing incentives or changes in quality metrics are intended to influence the tobacco-related behaviors of providers. The main threat to the successful execution of the organizational role of health care in controlling the epidemic is the tendency of people and organizations under uncertain or difficult conditions to identify only a satisfactory solution to a complex problem, not necessarily the optimum one [59]. This principle, termed 'satisficing', has been identified as the dominant process at play in response to a number of implementation challenges. For example, it is clear that managers who work in publicly funded health care institutions first consider their first-hand knowledge of organizational idiosyncrasies when engineering responses to regulatory mandates, and only later integrate external knowledge such as research and guidelines [60, 61]. Satisfied solutions encourage continuation of behaviors that fall short of optimal effectiveness [62, 63]. In a stark example of the concept, efforts to increase the rates at which smoking status was identified among hospitalized patients, with counseling delivered to current smokers, were dramatically successful in terms of the number of organizations that met this quality metric but disappointing in terms of the impact on smoking status [64, 65].

With this in mind, the professional's organizational role becomes ensuring that systems are built that not only allow the organization to claim compliance with regulatory requirements but also align with the professional goals of reducing tobacco use prevalence. Governments play an important role in protecting our health, yet there is no substitute for clinician leadership in ensuring that the spirit of the selected regulatory response remains firmly aimed at improving patient-centered outcomes [66, 67]. Models of organizational responsibility that link reimbursement schemes to disease-specific quality metrics within the population served by the organization show promise [68, 69]. However, it remains unclear how prepared the system is to achieve population-based goals in contrast to its ability to meet process goals [70].

The Professional's Institutional Role

Consider for a moment the set of professional norms and cooperative relationships that govern the behavior of individuals within the community of health care. These mechanisms of social order reflect our professional values and are a direct expression of our desire to maximize the health benefits derived by the patients we serve [71]. Both the norms and the relationships align with our social purpose, and transcend individual or organizational goals. An analogy may help to make the point. Once we have identified hypertension as a threat to well-being, for example, the inherent values of the institution of health care would naturally compel members to (1) create evidence-based clinical systems, which are designed to address the problem using methods derived from insights into pathophysiology; (2) identify the individual role and responsibilities of various members of the health care team, and define the functional relationships between members accordingly, in a manner that maximizes effectiveness; (3) ensure that appropriate resources and services were made available to people who need them; (4) transmit accumulated knowledge from one generation to the next in order to ensure impact permanence, and (5) provide for quality improvement efforts in order to refine systems of care and improve outcomes. A hypothetical professional who settled for hypertension interventions that exist outside of these norms, for example an exclusive reliance on self-help materials or the im-

Table 3. Comparison of current health care culture surrounding prevalent chronic illnesses

	Hypertension	Tobacco dependence
Context of care		
Screening	+	+
Initiate pharmacotherapy	+	±
Multidisciplinary coordination	+	
Subspecialty care	+	
Inpatient care	+	±
Transition management	+	
Training models		
Undergraduate curriculum	+	±
Postgraduate training	+	
Role definitions	+	
Professional society standards	+	±
Demonstrated competence	+	
Research		
Transtheoretical coherence	+	±
Integration into theory of practice	+	±
Professional society standards	+	
Subspecialty training	+	
Policy integration		
Dissemination of information	+	±
Community member involvement		±
Integrate with other institution goals		±
Outcome accountability	±	±

passioned admonition to 'get better', would likely be viewed by peers as 'different' and be subject to cultural pressures to behave more appropriately. As is the case for most chronic illnesses, institutional norms related to hypertension would not allow for excessive flexibility in either the individual or organizational roles to an extent that allows our fiduciary responsibilities to the patient to be sacrificed. Analogously, the health care professional's institutional responsibility to affect the tobacco epidemic involves ensuring the application of these same norms and relationships to the problem of tobacco dependence, vis-à-vis the same established models employed to tackle other chronic illnesses (table 3).

The central activity of the institution of health care involves providing the context for care – the functional framework within which professionals assume their varied individual roles. In the outpatient care arena, for example, institutional norms include resources for the provision of both primary and specialty care, each delivered by means of the cooperative relationships between professionals from various disciplines, such as social work, nursing, medicine and behavioral health, among others. No single element of the framework is responsible for the whole of outpatient care, nor is every element expected to perform the same role. It is the functional relationships between entities that define the comprehensive nature of care. The context for the provision of tobacco dependence treatment has not yet reached this level of institutional integration, despite being recognized as a singularly prevalent cause of death and disability [72]. Imagine a set of cultural norms for tobacco use treatment that mirrors the context of care for other chronic illnesses, a context of care within which primary care clinicians are responsible for identifying tobacco dependence, initiating care, coordinating the execution of a comprehensive care plan that includes input from various disciplines and referring the subset of particularly complex patients to specialty providers, themselves prepared with more highly specific resources aimed at the longitudinal control of tobacco dependence.

The context also naturally involves the care of hospitalized smokers. However, despite being perceived by health care professionals as an ideal time to intervene on dependence, opportunities are frequently foregone in instances where the reason for admission was unrelated to smoking or when patients are perceived as unreceptive to advice [73, 74]. The need to avoid alienating patients paradoxically leads providers to avoid interacting with the very patients who show the cardinal signs of disease.

A core feature of the institutional norms guiding our role in chronic illness management is the requirement for specialized training. Health care professionals are allowed preeminent authority over the practice of health care by the community, but this social contract requires demonstrated mastery of content, state licensure or some other tangible means of assuring professional standing. Undergraduate and postgraduate training settings are the responsibility of professional schools, academic medical centers and professional societies, which together ensure that curricula are aligned with current scientific understanding of pathogenesis, treatment and system implementation. Training objectives and methods are designed to be delivered incrementally, within a system of graded responsibility, and consistent with the role and education level of the trainee. Tobacco dependence is a chronic illness in desperate need of similar educational formalization [75–78]. Health care disciplines that already have certification processes in place, such as medicine and nursing, should include metrics that reflect mastery of the most current understanding of the disorder, and in disciplines that do not yet have a formal state certification process, tobacco treatment specialists, for example, should continue to work toward that goal. In this manner, the treatment of tobacco dependence would achieve generational continuity within the community of health care professionals and ensure patients that our social contract with them remains intact, even if they smoke.

The institutional role of the health care professional also includes the dissemination of our understanding of illness causation, cure and prevention into the community at large. Dissemination takes several forms, including policy development, direct involvement of community members in pursuit of the health care mission, integration of the goals of other institutions' (e.g. the institutions of business or education) and efforts to improve the outcome accountability of health care to the community at large [79, 80]. The tobacco epidemic is a perfect example of a problem that requires high-level cooperation between various agents, including departments of health, community leadership organizations, local businesses, charitable organizations and payor groups, in order to simultaneously address the social, environmental and biological determinants of the epidemic [8, 81].

Conclusion

While the lay public's perspectives on tobacco use may not differ substantially from the 17th century opinion of King James I, the scientific community's understanding of the problem has evolved dramatically over the last 100 years. Insights into the biological mechanisms by which the brain translates into the mind have given us new tools with which to impact one of the major preventable public health disasters in history. When considering the role of health care, it is useful to consider the three interwoven cardinal perspectives separately. Providers might explore their individual responsibilities by expanding their definitions of success, becoming more intimately familiar with their levers for effecting change and focusing their tobacco-related efforts on achieving long-term control over the compulsion to smoke. The emphasis on restricting interventions to the subset of patients found 'willing' at the moment of interaction has the unfortunate effect of leaving the vast majority of patients without access to care for their disease of the brain. Organizational efforts are being brought to bear on the problem, increasing the chances that the health care professional might impact the prevalence of illness in a meaningful way. There is no substitute for the health care professional's leadership in ensuring that organizational interventions remain targeted at improving patient-centered outcomes and that satisficed solutions are avoided.

Institutional norms related to tobacco dependence, by virtue of their fundamental power to supersede the influence of individual and organizational responsibilities, must be systematically reexamined for health care professionals to begin making a substantive impact on the epidemic. Despite, or perhaps because of, its prevalence, tobacco dependence seems to have been excluded from the very same institutional structures that have evolved over the modern era of health care, which make us effective at dealing with chronic illness. Imagine how much more effective health care professionals would be if the norm was for tobacco-related roles and responsibilities to be both horizontally integrated across disciplines and vertically integrated across levels of specialization. Imagine what an impact we might have if our cultural expectation was for every health care trainee, of every discipline impacted by tobacco, to be required to demonstrate proficiency in handling reluctance, the cardinal sign of dependence, prior to certification in their respective field. Imagine, finally, where we might be today if the institutional mission of health care had been to destigmatize purposefully the illness of tobacco dependence in a manner analogous to our approach to other stigmatized conditions, encouraging the afflicted to engage with us without fear of judgment or shame.

While the role of population-based interventions remains unquestioned, the role of the health care professional in reducing the toll of the tobacco epidemic has been less clear. Though many have concluded that the reach of health care professionals is limited due to the necessary one-on-one nature of their interactions with smokers, practitioners interact with patients on over 1.1 billion annual instances in the United States alone [82]. The potential impact of this level of access to dependent patients is enormous.

Given that tobacco smoking is responsible for a major portion of preventable death and disability, imagine what health care can accomplish with a few hundred million chances to make an impact.

Key Points

- Nicotine activates cholinergic receptors in the survival centers of the brain, creating a powerful but artificial safety signal and 'hijacking' fundamental survival functions.
- Nicotine addiction is a primary, chronic disorder of the reward, motivation and memory circuits of the brain, manifesting as altered motivational hierarchies that can be both confusing and frustrating to the patient and the clinician.
- The role of the health care professional can be conceptualized as providing for long-term control over the compulsion to smoke in this relapsing and remitting, chronic illness of the brain.
- *Individual* professional responsibilities include providing evidence-based treatments, ensuring follow-up visits are arranged, assessing the response to therapy, managing factors that place the patient at risk for relapse and reasserting control at the earliest stages of illness exacerbation.
- *Organizational* professional responsibilities include ensuring systems are in place that encourage the reduction of tobacco use prevalence in the community.
- *Institutional* professional responsibilities include the full integration of tobacco use treatment into the existing norms and relationships of health care.

Acknowledgements

This work was supported in part by grants derived from the Pennsylvania Master Settlement Agreement through the Pennsylvania Department of Health and the National Institutes of Health (R01 CA136888 and P30 CA016520).

References

1 King James I (England). A counterblaste to tobacco. London, R.B., 1604, p 38, http://books.google.co.uk/books?id=EasUAAAAYAAJ&ots=QUl7Wbc KAz&dq=a%20counterblaste%20to%20tobacco&pg=PT6#v=onepage&q&f=false.

2 Johnston LM, Glasg MB: Tobacco smoking and nicotine. Lancet 1941;i:867.

3 Finnegan JK, Larson PS, Haag HB: The role of nicotine in the cigarette habit. Science 1945;102: 94–96.

4 Henningfield JE, Miyasato K, Jasinski DR: Abuse liability and pharmacodynamic characteristics of intravenous and inhaled nicotine. J Pharmacol Exp Ther 1985;234:1–12.

5 Hughes JR, Hatsukami D: Signs and symptoms of tobacco withdrawal. Arch Gen Psychiatry 1986;43: 289–294.

6 US Department of Health and Human Services: The Health Consequences of Smoking: Nicotine Addiction: A Report of the Surgeon General (1988). http://profiles.nlm.nih.gov/NN/B/B/Z/D/ (accessed August 7, 2014).

7 Brady JV, Lukas SE (eds): Testing Drugs for Physical Dependence Potential and Abuse Liability. Rockville, Department of Health and Human Services, National Institute of Drug Abuse, 1984, http://archives.drugabuse.gov/pdf/monographs/52.pdf (accessed August 7, 2014).

8   US Department of Health and Human Services: The Health Consequences of Smoking – 50 Years of Progress: A Report of the Surgeon General. Atlanta, US Department of Health and Human Services, Centers for Disease Control and Prevention, National Center for Chronic Disease Prevention and Health Promotion, Office on Smoking and Health, 2014, http://www.ncbi.nlm.nih.gov/books/NBK179276/ (accessed April 13, 2014).

9   US Department of Health and Human Services: How Tobacco Smoke Causes Disease: The Biology and Behavioral Basis for Smoking-Attributable Disease: A Report of the Surgeon General. Atlanta, US Department of Health and Human Services, Centers for Disease Control and Prevention, National Center for Chronic Disease Prevention and Health Promotion, Office on Smoking and Health, 2010, http://www.ncbi.nlm.nih.gov/books/NBK53017/ (accessed April 14, 2014).

10 Leone FT, Evers-Casey S: Behavioral interventions in tobacco dependence. Prim Care 2009;36:489–507.

11 Henningfield J: Behavioral pharmacology of cigarette smoking. Adv Behav Pharmacol 1984;4:131–210.

12 Stolerman I: Animal Models for Nicotine Dependence. Understanding Nicotine and Tobacco Addiction. Chichester, Wiley, 2006, pp 17–35.

13 Hyman SE: Addiction: a disease of learning and memory. Am J Psychiatry 2005;162:1414–1422.

14 American Society of Addiction Medicine: Definition of Addiction. http://www.asam.org/for-the-public/definition-of-addiction (accessed August 7, 2014).

15 Leone FT, Evers-Casey S, Toll BA, Vachani A: Treatment of tobacco use in lung cancer: diagnosis and management of lung cancer, 3rd ed: American College of Chest Physicians evidence-based clinical practice guidelines. Chest 2013;143(5 suppl):e61S–e77S.

16 Roberts DC, Koob GF: Disruption of cocaine self-administration following 6-hydroxydopamine lesions of the ventral tegmental area in rats. Pharmacol Biochem Behav 1982;17:901–904.

17 Gong W, Neill D, Justice JB: 6-Hydroxydopamine lesion of ventral pallidum blocks acquisition of place preference conditioning to cocaine. Brain Res 1997;754:103–112.

18 Kandel ER, Kandel DB: A molecular basis for nicotine as a gateway drug. N Engl J Med 2014;371:932–943.

19 Centers for Disease Control and Prevention (CDC): Cigarette smoking among adults and trends in smoking cessation – United States, 2008. MMWR Morb Mortal Wkly Rep 2009;58:1227–1232.

20 García-Rodríguez O, Secades-Villa R, Flórez-Salamanca L, Okuda M, Liu S-M, Blanco C: Probability and predictors of relapse to smoking: results of the National Epidemiologic Survey on Alcohol and Related Conditions (NESARC). Drug Alcohol Depend 2013;132:479–485.

21 Pascual MM, Pastor V, Bernabeu RO: Nicotine-conditioned place preference induced CREB phosphorylation and Fos expression in the adult rat brain. Psychopharmacology (Berl) 2009;207:57–71.

22 Aguilar MA, Rodríguez-Arias M, Miñarro J: Neurobiological mechanisms of the reinstatement of drug-conditioned place preference. Brain Res Rev 2009;59:253–277.

23 Rose G: Sick individuals and sick populations. Int J Epidemiol 1985;14:32–38.

24 Doyle YG: Sick individuals and sick populations: 20 years later. J Epidemiol Community Health 2006;60:396–398.

25 Fiore M, Jaén C, Baker T, et al: Treating Tobacco Use and Dependence: 2008 Update – Clinical Practice Guideline. Rockville, US Department of Health and Human Services, Public Health Service, Agency for Healthcare Research and Quality, 2008.

26 Russell MA, Wilson C, Taylor C, Baker CD: Effect of general practitioners' advice against smoking. Br Med J 1979;ii:231–235.

27 Kottke TE, Battista RN, DeFriese GH, Brekke ML: Attributes of successful smoking cessation interventions in medical practice. A meta-analysis of 39 controlled trials. JAMA 1988;259:2883–2889.

28 Silagy C, Muir J, Coulter A, Thorogood M, Yudkin P, Roe L: Lifestyle advice in general practice: rates recalled by patients. BMJ 1992;305:871–874.

29 Ashenden R, Silagy C, Weller D: A systematic review of the effectiveness of promoting lifestyle change in general practice. Fam Pract 1997;14:160–176.

30 Evers-Casey S: Tobacco-Related Knowledge and Attitudes Do Not Relate to Provider Self-Efficacy. Scottsdale, Society for Research on Nicotine and Tobacco, 2004.

31 Association of American Medical Colleges: Physician Behavior and Practice Patterns Related to Smoking Cessation. Washington, Association of American Medical Colleges, 2007.

32 An L: Treatment of tobacco use as a chronic medical condition: primary care physicians' self-reported practice patterns. Prev Med 2004;38:574–585.

33 Leone FT, Evers-Casey S: Developing a rational approach to tobacco use treatment in pulmonary practice: a review of the biological basis of nicotine addiction. Clin Pulm Med 2012;19:53–61.

34 Sachs D, Leone F, Farber H, Bars M, Prezant D, Schane R, et al: ACCP Tobacco Dependence Treatment Toolkit. American College of Chest Physicians Tobacco-Dependence Treatment Tool Kit, ed 3. http://tobaccodependence.chestnet.org (accessed November 8, 2010).

35 The Philadelphia COPD Initiative. http://www.phillycopd.com (accessed December 12, 2012).

36 Thomson P, Jones J, Browne M, Leslie SJ: Why people seek complementary and alternative medicine before conventional medical treatment: a population based study. Complement Ther Clin Pract 2014, Epub ahead of print.

37 Walji R, Boon H: Redefining the randomized controlled trial in the context of acupuncture research. Complement Ther Clin Pract 2006;12:91–96.

38 White AR, Rampes H, Liu JP, Stead LF, Campbell J: Acupuncture and related interventions for smoking cessation. Cochrane Database Syst Rev 2014;1:CD000009.

39 Barnes J, Dong CY, McRobbie H, Walker N, Mehta M, Stead LF: Hypnotherapy for smoking cessation. Cochrane Database Syst Rev 2010;10:CD001008.

40 Guirguis AB, Ray SM, Zingone MM, Airee A, Franks AS, Keenum AJ: Smoking cessation: barriers to success and readiness to change. Tenn Med 2010;103:45–49.

41 Davis MF, Shapiro D, Windsor R, Whalen P, Rhode R, Miller HS, et al: Motivational interviewing versus prescriptive advice for smokers who are not ready to quit. Patient Educ Couns 2011;83:129–133.

42 Lai DT, Cahill K, Qin Y, Tang J-L: Motivational interviewing for smoking cessation. Cochrane Database Syst Rev 2010;1:CD006936.

43 Grove JR: Attributional correlates of cessation self-efficacy among smokers. Addict Behav 1993;18:311–320.

44 National Institute on Drug Abuse, US Department of Health and Human Services: Principles of Drug Addiction Treatment: A Research-Based Guide, ed 2. Rockville, National Institute on Drug Abuse, US Department of Health and Human Services, 2009, NIH Publ No 09–4180.

45 Cromwell J, Bartosch WJ, Fiore MC, Hasselblad V, Baker T: Cost-effectiveness of the clinical practice recommendations in the AHCPR guideline for smoking cessation. Agency for Health Care Policy and Research. JAMA 1997;278:1759–1766.

46 Mowat DL, Mecredy D, Lee F, Hajela R, Wilson R: Family physicians and smoking cessation. Survey of practices, opinions, and barriers. Can Fam Physician 1996;42:1946–1951.

47 Wechsler H, Levine S, Idelson RK, Schor EL, Coakley E: The physician's role in health promotion revisited – a survey of primary care practitioners. N Engl J Med 1996;334:996–998.

48 McEwen A, Akotia N, West R: General practitioners' views on the English national smoking cessation guidelines. Addiction 2001;96:997–1000.

49 McEwen A, West R, Owen L: General practitioners' views on the provision of nicotine replacement therapy and bupropion. BMC Fam Pract 2001;2:6.

50 Vogt F, Hall S, Marteau TM: General practitioners' and family physicians' negative beliefs and attitudes towards discussing smoking cessation with patients: a systematic review. Addiction 2005;100:1423–1431.

51 Park E, Eaton CA, Goldstein MG, DePue J, Niaura R, Guadagnoli E, et al: The development of a decisional balance measure of physician smoking cessation interventions. Prev Med 2001;33:261–267.

52 Smolders M, Laurant M, Verhaak P, Prins M, van Marwijk H, Penninx B, et al: Which physician and practice characteristics are associated with adherence to evidence-based guidelines for depressive and anxiety disorders? Med Care 2010;48:240–248.

53 Price RA: Association between physician specialty and uptake of new medical technologies: HPV tests in Florida Medicaid. J Gen Intern Med 2010; 25:1178–1185.

54 Evidence-based care: 1. Setting priorities: how important is the problem? Evidence-Based Care Resource Group. CMAJ 1994;150:1249–1254.

55 Eisenberg JM: Physician utilization: the state of research about physicians' practice patterns. Med Care 2002;40:1016–1035.

56 Weiner B: On sin versus sickness. A theory of perceived responsibility and social motivation. Am Psychol 1993;48:957–965.

57 Brewin CR: Perceived controllability of life-events and willingness to prescribe psychotropic drugs. Br J Soc Psychol 1984;23:285–287.

58 Lutfey KE, Eva KW, Gerstenberger E, Link CL, McKinlay JB: Physician cognitive processing as a source of diagnostic and treatment disparities in coronary heart disease: results of a factorial priming experiment. J Health Soc Behav 2010;51:16–29.

59 Leone F, Evers-Casey S, Halenar M, O'Connell K: Potential social, environmental, and regulatory threats to the effectiveness of EHR-supported tobacco treatment in healthcare. J Smok Cessat 2013;15:1–9.

60 Macdonald J, Bath PA, Booth A: Healthcare managers' decision making: findings of a small scale exploratory study. Health Informatics J 2008;14:247–258.

61 Bate L, Hutchinson A, Underhill J, Maskrey N: How clinical decisions are made. Br J Clin Pharmacol 2012;74:614–620.

62 Ben-Haim Y: Doing our best: optimization and the management of risk. Risk Anal 2012;32:1326–1332.

63 Fiore MC, Goplerud E, Schroeder SA: The Joint Commission's new tobacco-cessation measures – will hospitals do the right thing? N Engl J Med 2012;366:1172–1174.

64 The Joint Commission: Specifications Manual for National Hospital Inpatient Quality Measures. http://www.jointcommission.org/specifications_manual_for_national_hospital_inpatient_quality_measures.aspx.

65 Reeves GR, Wang TY, Reid KJ, Alexander KP, Decker C, Ahmad H, et al: Dissociation between hospital performance of the smoking cessation counseling quality metric and cessation outcomes after myocardial infarction. Arch Intern Med 2008;168:2111–2117.

66 Frieden TR: Government's role in protecting health and safety. N Engl J Med 2013;368:1857–1859.

67 Angood P, Birk S: The value of physician leadership. Physician Exec 2014;40:6–20.

68 Jaffe HW, Frieden TR: Improving health in the USA: progress and challenges. Lancet 2014;384:3–5.

69 Colla CH, Fisher ES: Beyond PCMHs and accountable care organizations: payment reform that encourages customized care. J Gen Intern Med 2014;29:1325–1327.

70 Berkowitz SA, Pahira JJ: Accountable care organization readiness and academic medical centers. Acad Med 2014;89:1210–1215.

71 Freidson E: Profession of Medicine: A Study of the Sociology of Applied Knowledge. New York, Dodd, Mead, 1970.

72 Bernstein SL, Yu S, Post LA, Dziura J, Rigotti NA: Undertreatment of tobacco use relative to other chronic conditions. Am J Public Health 2013;103:e59–e65.

73 McCarty MC, Hennrikus DJ, Lando HA, Vessey JT: Nurses' attitudes concerning the delivery of brief cessation advice to hospitalized smokers. Prev Med 2001;33:674–681.

74 McCarty MC, Zander KM, Hennrikus DJ, Lando HA: Barriers among nurses to providing smoking cessation advice to hospitalized smokers. Am J Health Promot 2001;16:85–87, ii.

75 Lancaster T, Silagy C, Fowler G: Training health professionals in smoking cessation. Cochrane Database Syst Rev 2000;3:CD000214.

76 Leone FT, Evers-Casey S, Veloski J, Patkar AA, Kanzleiter L; Pennsylvania Continuum of Tobacco Education Work Group: Short-, intermediate-, and long-term outcomes of Pennsylvania's continuum of tobacco education pilot project. Nicotine Tob Res 2009;11:387–393.

77 Sheffer CE, Barone CP, Anders ME: Training health care providers in the treatment of tobacco use and dependence: pre- and post-training results. J Eval Clin Pract 2009;15:607–613.

78 Geller AC, Hayes RB, Leone F, Churchill LC, Leung K, Reed G, et al: Tobacco dependence treatment teaching by medical school clerkship preceptors: survey responses from more than 1,000 US medical students. Prev Med 2013;57:81–86.

79 Institute of Medicine: Crossing the Quality Chasm: A New Health System for the 21st Century. Washington, National Academy Press, 2014, http://www.nap.edu/openbook.php?isbn=0309072808.

80 Kohn LT, Corrigan JM, Donaldson MS (eds); Committee on Quality of Health Care in America, Institute of Medicine: To Err Is Human: Building a Safer Health System. Washington, National Academy Press, 1999.

81 Determinants of Health – Healthy People 2020. http://www.healthypeople.gov/2020/about/DOHAbout.aspx (accessed August 15, 2014).

82 Schappert SM, Rechtsteiner EA: Ambulatory medical care utilization estimates for 2006. Natl Health Stat Report 2008;8:1–29.

Assoc. Prof. Frank T. Leone, MD, MS
Comprehensive Smoking Treatment Program, University of Pennsylvania
51 North 39th Street, Suite 251 Wright-Saunders Bldg
Philadelphia, PA 19104 (USA)
E-Mail frank.tleone@uphs.upenn.edu

Loddenkemper R, Kreuter M (eds): The Tobacco Epidemic, ed 2, rev. and ext.
Prog Respir Res. Basel, Karger, 2015, vol 42, pp 229–242 (DOI: 10.1159/000369502)

Pharmacotherapy: Nicotine Replacement Therapy and Other Drugs in Smoking Cessation (Including Vaccination)

Philip Tønnesen

Danish Centre for Sleep Medicine, Department of Clinical Neurophysiology, Glostrup Hospital, Glostrup, Denmark

Abstract

The basic principles in quitting smoking are to set a target quit day and try to cut down to zero cigarettes in a few weeks – but best at target quit day – and then use one of the primary drugs for smoking cessation for 2–3 months. In this period, the ex-smoker has to break the psychological addiction as well as the nicotine dependence. Using one of the primary drugs reduces the withdrawal symptoms. Any support will increase quit rate and counselling should be used in combination with one of the primary drugs, i.e. varenicline, nicotine replacement treatment (NRT) and bupropion SR. Varenicline and the combination of two NRT formulations is equally effective, while varenicline is more effective than either single NRT or bupropion SR. NRTs are especially safe. All three drugs have also been shown to be especially effective in patients with chronic obstructive pulmonary disease and in patients with cardiovascular disorders; the main reason for the larger effect in this subgroup is the low quit rate among placebo-treated subjects. There is extensive and solid scientific proof that underlines the efficacy of these three primary drugs in smoking cessation as well as the very high cost-effectiveness of smoking cessation. Vaccines against nicotine have not been effective until now.

© 2015 S. Karger AG, Basel

The aims of this chapter are to summarise the state of the art in smoking cessation with the three first-line drugs, i.e. nicotine replacement therapy (NRT), varenicline and bupropion SR, as well as a short review of the second-line drugs and also the present state of nicotine vaccination. Special focus will be on NRT as NRT is the most used approach for smoking cessation. After reading this chapter, the clinician should have the necessary background information to be able to use and select among the three primary drugs in smoking cessation.

Benefits of Smoking Cessation

Long-term smoking is the main causal reason for chronic obstructive pulmonary disease (COPD) and lung cancer, and to approximately one third of cases of cardiovascular disorders. Compared to never smokers, long-term daily cigarette smoking is associated with higher early mortality from smoking-induced diseases, and ex-smokers have a longer average survival than continuing smokers [1] (see also chapters 7 and 8). Particularly convincing evidence comes from a longitudinal study of UK male doctors who were followed for more than 50 years [1, 2]. It was found that the mortality of the smokers was almost double (1.8 times) that of never smokers and that COPD was approximately 13 times more prevalent and lung cancer approximately15 times more prevalent among smokers compared with never smokers. After a 50-year observation, it was concluded that smokers die 10 years younger than non-smokers. Cessation at ages 60, 50, 40 or 30 years gains about 3, 6, 9 or 10 years of life expectancy, respectively. Among UK women, two thirds of all deaths of smokers in their 50s, 60s and 70s are caused by smoking; smokers lose at least 10 years of lifespan [3]. Smoking is also a strong risk factor for cardiovascular events even at older age. Smoking cessation is highly and rapidly beneficial also at advanced age [4].

However, to prove a causal relationship with tobacco smoking, an intervention study is necessary in order to get smokers to quit and observe the outcome. One of the best studies is the US Lung Health Study, a large randomised controlled trial (RCT) in 5,587 patients with mild COPD, which showed that repeated smoking cessation during 5 years resulted in a quit rate of 37%, and after 14.5 years the quitters had appreciably better lung function (+380 ml in forced expiratory volume in 1 s, FEV_1) and a higher survival rate compared to COPD patients who continued to smoke [5]. In another study, the quality of life of patients with moderate or severe COPD 1 year after quitting was significantly better than that of continuing smokers, in contrast to what many COPD patients believe [6].

Nicotine Addiction and Smoking

It is important to know that when treating an addictive disorder like smoking one cannot expect to get a 100% cure. A typical finding in most smoking cessation studies is that with adequate support and pharmacological therapy it is possible to achieve an initial quit rate of ~50–60% during the first 3 months in the so-called 'cessation period'. From 3 months up to 12 months, almost 50% of the subjects relapse to smoking in the so-called 'relapse period' ending up with a 1-year quit rate around 25–35%. To stop smoking is to break a complex habit and addiction, and to achieve reasonable quit rates, it is necessary to administer behavioural support, i.e. counselling combined with pharmacological drugs [7–9]. A special subgroup are pregnant smokers in whom smoking cessation is an essential aim to prevent negative health consequences for the unborn child (see also chapters 9 and 10). Recently, two Cochrane reviews have been published on pharmacological and psychological interventions during pregnancy [Chamberlain C, O'Mara-Eves A, Oliver S, Caird JR, Perlen SM, Eades SJ, Thomas J: Psychosocial interventions for supporting women to stop smoking in pregnancy. Cochrane Database Syst Rev 2013;10:CD001055] [Coleman T, Chamberlain C, Davey MA, Cooper SE, Leonardi-Bee J: Pharmacological interventions for promoting smoking cessation during pregnancy. Cochrane Database Syst Rev 2012;9:CD010078]. Nicotine addiction is dealt with in detail in chapters 5, 6, 18 and 19.

Smoking Cessation Treatments

It is important to underline that to achieve a reasonable quit rate in smoking cessation it is necessary to provide behavioural support combined with pharmacological drugs. When NRT is used in unsupported quit attempts, some data suggest that there is no effect from NRT.

Several high-quality meta-analyses have been performed regarding smoking cessation evaluating different interventions for smoking cessation, i.e. the Cochrane Database, the Fiore AHCPR (US Agency for Healthcare Policy and Research) publication from US, the NICE (National Institute for Clinical Excellence) guidelines from the UK and several others [7–12]. The Cochrane Library and AHCPR have included almost the same 300 studies in their meta-analyses and published clinical guidelines.

First-line pharmacological drugs for smoking cessation are nicotine replacement products (patch, gum, inhaler, nasal spray, lozenge/tablets and oral spray), and treatment with varenicline and bupropion SR with scientific well-documented efficacy when used for 2–3 months (tables 1, 2) [7, 9–12].

The above-named medications in combination with counselling have also shown to be effective for smokers with COPD and cardiovascular disorders, which often seem more difficult to get to quit smoking [13]. I will address three studies in COPD patients: each of them used one of the first-line medications.

Table 1. First-line drugs in smoking cessation: efficacy data from a meta-analysis from the Cochrane Register [modified from ref. 9–11]

	Sustained quit rates for 6–12 months, RR (95% CI)
Any type of NRT vs. placebo (117 studies; 50,000 smokers)	1.60 (1.53–1.68)
Bupropion SR vs. placebo (44 studies; 13,728 smokers)	1.62 (1.49–1.76)
Varenicline vs. placebo (14 studies; 6,166 smokers)	2.27 (2.02–2.55)

Table 2. First-line drugs for smoking cessation: efficacy figures (1-year quit rates) from the US clinical guidelines [modified from ref. 9][1]

	OR (95% CI)	Abstinence rate, %
Placebo	1.0	13.8
Monotherapies		
Varenicline	3.1 (2.5–3.8)	33.2
High-dose nicotine patch	2.3 (1.7–3.0)	26.5
Nicotine gum (>14 weeks)	2.2 (1.5–3.2)	26.1
Bupropion SR	2.0 (1.8–2.2)	24.2
Combination therapies		
Patch + ad libitum NRT	3.6 (2.5–5.2)	36.5
Patch + bupropion SR	2.5 (1.9–3.4)	28.9
Patch + nicotine inhaler	2.2 (1.3–3.6)	25.8

[1] A meta-analysis of data from placebo-controlled trials in smoking cessation reporting 1-year quit rates with the above drugs for smoking cessation used for 3 months in combination with counselling. The comparator is the placebo arm without drug but with counselling. The results are shown as ORs and as 1-year quit rates. OR = Odds ratio.

versus placebo came out with an OR of 3.1 (95% CI 2.5–3.8) and a quit rate of 33 and 13.8% in the placebo groups [9].

These findings support my theoretical thoughts about how to use NRT: Use a patch to attain a high basal nicotine substitution and then, when a subject experiences break-through withdrawal symptoms, add on an acute form of NRT according to the patient's preference. The same principle is also applied when treating pain in lung cancer patients, i.e. a long-acting morphine preparation (possibly a patch) and then, when break-through pain occurs, use an acute form of morphine tablets. I myself find this algorithm useful when I explain the above principle for physicians, and smokers might more clearly understand the need for medication when quitting smoking.

A dose-response effect has been observed with both the nicotine gum and the patch, and even 22- and 44-mg patches have been tested with promising results after 4 weeks of treatment, i.e. success rates of 45 and 68%, respectively [19]. In two studies, the degree of nicotine substitution was compared to outcome, and in both higher success rates were found with increasing degree of substitution [19].

In the CEASE study comprising 3,575 subjects, a higher success rate was achieved with patches of 25 mg/16 h compared with 15-mg nicotine patches [19].

NRT has been shown to be effective in different settings, such as smoking cessation specialist clinics and in general practice combined with minimal counselling, in 'healthy' smokers and patients with COPD. The adverse events are mostly mild and transient, and the most common side effects are local nicotine-induced irritation of the skin, mouth and throat and seldom nicotine 'overdose' symptoms. NRT has been found safe in patients with cardiovascular disorders [21].

NRT are available over the counter without the possible barrier of getting a prescription from the physician.

Overall, in clinical use, combinations of different NRT administration forms seem safe with few side effects. Also, concomitant use of NRT and cigarette smoking seems to be safe with similar nicotine concentrations as during normal cigarette smoking [7, 27].

A head-to-head comparison with varenicline and nicotine transdermal patches has recently been published in *Thorax* with the conclusion that varenicline demonstrated a greater abstinence rate than nicotine patches at the end of treatment [30]. In this multi-national 24-centre study, 376 and 370 smokers were randomly allocated to varenicline for 12 weeks and nicotine patches (21 mg/24 h) for 10 weeks in an open-label trial. There were weekly visits during the first 12 weeks followed by 7 clinic visits and 5 telephone calls in the follow-up period from months 3 to 12. The quit rates

were higher for varenicline versus NRT at the end of therapy weeks 9–12 and 8–11, i.e. 55.9 versus 43.2% (OR 1.70, 95% CI 1.26–2.28). Continuous quit rates at weeks 8 (9) to 24 were higher for varenicline than NRT but not statistically significant. The continuous quit rates at weeks 8 (9) to 52 were 26.1% for varenicline versus 20.3% for NRT (p = 0.056), but when including all randomised subjects the difference reached significance. There was no significant difference in the 7-day point prevalence after 24 and 52 weeks.

Taking all this potential serious limitations and bias into account and also that the 1-year abstinence rate did not reach statistical significance, this trial is not adequate to conclude that varenicline is superior to NRT. The positive message from this trial is that we can expect a 1-year continuous quit rate between 20 and 26% and a 1-year point prevalence of 31–35%, i.e. 1 in 3 were quitters after 1 year.

An indirect comparison by NICE reported that varenicline was more effective than bupropion SR (OR 1.58, 95% CI 1.22–2.05) and NRT (OR 1.66, 95% CI 1.17–2.36); similar results were reported by others [31].

Another study from a smoking cessation clinic in London compared quit rates with varenicline versus NRT in routine treatment with historical controls before the introduction of varenicline. They found 4-week quit rates of 61% with NRT and 72% with varenicline, but longer follow-up data were not reported [32].

Smoking Reduction and Intermittent Use of Nicotine Replacement Products

Many smokers would prefer to reduce the number of cigarettes smoked daily instead of complete quitting (see also chapter 23). The aim of smoking reduction is to widen access to cessation by including smokers not currently able or willing to stop abruptly, wanting to reduce smoking, but unable or unwilling to quit. As shown below by the concept of smoking reduction, it is possible to recruit a new group of smokers, who are not interested in abrupt cessation. The reduction process should be looked at as a gateway to complete cessation.

The definition of smoking reduction is a decrease in the number of cigarettes (or tobacco) smoked daily. A 50% reduction or more in daily cigarettes has been chosen arbitrarily in most studies.

Several RCTs have been published [7, 9, 33]. In 8 studies, 2 using nicotine inhalers and 6 using nicotine chewing gums for 0.5–1 year, comprising 2,424 smokers, a reduction in smoking (>50%) was reported in 15.9% of smokers using NRTs compared with 6.7% of placebo users. Surprisingly, after 1 year, a smoking cessation rate of 8.4% was found among nicotine users versus 4.1% in placebo users. A reduction of more than 50% after 3–4 months had a strong predictive value with quitting at 1 year [34].

Also, participation in reduction trials increased motivation to quit smoking thus not undermining the motivation to stop smoking completely.

The smoking reduction concept should be offered to smokers who are not motivated to quit. They should be prescribed NRT – nicotine gums or inhalers – for 3 months and recommended to reduce the number of cigarettes by at least 50% during the first 1–2 weeks and then try to reduce further. If the smoker has not reduced more than 50% after 3 months, NRT should be stopped as the chance of quitting is then low. In smokers that have reduced more than 50%, NRT should be continued for up to 1 year, and after 6 months they should be recommended to try to stop smoking completely [33, 34].

In summary, smoking reduction seems to have a role for smokers not motivated or able to quit, paving the way to complete cessation.

Use of NRT during work hours and during longer travels seems to increase, as public ban of smoking is implemented in more and more places. All the acute NRT formulations can be used for this purpose, but due to local side effects the nasal and the mouth spray should not be recommended. It is often useful to instruct smokers to try a piece of gum/inhaler a few hours before the travel starts.

Long-Term Nicotine Replacement Therapy

Long-term NRT can arbitrary be defined as NRT use after 12 months. The prevalence is not very precise from data in the literature and has been reported as low as 1–2% up to 25%. On average, ~5–10% of abstainers still use NRT after 12 months [9]. It is not a new nicotine dependence on NRT but rather that ex-smokers have not been able to break the addiction to nicotine already existing. It is the acute formulations of NRT that are used in the long term, i.e. mainly gums, sublingual tablets and inhalers, while nobody misuses the patch.

In formal studies, it has been possible to get ~50% to stop the use of NRT by counselling.

In a recent RCT, we used varenicline and placebo for 3 months in combination with counselling in 139 long-term users (6–7 years) of mainly nicotine chewing gums [35]. After 3 months, the quit rate from NRT was 64% in the varenicline group and 41% in the placebo group, and after 12 months 43 versus 36% (the study was not powered for 12 months), respectively; however, the overall OR was 1.83 in favour of var-

Table 6. Efficacy of smoking cessation (prolonged abstinence (after 6–12 months) from a meta-analysis of 8 smoking cessation trials in 7,372 COPD patients [modified from ref. 33].

Therapy	OR (95% CI)	p value
Nothing/usual care	1	
Counselling alone	1.82 (0.96–3.34)	0.07
Counselling + antidepressants	3.32 (1.53–7.21)	0.002
Counselling + NRT	5.08 (4.32–5.97)	<0.001
Counselling + varenicline (1 study only)	4.04 (2.13–7.67)	<0.001

enicline. A proposed schedule for weaning long-term users of NRT could be: Combine counselling visits with varenicline for 3 months (4–5 visits). Stop using NRT after 1–2 weeks of therapy with varenicline. Expect a 1-year success rate of 35% and also expect a weight gain of 2–4 kg after 1 year.

Treatment of Patients with Respiratory Disorders Who Smoke

In patients with coronary heart disease, smoking cessation is more efficient than statin and anti-hypertensive treatment [36] (see chapter 8). Regarding COPD patients, many smokers quit when they get the diagnosis of COPD (see also chapter 7); this leaves smokers who are less motivated and more dependent behind. We published guidelines on smoking cessation in patients with respiratory disorders a few years ago [37].

A new way of thinking about smoking cessation in COPD patients has been inspired by a study from Sweden, where smokers with COPD were hospitalised for 11 days with the only reason to quit smoking. In this RCT, 247 hospitalised COPD patients were compared to 231 patients receiving usual care. Their mean age was 52 years and their mean FEV_1 was 75% of predicted. The 3rd day was the target quit day and they were offered NRT and daily exercise. Counselling consisted of 1-hour daily meetings with trained smoking cessation nurses and an educational program followed by weekly telephone calls by nurses. After 2–3 months, they were to spend 2–4 days in hospital together with their spouses.

The quit rate after 1 year was 52% for hospitalised patients and 7% for patients receiving usual care, and, after 3 years, the figures were 38 versus 10%, respectively. These very high abstinence rates and the high cost-effectiveness of this treatment encourage the need for re-thinking the level of intervention for COPD patients regarding smoking cessation [38].

A recent meta-analysis included 8 trials involving 7,372 COPD patients receiving treatment for smoking cessation

Table 7. Three double-blind, placebo-controlled, randomised smoking cessation studies with nicotine sublingual tablets, varenicline and bupropion SR in patients with COPD [data from ref. 48, 56, 69]

Medication	n	Sustained quit rates for 1 year, %			p value
		median FEV$_1$, % pred.	active	placebo	
Varenicline	505	70	18.6	5.6	<0.0001
Bupropion SR	404	72	10	8	n.s.
NRT	370	56	14	5	<0.001

[13]. As shown in tables 6 and 7, counselling and all three treatments for smoking cessation (i.e. NRT, bupropion SR and varenicline) were all highly effective in COPD with an OR of 5.08 for NRT versus placebo. This underlines the importance of prescribing NRT to COPD patients when they start to quit smoking.

Nicotine Replacement Therapy in Patients with Chronic Obstructive Pulmonary Disease

In COPD patients, NRTs seem to be especially effective, as shown in the study that evaluated the effect of sublingual nicotine and two levels of counselling in a double-blind trial in Denmark [6]. To evaluate the efficacy of sublingual nicotine tablets and two levels of support for smoking cessation in COPD outpatients, we enrolled 370 COPD patients who smoked a mean of 19.6 cigarettes/day (mean, 42.7 pack-years; mean FEV$_1$, 56% of predicted). Three-month treatment with 2-mg sublingual nicotine tablets or placebo were combined with either low (4 visits plus 6 telephone calls) or high support (7 visits plus 5 telephone calls) provided by nurses.

Smoking cessation rates were statistically significantly superior with sublingual nicotine compared to placebo for all measures of abstinence: 6-month point prevalence, 23 versus 10%, and 12-month point prevalence, 17 versus 10%, respectively. There was no significant difference in the effect of low versus high behavioural support. The St. George's Respiratory Questionnaire score improved significantly in abstainers versus non-abstainers; the changes in mean scores were –10.9 versus –2.9 for total score, and –28.6 versus –2.3 for symptom score, respectively. This is a little surprising but very positive finding that should be used to motivate COPD smokers in the process of smoking cessation. This trial demonstrated the long-term efficacy of NRT for smoking cessation for the general population of COPD smokers, regardless of daily cigarette consumption. Cessation success

rates were in the same range as in healthy smokers, and abstinence improved St. George's Respiratory Questionnaire scores. NRT should be used to aid cessation in all smokers with COPD, regardless of disease severity and the number of cigarettes smoked [13].

Weight Gain

A weight gain of 3–6 kg for abstainers after 1 year is found in most studies (see also chapters 6 and 18) [7, 9, 39, 40].

In 10% of males and 13% of females, the weight increases more than 14 kg i.e. super gainers. About half of the participants are afraid of gaining weight and it may be a more prominent problem for females.

Weight gain can be regarded as a withdrawal symptom due to increased hunger and increased caloric intake. NRTs are only partially able to reduce the weight gain after smoking cessation, while bupropion has a more favourable effect, i.e. a reduction in weight gain of 2–3 kg after cessation [7]. To prevent or reduce the weight gain after cessation, compensatory exercise can be recommended [41, 42]. In high-risk patients – especially in overweight smokers and in smokers with an increased risk of developing diabetes mellitus – interventions aimed at preventing weight gain after smoking cessation should be considered, because a weight gain may increase the risk of developing diabetes mellitus [43].

For patients suffering from COPD or lung cancer, the weight increase might be an advantage if underweight. Also, an increase in appetite might also be an advantage in patients with decreased appetite.

Varenicline

Varenicline affects central nicotine receptors in the brain by binding to specific nicotine receptors. In contrast to NRT, varenicline can be taken as tablets [7, 10]. In combination with counselling, varenicline increases long-term quit rates two- and threefold compared to no-drug treatment [10, 44–46].

The average 1-year success rate reported in most studies is around 33%, or the relative increase in quit rate compared to placebo is approximately 127% (relative risk) [7, 10]. In COPD patients and patients with cardiovascular disorders [47], varenicline has shown to be particular effective. It is a good idea to taper the number of cigarettes during the 1st week of therapy, waiting for the concentration of varenicline to build up in the brain, and then, after 1–2 weeks, set a target quit day where the smoker stops completely cigarette smoking.

Varenicline in Patients with Chronic Obstructive Pulmonary Disease

In a 27-centre, double-blind, multinational study, 504 patients with mild-to-moderate COPD (post-bronchodilator FEV_1/forced vital capacity, <70% of predicted; normal value ≥50%) were randomised to receive varenicline (n = 250) or placebo (n = 254) for 3 months with a 40-week non-treatment follow-up [48]. The continuous abstinence rate for weeks 9–52 was significantly higher for patients treated with varenicline than placebo (18.6 vs. 5.6%, respectively; OR 4.04, 95% CI 2.13–7.67; p < 0.0001). Nausea, abnormal dreams, upper-respiratory-tract infection and insomnia were the most commonly reported adverse events for patients in the varenicline group. Serious adverse events were infrequent in both treatment groups. Two patients in the varenicline group and 1 patient in the placebo group died during the study. Reports of psychiatric adverse events were similar for both treatment groups.

Overall, varenicline was more efficacious than placebo regarding smoking cessation in patients with mild-to-moderate COPD and demonstrated a safety profile consistent with that observed in previous trials.

Varenicline and Serious Adverse Events

There have been reports about depression, suicidal behaviour and myocardial infarction with the use of varenicline, and present depression is a relative contraindication [7, 10, 49–52]. However, there is no clear evidence that these side effects are causally related to the drug.

In a recent meta-analysis from the Cochrane Database it was stated that the main adverse effect of varenicline was nausea, which was mostly mild to moderate and tended to subside over time; however, it cannot be ruled out that varenicline has possible links with serious adverse events, including serious psychiatric or cardiovascular events [10].

A large treatment database from general practices in primary care in the UK included 80,660 men and women aged 18–95 years who were prescribed a new course of a smoking cessation product between September 1, 2006, and May 31, 2008: NRTs (n = 63,265), varenicline (n = 10,973) and bupropion (n = 6,422). There was no clear evidence that varenicline was associated with an increased risk of fatal (n = 2) or non-fatal (n = 166) self-harm, although a twofold increased risk cannot be ruled out on the basis of the upper limit of the 95% CI. Compared with NRTs, the hazard ratios for self-harm among patients prescribed varenicline and bupropion were 1.12 (95% CI 0.67–1.88) and 1.17 (0.59–2.32), respectively. There was no evidence that varenicline was associated with an increased risk of depression (n = 2,244; hazard ratio 0.88, 95% CI 0.77–1.00) or suicidal thoughts (n = 37; hazard ratio 1.43, 95% CI 0.53–3.85) [50].

In conclusion, although a twofold increased risk of self-harm with varenicline cannot be ruled out, these findings provide some reassurance concerning its association with suicidal behaviour.

Another new meta-analysis including all trials published to date, which focused on events occurring during drug exposure and analysed findings using four summary estimates, found no significant increase in serious cardiovascular adverse events associated with varenicline use [53].

For rare outcomes, summary estimates based on absolute effects are recommended and estimates based on the Peto OR should be avoided. A detailed analysis of adverse events of varenicline can be found on the FDA home page [54].

Thus far, surveillance reports and secondary analyses of trial data are inconclusive, but the possibility of a link between varenicline and serious psychiatric or cardiovascular events cannot be ruled out. In my opinion, based on the above data, there is no clear evidence that varenicline is casually linked to either cardiovascular or psychiatric adverse events. Overall, varenicline is the most effective drug for smoking cessation [7, 10].

Also, varenicline tends to be more effective than bupropion and single NRT but has similar effectiveness as a combination of two NRTs. In my opinion, taking into account that varenicline is very effective and that there is no evidence of a causal relationship between the above-mentioned severe adverse events and varenicline, it can also be recommended as a first-line agent for smoking cessation in COPD patients. This is also the recommendation in several guidelines for smoking cessation [7, 10].

Bupropion SR

Bupropion SR (tablets) is an older antidepressant, drug but its effect on smoking cessation is not related to its antidepressive effect [11, 55, 56].

The average 1-year success rate reported in most studies is about 24% or a relative increase in quit rate compared to placebo of ~69% (relative risk) [11]. In COPD patients, bupropion has been shown to be particular effective. The combination of bupropion SR and NRT is more effective than either alone. Similar to the use of varenicline, it is a good idea to taper the number of cigarettes during the 1st week of therapy waiting for the concentration of bupropion to build up in the brain, and then, after 1–2 weeks, to set a target quit day where the smoker stops completely smoking cigarettes.

Bupropion SR in Patients with Chronic Obstructive Pulmonary Disease

In a multicentre study (11 centres in the USA), 404 COPD patients (15+ cigarettes/day) were allocated to bupropion SR for 3 months or placebo in a design with moderate intensive support (i.e. 10 visits) with weekly individual sessions during the first 7 weeks [57]. Most patients had mild COPD (stage I: FEV_1 >50%) and 15% were in stage II (FEV_1: 35–49%) with a cigarette consumption of 28 cigarettes/day and 52 pack-years and a Fagerström score of 7 (maximal score 11). Abstinence rate was significantly higher up to 6 months in the bupropion group compared with the placebo group (16 vs. 9%, respectively).

The most common adverse events of bupropion are insomnia and dry mouth. The most serious adverse events are major motor seizures, which have been reported in 0.1% of patients treated with bupropion, as well as allergic reactions (1–2%), including serious cases of hypersensitivity (0.1%). There are also many contraindications to the use of bupropion [7, 10, 51, 55].

In summary, bupropion SR is of similar efficacy as NRT. Compared with NRT and varenicline, bupropion has more serious side effects and more contraindications.

Overall, NRT, varenicline and bupropion SR have shown higher relative efficacy in COPD patients than in smokers without comorbidity. These studies have also reported a very low quit rate among COPD patients using placebo, probably because these smokers are more nicotine dependent and not able to quit without the support of smoking cessation medication.

Apart from the two most effective treatments for smoking cessation today, i.e. varenicline and a combination of two NRTs, the future development of novel drugs may broaden the spectrum of drugs available for effective treatment of nicotine dependence and may render it possible to tailor drug therapy to the need of the individual smoker. Recently, a vaporiser has been marketed that may deliver nicotine at alveolar level to the lungs like cigarettes. Medicinal electronic cigarettes will probably also be on the market in a few years, while we have to wait for clinical trials of ongoing research with new nicotine vaccines [58].

Secondary Drugs for Smoking Cessation

Cytisine
Cytisine is a natural drug extracted from the seeds of the plant Golden Rain and is a nicotine receptor partial agonists as the synthetic drug varenicline. It is available in some former Eastern European countries and over the Internet. Seven trials have been published, but only two high-quality studies were included in two meta-analyses with an RR of 3.98 (95% CI 2.01–7.87) for cytisine versus placebo [59, 60]. In both trials, cytisine was used for only 4 weeks and with relative little behavioural support in contrast to all studies with varenicline, where weekly visits were scheduled during the first 12 weeks. The absolute quit rate in the largest study with 749 smokers was modest (i.e. 12-month sustained quit rate 8.4 versus 2.4% after 12 months for cytisine versus placebo, respectively). There was no difference in overall adverse events between the two groups although gastrointestinal side effects were higher in the cytisine group [61]. Another advantage is the very low cost of cytisine, thus it could be a drug of choice in low- and middle-income countries. However, further studies are needed with extended use of cytisine and more intensive behavioural support to evaluate the absolute quit rates and adverse events. In a recent large randomized, controlled trial cytisine for 25 days showed superiority to nicotine patches for 8 weeks after 1 and 6 months [71]. Thus cytisine seems a much cheaper alternative to current pharmacotherapies which are often unavailable to so many smokers – especially those in low-income and middle-income countries [72].

Nortriptyline
Nortriptyline, a tricyclic antidepressant, is the only other antidepressant (i.e. bupropion SR) that has demonstrated evidence of efficacy for smoking cessation. The dose of nortriptyline for smoking cessation is 75–150 mg/day. A Cochrane meta-analysis of six trials found an RR of 2.03 (95% CI 1.5–2.8) for 1-year quit rates for nortriptyline versus placebo [11]. However, there are many contraindications to nortriptyline, including common anti-cholinergic side effects and particularly cardiac conduction disturbances and orthostatic blood pressure decreases. However, current evidence suggests that nortriptyline, at doses between 75 and 100 mg, is not significantly associated with serious adverse events when administered in patients without underlying cardiovascular disease. One advantage of nortriptyline is the very low cost.

Clonidine

Clonidine, an imidazoline drug previously used in the management of hypertension, has limited efficacy as smoking cessation therapy. It has been recommended as second-line therapy in US smoking cessation guidelines. To reduce adverse events, a patch formulation has been marketed. A Cochrane meta-analysis included six trials (3 with oral and 3 with transdermal patches) and showed an OR for clonidine versus placebo of 1.89 (95% CI 1.30–2.7) [62]. However, adverse effects associated with clonidine, such as drowsiness, fatigue and dry mouth, were reported with a high incidence and may limit its use. Most experts considered clonidine as obsolete. The oral dose used is 100–300 μg once daily, but in my experience the optimal dose is around 100–150 μg.

Nicotine Vaccination

Smokers have no antibodies to nicotine as it is a small molecule.

The rationale for nicotine vaccination is that the vaccine (nicotine bound to a hapten) will induce antibodies against nicotine, and as the nicotine from tobacco is bound in the blood by these antibodies, less nicotine will reach the brain. Phase I and II studies have evaluated three different vaccines, NicVAX, NicQb and TA-NIC [63–65]. Dosing has been 2–6 injections at intervals of 2–4 weeks and a later booster dose. Marked inter-individual variability has been observed in antibody levels, and antibody levels decreased by 50% over 6–8 weeks. The vaccines have been well tolerated. Only mild local reactions and systemic (flu-like) reactions have been reported.

In the NicQb study including 133 smokers, 57% of subjects with the highest antibody levels and 31% of controls quit smoking [63]. In the TA-NIC study, 38% of smokers who got the highest dose and 8% of controls quit smoking [64]. In the NicVAX study including 68 smokers, 40% of subjects who got the highest dose and 8% of controls quit smoking, although no support was delivered to encourage participants to quit smoking [65].

Few trials have been published, but both a Cochrane meta-analysis from 2012 including four trials [66] and another recent review [67] found no effect of nicotine vaccines compared with placebo both for smoking cessation and for relapse prevention and with varenicline used to induce smoking cessation.

We have to wait for potential more effective nicotine vaccines before this very interesting principle is totally discharged [67, 68].

Conclusion

Varenicline, NRT and bupropion SR increase 1-year cessation outcomes by ~50%, and combined with counselling and behavioural strategies they are important adjuncts for maintaining long-term smoking cessation.

The first-line drugs are a combination NRT or varenicline, and alternatively bupropion SR. Regarding NRT, a patch and another NRT formulation should be used in combination for ~3 months with individual variations. All three primary drugs are very cost-effective treatments compared with several other common medical treatments and should be much more widely implemented in the future. As COPD patients and patients with cardiovascular disorders might be more nicotine dependent and have more difficulty in stopping smoking, a more aggressive therapeutic approach should be used, i.e. higher doses of NRT, a combination of two NRT formulations, varenicline plus NRT, bupropion SR plus NRT, longer durations of therapy (6–12 months) and more support visits. Family members who smoke should also be enrolled in the cessation program.

Most COPD patients and patients with cardiovascular disorders have used NRT previously, and then varenicline might be the drug of choice as it is safe, with almost no contraindications or interactions. Also, varenicline tends to be more effective than bupropion SR.

NRT seems to have the following advantages compared to varenicline and bupropion SR: the most extensive scientific documentation, effective in healthy and sick smokers, effective with both low and high support and in general practice, safe with almost no contraindications and available without prescription. NRT delivers nicotine in lower doses than during smoking without introducing a new drug.

Consequently, I recommend NRT as the first choice in naïve smokers without smoking-induced disorders without prior NRT or properly implemented NRT. When only minimal support is administered, NRT is the drug of choice, as varenicline has not been tested in such a condition.

One of the problems with NRT is underdosing. Pre-loading can optimise NRT as well as a combination of two NRT formulations securing that proper instruction is delivered. The problems with both varenicline and bupropion SR are that a majority of smokers do not use the drugs long enough, mostly due to costs. Many insurance companies do not cover drugs for smoking cessation.

Key Points

- The primary drugs to be used for smoking cessation are varenicline, nicotine replacement products (NRTs) and bupropion SR.
- Varenicline and a combination of two NRT formulations is equally effective.
- Varenicline is more effective than either single nicotine replacement treatment (NRT) or bupropion SR.
- NRT is especially safe.
- All three drugs have also been shown to be especially effective in patients with chronic obstructive pulmonary disease and cardiovascular disorders.
- In the future, cytisine may become an alternative to current pharmacotherapies which are often unavailable to so many smokers – especially those in low-income and middle-income countries – because of their high cost.
- Smoking cessation treatment, i.e. counselling in combination with drugs, is one of the most cost-effective interventions in medicine.
- Smoking cessation treatment should be used more widely and its costs should be re-imbursed.

References

1 Jha P, Ramasundarahettige C, Landsman V, Rostron B, Thun P, Peto R: 21st-century hazards of smoking and benefits of cessation in the United States. N Engl J Med 2013;368:341–350.
2 Doll R, Peto R, Boreham J, Sutherland I: Mortality from cancer in relation to smoking: 50 years observations on British doctors. Br J Cancer 2005;14: 426–429.
3 Pirie K, Peto R, Reeves GK, Green J, Beral V; Million Women Study Collaborators: The 21st century hazards of smoking and benefits of stopping: a prospective study of one million women in the UK. Lancet 2013;381:133–141.
4 Gellert C, Schottker B, Muller H, Holleczek B, Brenner H: Impact of smoking and quitting on cardiovascular outcomes and risk advancement periods among older adults. Eur J Epidemiol 2013; 28:649–658.
5 Anthonisen NR, Skeans MA, Wise RA, Manfreda J, Kanner RE, Connett JE; Lung Health Study Research Group: The effects of a smoking cessation intervention on 14.5-year mortality. Ann Intern Med 2005;142:233–239.
6 Tønnesen P, Mikkelsen K, Bremann L: Nurse-conducted smoking cessation in patients with COPD using nicotine sublingual tablets and behavioral support. Chest 2006;130:334–342.
7 Fiore MC, Bailey WC, Cohen SJ, Dorfman SF, Goldstein MF, Gritz ER, et al: Treating Tobacco Use and Dependence: Clinical Practice Guideline. Rockville, US Department of Health and Human Services, Public Health Service, 2000.
8 National Institute for Clinical Excellence (NICE): Guidance on the use of nicotine replacement therapy (NRT) and bupropion for smoking cessation. National Institute for Clinical Excellence Technology Appraisal Guidance No 39, 2002, http://www.healthcareimprovementscotland.org/programmes/nice_guidance_and_scotland/stas/appraisal_39.aspx.
9 Stead LF, Perera R, Bullen C, Mant D, Hartmann-Boyce J, Cahill K, Lancaster T: Nicotine replacement therapy for smoking cessation. Cochrane Database Syst Rev 2012;11:CD000146.
10 Cahill K, Stead LF, Lancaster T: Nicotine receptor partial agonists for smoking cessation. Cochrane Database Syst Rev 2012;4:CD006103.

11 Hughes JR, Stead LF, Hartmann-Boyce J, Cahill K, Lancaster T: Antidepressants for smoking cessation. Cochrane Database Syst Rev 2014;1: CD000031.
12 Cahill K, Stevens S, Perera R, Lancaster T: Pharmacological interventions for smoking cessation: an overview and network meta-analysis. Cochrane Database Syst Rev 2013;5:CD009329.
13 Strassmann R, Bausch B, Spaar A, Kleijnen J, Braendli O, Puhan MA: Smoking cessation interventions in COPD: a network meta-analysis of randomised trials. Eur Respir J 2009;34:634–640.
14 Cromwell J, Bartosch WJ, Fiore MC, Hasselblad V, Baker T: Cost-effectiveness of the clinical practice recommendations in the AHCPR guideline for smoking cessation. Agency for Health Care Policy and Research. JAMA 1997;278:1759–1766.
15 Parrott S, Godfrey C, Raw M, West R, McNeill A: Guidance for commissioners on the cost effectiveness of smoking cessation interventions. Thorax 1998;53(suppl 5):S1–S38.
16 NHS Centre for Reviews & Dissemination: A Rapid and Systematic Review of the Clinical and Cost Effectiveness of Bupropion SR and Nicotine Replacement Therapy (NRT) for Smoking Cessation. York, NHS Centre for Reviews & Dissemination, 2002.
17 Tønnesen P, Fryd V, Hansen M, Helsted J, Gunnersen AB, Forchammer H, Stockner M: Effect of nicotine chewing gum in combination with group counseling on the cessation of smoking. N Engl J Med 1988;318:15–18.
18 Tønnesen P, Nørregaard J, Mikkelsen K, Jørgensen S, Nilsson F: A double-blind trial of a nicotine inhaler for smoking cessation. JAMA 1993; 269:1268–1271.
19 Tønnesen P, Paoletti P, Gustavsson G, Russell MA, Saracci R, Gulsvik A, Rijcken B, Sawe U: Higher dosage nicotine patches increase one-year smoking cessation rates: results from the European CEASE trial. Collaborative European Anti-Smoking Evaluation. European Respiratory Society. Eur Respir J 1999;13:238–246.
20 García-Rodríguez O, Secades-Villa R, Flórez-Salamanca L, Okuda M, Liu SM, Blanco C: Probability and predictors of relapse to smoking: results of the National Epidemiologic Survey on Alcohol and Related Conditions (NESARC). Drug Alcohol Depend 2013;132:479–485.

21 Murray RP, Bailey WC, Daniels K, Bjornson WM, Kurnow K, Connett JE, Nides MA, Kiley JP: Safety of nicotine polacrilex gum used by 3,094 participants in the Lung Health Study. Lung Health Study Research Group. Chest 1996;109:438–445.
22 Russell MAH, Stableton JA, Feyerabend C, Wiserman SM, Guvtavsson G, Säwe U, Connor P: Targeting heavy smokers in general practice: randomized controlled trial of transdermal nicotine patches. Br Med J 1993;306:1308–1312.
23 Sutherland G, Stapleton JA, Russell MAH, Jarvis MJ, Hajek P, Belcher M, Feyerabend C: Randomised controlled trial of a nasal nicotine spray in smoking cessation. Lancet 1992;340:324–329.
24 Wallström M, Nilsson F, Hirch JM: A randomized, double-blind, placebo-controlled clinical evaluation of a nicotine sublingual tablet in smoking cessation. Addiction 2000;95:1161–1171.
25 Daughton DM, Fortmann SP, Glover ED, Hatsukami DK, Heatley SA, Lichtenstein E, Repsher L, Millatmal T, Killen JD, Nowak RT, Ullrich F, Patil KD, Rennard SI: The smoking cessation efficacy of varying doses of nicotine patch delivery systems 4 to 5 years post-quit day. Prev Med 1999;28:113–118.
26 Imperial Cancer Research Fund General Practice Research Group: Effectiveness of a nicotine patch in helping people to stop smoking: results of a randomized trial in general practice. Br Med J 1993;306:1304–1308.
27 Fagerström KO, Säwe U, Tønnesen P: Therapeutic use of nicotine patches: efficacy and safety. J Smoking Relat Disord 1992;3:247–261.
28 Schneider NG, Olmstead RE, Franzon MA, Lunell E: The nicotine inhaler: clinical pharmacokinetics and comparison with other nicotine treatments (review). Clin Pharmacokinet 2001;40:661–684.
29 Tønnesen P, Lauri H, Perfekt R, Mann K, Batra A: Efficacy of a nicotine mouth spray in smoking cessation: a randomised, double-blind trial. Eur Respir J 2012;40:548–554.
30 Aubin JH, Bobak A, Britton JR, Oncken C, Billing CB, Gong J, Williams KE, Reeves KR: Varenicline versus transdermal nicotine patch for smoking cessation: results from a randomized, open-label trial. Thorax 2008;63:717–724.
31 Hartmann-Boyce J, Stead LF, Cahill K, Lancaster T: Efficacy of interventions to combat tobacco addiction: Cochrane update of 2013 reviews. Addiction 2014;109:1414–1125.

32 Stableton AJ, Watson L, Spirling LI, Smith R, Milbrandt A, Ratcliffe M, Sutherland G: Varenicline in the routine treatment of tobacco dependence: a pre-post comparison with nicotine replacement therapy and an evaluation in those with mental illness. Addiction 2007;103:146–154.

33 Wennike P, Danielsson T, Landfeldt T, Westin Å, Tønnesen P: Smoking reduction promotes smoking cessation: results from a double blind, randomized, placebo-controlled trial of nicotine gum with 2-year follow-up. Addiction 2003;98:1395–1402.

34 Bolliger CT, Zellweger JP, Danielsson T, et al: Smoking reduction with oral nicotine inhalers: double blind, randomised clinical trial of efficacy and safety. BMJ 2000;321:329–333.

35 Tønnesen P, Mikkelsen K: Varenicline to stop long-term nicotine replacement use: a double-blind, randomized, placebo-controlled trial. Nicotine Tob Res 2013;15:419–427.

36 Unal B, Critchley JA, Capewell S: Modelling the decline in coronary heart disease deaths in England and Wales, 1981–2000: comparing contributions for primary prevention and secondary prevention. BMJ 2005;331:614.

37 Tønnesen P, Carrozzi L, Fagerström KO, Gratziou C, Jimenez-Ruiz C, Nardini S, Viegi G, Lazzaro C, Campell IA, Dagli E, West R: Smoking cessation in patients with respiratory diseases: a high priority, integral component of therapy. Eur Respir J 2007; 29:390–417.

38 Sundblad BM, Larsson K, Nathell L: High rate of smoking abstinence in COPD patients: smoking cessation by hospitalization. Nicotine Tob Res 2008;10:883–890.

39 Klesges RC, Winders SE, Meyers AW: How much weight gain occurs following smoking cessation? A comparison of weight gain using both continuous and point prevalence abstainers. J Consult Clin Psychol 1997;65:286–291.

40 Yang M, Mehta HB, Bhowmik D, Essien EJ, Abughosh SM: Predictors of smoking cessation medication use among nonobese and obese smokers. Subst Use Misuse 2014;49:752–761.

41 Ussher MH, Taylor AH, Faulkner GE: Exercise interventions for smoking cessation. Cochrane Database Syst Rev 2014;8:CD002295.

42 Gennuso KP, Thraen-Borowski KM, Schlam TR, LaRowe TL, Fiore MC, Baker TB, Colbert LH: Smokers' physical activity and weight gain one year after a successful versus unsuccessful quit attempt. Prev Med 2014;67C:189–119.

43 Stein JH, Asthana A, Smith SS, Piper ME, Loh WY, Fiore MC, Baker TB: Smoking cessation and the risk of diabetes mellitus and impaired fasting glucose: three-year outcomes after a quit attempt. PLoS One 2014;9:e98278.

44 Jorenby DE, Hays T, Rigotti NA, Azoulay S, Watsky EJ, Williams K, et al: Efficacy of varenicline, an α4, β2 nicotinic acetylcholine receptor partial agonist, vs placebo or sustained-release bupropion for smoking cessation: a randomized controlled trial. JAMA 2006;296:56–63.

45 Stapleton J, West R, Hajek P, Wheeler J, Vangeli E, Abdi Z, O'Gara C, McRobbie H, Humphrey K, Ali R, Strang J, Sutherland G: Randomized trial of nicotine replacement therapy (NRT), bupropion and NRT plus bupropion for smoking cessation: effectiveness in clinical practice. Addiction 2013;108: 2193–2201.

46 Koegelenberg CF, Noor F, Bateman ED, van Zyl-Smit RN, Bruning A, O'Brien JA, Smith C, Abdool-Gaffar MS, Emanuel S, Esterhuizen TM, Irusen EM: Efficacy of varenicline combined with nicotine replacement therapy vs varenicline alone for smoking cessation: a randomized clinical trial. JAMA 2014;312:155–161.

47 Ockene I, Salmoirago-Blotcher E: Varenicline for smoking cessation in patients with coronary heart disease. Circulation 2010;121:188–190.

48 Tashkin DP, Rennard S, Hays JT, Ma W, Lawrence D, Lee TC: Effects of varenicline on smoking cessation in patients with mild to moderate COPD: a randomized controlled trial. Chest 2011;139:591–599.

49 Mills EJ, Thorlund K, Eapen S, Wu P, Prochaska JJ: Cardiovascular events associated with smoking cessation pharmacotherapies: a network meta-analysis. Circulation 2014;129:28–41.

50 Prochaska JJ, Hilton JF: Risk of cardiovascular serious adverse events associated with varenicline use for tobacco cessation: systematic review and meta-analysis (review). BMJ 2012;344:e2856.

51 Gunnell D, Irvine D, Wise L, Davies C, Martin RM: Varenicline and suicidal behaviour: a cohort study based on data from the General Practice Research Database. BMJ 2009;339:b3805.

52 Thomas KH, Martin RM, Davies NM, Metcalfe C, Windmeijer F, Gunnell D: Smoking cessation treatment and risk of depression, suicide, and self harm in the Clinical Practice Research Datalink: prospective cohort study. BMJ 2013;347:f5704.

53 Chelladurai Y, Singh S: Varenicline and cardiovascular adverse events: a perspective review. Ther Adv Drug Saf 2014;5:167–172.

54 US Food and Drug Administration: FDA Drug Safety Communication: Safety Review Update of Chantix (Varenicline) and Risk of Cardiovascular Adverse Events. http://www.fda.gov/Drugs/DrugSafety/ucm330367.htm.

55 David SP, Strong DR, Munafo MR, Brown RA, Lloyd-Ricardson EE, Wileyto PE, Evins EA, Shields PG, Lerman C, Niaura R: Bupropion efficacy for smoking cessation is influenced by DRD2 Taq1A polymorphism: analysis of pooled data from two clinical trials. Nicotine Tob Res 2007;9:1251–1257.

56 Hays JT, Hurt RD, Rigelli NA: Sustained-release bupropion for pharmacological relapse prevention after smoking cessation, a randomised, controlled trial. Ann Intern Med 2001;135:423–433.

57 Tashkin DP, Kanner R, Bailey W, Buist S, Anderson P, Nides MA, Gonzales D, Dozier G, Patel MK, Jamerson BD: Smoking cessation in patients with chronic obstructive pulmonary disease: a double-blind, placebo-controlled, randomized trial. Lancet 2001;357:1571–1575.

58 Elrashidi MY, Ebbert JO: Emerging drugs for the treatment of tobacco dependence: 2014 update. Expert Opin Emerg Drugs 2014;19:243–260.

59 Leaviss J, Sullivan W, Ren S, Everson-Hock E, Stevenson M, Stevens JW, Strong M, Cantrell A: What is the clinical effectiveness and cost-effectiveness of cytisine compared with varenicline for smoking cessation? A systematic review and economic evaluation. Health Technol Assess 2014;18:1–120.

60 Hajek P, McRobbie H, Myers K: Efficacy of cytisine in helping smokers quit: systematic review and meta-analysis. Thorax 2013;68:1037–1042.

61 West R, Zatonski W, Cedzynska M, Lewandowska D, Pazik J, Aveyard P, Stapleton J: Placebo-controlled trial of cytisine for smoking cessation. N Engl J Med 2011;365:1193–1200.

62 Gourlay SG, Stead LF, Benowitz NL: Clonidine for smoking cessation. Cochrane Database Syst Rev 2004;3:CD000058.

63 Cornuz J, Zwahlen S, Jungi WF, Osterwalder J, Klingler K, van Melle G, Bangala Y, Guessous I, Müller P, Willers J, Maurer P, Bachmann MF, Cerny T: A vaccine against nicotine for smoking cessation: a randomized controlled trial. PLoS One 2008;3:e2547.

64 Wagena EJ, de Vos A, Horwith G, van Schayck CP: The immunogenicity and safety of a nicotine vaccine in smokers and nonsmokers: results of a randomized, placebo-controlled phase 1/2 trial. Nicotine Tob Res 2008;10:213–218.

65 Hatsukami DK, Jorenby DE, Gonzales D, Rigotti NA, Glover ED, Oncken CA, Tashkin DP, Reus VI, Akhavain RC, Fahim RE, Kessler PD, Niknian M, Kalnik MW, Rennard SI: Immunogenicity and smoking-cessation outcomes for a novel nicotine immunotherapeutic. Clin Pharmacol Ther 2011;89: 392–399.

66 Hartmann-Boyce J, Cahill K, Hatsukami D, Cornuz J: Nicotine vaccines for smoking cessation. Cochrane Database Syst Rev 2012;8:CD007072.

67 Wolters A, de Wert G, van Schayck OC, Horstman K: Vaccination against smoking: an annotated agenda for debate. A review of scientific journals, 2001–2013. Addiction 2014;109:1268–1273.

68 Raupach T, Hoogsteder PH, Onno van Schayck CP: Nicotine vaccines to assist with smoking cessation: current status of research. Drugs 2012;72:10–16.

69 Hughes JR, Gust SW, Keenan R, Fenwick JW, Skoog K, Higgins ST: Long-term use of nicotine vs. placebo gum. Arch Intern Med 1991;151:1993–1998.

70 Balfour DJK, Fagerström KO: Pharmacology of nicotine and its therapeutic use in smoking cessation and neurodegenerative disorders. Pharmacol Ther 1996;72:51–81.

71 Walker N, Howe C, Glover M, McRobbie H, Barnes J, Nosa V, Parag V, Bassett B, Bullen C: Cytisine versus nicotine for smoking cessation. N Engl J Med 2014;371:2353–2362.

72 Rigotti NA: Cytisine – a tobacco treatment hiding in plain sight. N Engl J Med 2014;371:2429–2430.

Philip Tønnesen, MD, Senior Consultant
Danish Centre for Sleep Medicine
Department of Clinical Neurophysiology
Glostrup Hospital, Nordre Ringvej
DK-2600 Glostrup (Denmark)
E-Mail philipt@dadlnet.dk

Loddenkemper R, Kreuter M (eds): The Tobacco Epidemic, ed 2, rev. and ext.
Prog Respir Res. Basel, Karger, 2015, vol 42, pp 243–251 (DOI: 10.1159/000369503)

Smokeless Tobacco – Health Hazards or Less Harm?

Gunilla Bolinder[a] · Hans Gilljam[b]

Departments of [a]Medicine and [b]Public Health Sciences, Karolinska Institutet, Stockholm, Sweden

Abstract

The long-term use of smokeless tobacco has led to severe health consequences in countries like India, Pakistan and Sudan, whereas the products used in Scandinavia and USA are less hazardous. Both the type of product and the general health of the population determine the outcome. All tobacco products contain carcinogenic substances and substantial quantities of nicotine. Nicotine has, apart from its psychoactive properties, abundant vasoregulatory effects through the mediation of cholinergic as well as adrenergic stimuli. Studies of the effects of snuff or snus use in developed countries have shown a moderate risk for cancer, cardiovascular mortality and metabolic diseases, such as type II diabetes. Also, snus use during pregnancy has been found to be a health risk for the newborn baby. The evidence, therefore, suggests that although snuff and snus are less hazardous than smoked tobacco, the most deadly of all consumer products, there is indeed reason to be cautious about the use of smokeless tobacco.

© 2015 S. Karger AG, Basel

Historical and Present Use

During the 17th and 18th centuries, the use of smokeless tobacco, both in the form of nasal snuff and as chewing tobacco, was widespread, especially in the upper social classes in Europe [1] (see chapter 1). A decline in smokeless tobacco use occurred during the first years of the 20th century, mainly due to the prohibition of spitting, in order to prevent the dissemination of tuberculosis [2]. At the same time, cigarette smoking increased in popularity. The use of smokeless tobacco remained, however, common in many parts of the world, both in developed countries like the US and Sweden (with the highest prevalence per capita in Europe) and in developing countries in Central and Southeast Asia [3, 4].

In 1992, the European Union (EU) prohibited the sale of snus (moist snuff) in all EU countries except Sweden, where the use of snus was regarded as 'traditional'. As the use of snus is not forbidden in the EU, it is still possible to buy the products through the Internet. Other smokeless tobacco products not embraced by the restrictions, such as dry snuff, chewing tobacco and a plethora of products consumed in the Indian subcontinent, are freely available. While cigarette smoking has declined during the past 4 decades in most western countries, the consumption of smokeless tobacco has varied in the countries with significant use. In the US, the total use of smokeless tobacco products has been stable at around 3.5% (equivalent to 12 million, almost exclusively male users) from 1987 to 2010, with large differences between ethnic groups and between states [3]. An increased use among white, non-Hispanic adolescents and young males is, however, a matter of concern [3]. In Sweden, where snus is the dominant smokeless product (99%), the prevalence of use among males peaked in 2004, and has since fallen with approximately 20% to the 2013 level of 18% daily users according to national surveys [5]. The daily use among females has been steady at about 3.5%. Occasional use is stable at 5 and 3%, respectively. Daily smoking habits in 2013 were 11% for both men and women. The snus habit has strong support among young male athletes, especially in team sports like baseball (US) and ice hockey (Sweden). The use of snus among young women has prompted research regarding fecundity, hormonal effects associated with contraceptives and possible effects on offspring. This presentation will mainly deal with the modern industrially manufactured smokeless tobacco products used in the US and Europe, and not with the vast supply of different tobacco products consumed in developing countries (e.g. betel quid, ash, lime, nass, khaini, mishri, zarda or kiwam).

Categories of Products

Smokeless tobacco is mainly used as chewing tobacco or snuff/snus. Historically, dry snuff was more popular and is still in use in some countries. It is inhaled as a powder through the nostrils. In the US, chewing tobacco is marketed as loose leaf, plug or twist. Swedish snus is processed according to an industry standard (see Carcinogenicity) which may or may not be followed by US snuff brands. Snus, also called wet snuff, is finely cut or ground dark tobacco leaves, mixed with water and flavoring [6]. The 'pinch' is held in place between lip and gum without chewing. In recent years, sales of snus packaged in portion-sized pouches of cellulose fiber are more popular than loose-leaf snus on the Swedish and Norwegian markets. The pouches are also held under the upper lip. Snus is by far the predominant product in Scandinavia (fig. 1) and used by approximately 10% of the US smokeless tobacco users. Most smokeless tobacco products are made alkaline with different kinds of salt to facilitate nicotine absorption through the oral mucosa. Licorice, fruit and spices are typically used for flavoring.

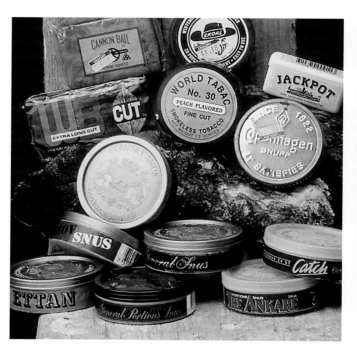

Fig. 1. Different snus products in Sweden.

Nicotine Absorption of Smokeless Tobacco

The absorption of nicotine through the buccal mucosa is less rapid than the almost momentary absorption by inhaling tobacco smoke into the lungs. Still, there is a rapid increase in blood nicotine level during the first 10 min after exposure [7]. The absorption is facilitated by increased pH, with most products having a pH between 7.5 and 8.5. The average blood nicotine levels are similar in habitual smokers and smokeless tobacco users [8, 9]. Smokeless tobacco users, however, seem to absorb a greater total amount of nicotine through the gastrointestinal mucosa by swallowing, followed by a first-pass metabolism of nicotine to pharmacologically inactive metabolites in the liver [7, 10]. This results in equal levels of blood nicotine, but significantly higher levels of cotinine in smokeless tobacco users than in smokers.

Nicotine Dependence

Nicotine is the substance in tobacco causing addiction, i.e. the compulsive craving for tobacco, deprived of voluntary control, irrespective of its form of administration, i.e. smoked or smokeless tobacco (see also chapter 5) [11]. Almost all regular tobacco users try to attain blood levels of nicotine sufficiently high to be associated with a positive experience of relaxation

and stimulation. Smokeless tobacco users tend to keep the blood levels at a constant level by changing the quid regularly during the day. The average usage in Sweden is 13 h/day, and a number of subjects use it also during sleep [12]. This continuous venous supply leads to a tonic nicotine concentration pattern, differing from smokers who obtain nicotine in a more wave motion pattern with high arterial peak concentrations of nicotine alternating with lower concentrations.

Potential Health Hazards Caused by Snus

The potential health consequences of using snus may affect several organs or functions. They are described in detail below and schematically depicted in figure 2.

Local Mucosal Effects in the Mouth
'Snuff dipper's lesion' is nowadays the most common term for the clinically observable changes in soft tissue morphology as a result of long-term smokeless tobacco use [13–16]. The lesion is characterized by a local thickening and hyperkeratosis of the epithelium [17], which is in most cases reversible when smokeless tobacco use is interrupted. Gingival recession and discoloration of the teeth are usual findings, and generally not reversible to the same extent as the epithelial lesions on discontinued tobacco use. The degree

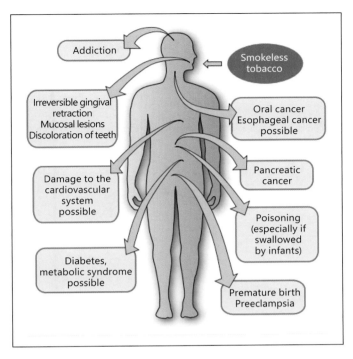

Fig. 2. Health damage caused by the consumption of snus [modified from ref. 90, 91].

of damage is related to increased pH, increased nicotine content and time of exposure (years and amount of tobacco use) [18]. The transformation of lesions into premalignant leukoplakias or into clinical squamous cell carcinoma seems to be rare, but this finding can only be considered valid for the Scandinavian products. Using snus did not seem to be a risk factor for periodontitis. Neither does tooth decay seem to increase with snus use, probably because of the relatively high pH of snus, as well as increased saliva secretion, which reduces the risk of acid attacks.

Cancerogenicity and Cancer Epidemiology
Scientific observations concerning the health effects of smokeless tobacco were first noted in 1761 by John Hill [19], a London physician observing that nasal cancer could develop as a consequence of snuff use [20]. During the last 10–20 years, a number of experimental and epidemiological studies have been performed in order to evaluate the role of smokeless tobacco use in the development of oral cancer and other forms of cancer. Expert reports based on all available scientific literature on the matter have been published both in the US and Europe without reaching any final conclusive statement of the evidence on carcinogenicity of smokeless tobacco use in humans [3, 6, 21–25]. The incidence of oral cancer varies greatly from 3 to 5% of all cancers in many in-

dustrialized countries, to 25% of all malignancies in Asian countries, such as India [4, 26]. It seems beyond doubt that the use of chewing tobacco together with different mixtures of flavoring, alkaline substances and a variety of natural products, when used in populations with poor mouth hygiene and inadequate nutritional status, is causally related to the development of oral cancer. In the Western World, one of the most cited investigations is a case-control study by Winn et al. [27] published in 1981 of women in the tobacco-cultivating areas of North Carolina, US, which did reveal a relative risk (RR) for white snuff users of 4.8 (for black women 1.5) to develop oral cancer compared with nonusers, and a positive dose-response relationship was found as well. On the other hand, most epidemiological investigations regarding smokeless tobacco use in populations of industrialized countries have failed to demonstrate a significantly increased cancer incidence [28]. Methodological problems in most studies regarding the classification of tobacco use, confounding from simultaneous or earlier smoking, alcohol use, differences in dietary habits, and duration and amount of tobacco used limit an unequivocal interpretation. However, regarding the role of exposure to chemicals in the development of oral cancer, smoking and alcohol consumption are the dominant risk factors in the Western World.

The content of nitrosamines in tobacco is supposed to account for the possible raised risk of cancer in smokeless tobacco users. Tobacco-specific nitrosamines in smokeless tobacco [N-nitrosonicotine and 4-(methylnitrosamino)-1-(3-pyridyl)-1-butone] have been shown to be potent carcinogens in animal tests [19]. The biological relevance of carcinogenicity is based on findings of mutations, micronuclei, sister chromatid exchanges and cell formation due to the exposure to extracts of smokeless tobacco [3, 21].

A limited number of investigations concerning cancer at other sites than the oral cavity (upper digestive tract and bladder) have been performed [3, 21], but the findings are inconclusive, with the possible exception of pancreatic cancer, where the evidence points to a double risk for regular snus users [23]. Otherwise, RR estimates seldom exceed 2.0, a common limit for good evidence of causality in carefully controlled studies in epidemiological research.

To sum up, all smokeless tobacco products contain potentially cancerogenic nitrosamines, although the content differs widely between products. Since about 15 years, manufacturing methods involving lower levels of nitrosamines and heavy metals together with cold storage might reduce the cancer risks even further. However, experimental and epidemiological studies and case reports mostly describe a consistent pattern of an increasing risk of cancer due to the use of smokeless tobacco with a dose-response pattern, i.e. the risk increases with longer duration and higher amounts of tobacco used.

Compared with the extremely high risk of developing cancer due to tobacco smoking (according to the WHO, 33% of all cancers in the industrialized world are caused by smoking), it seems as if the risks associated with the use of smokeless tobacco are obviously of minor importance. On the other hand, compared to the preparedness for precautions against other possible cancer risks in society, like the contents of food, the working environment, domestic chemicals, UV radiation and air pollution, smokeless tobacco use might be more harmful to health than any of these risk factors. One must consider that the use of smokeless tobacco is most often initiated at a very young age and to be continued for decades.

Gastrointestinal Effects

There is little knowledge of the local gastrointestinal mucosal effects of long-term smokeless tobacco use. Intravenously infused nicotine was shown to decrease pancreatic bicarbonate secretion in animals [29], supporting a connection between the increased incidence of peptic ulcer in smokers and nicotine exposure [30]. In a large-scale observational study of Swedish men, smokeless tobacco users had a significantly lower prevalence of heartburn (RR 0.9, 95% CI 0.8–0.9) and a similar prevalence of peptic ulcer (RR 1.1, 95% CI 0.9–1.2) compared with nonusers of tobacco, whereas smokers showed an almost threefold risk of peptic ulcer [31]. This finding was also confirmed in a clinical endoscopy study of healthy individuals with different tobacco habits. Snus users had increased basal cell hyperplasia in the esophagus, but the incidence of peptic ulcers was not increased, while smokers had a threefold risk compared with tobacco-free individuals. The higher levels of nitrate in the saliva of snus users may contribute to the release of nitric oxide in the stomach, which can reduce hydrochloric acid production [32].

Smoking has been negatively associated with the incidence of ulcerative colitis, but in a few studies no such correlation to smokeless tobacco or transdermal nicotine use has been found [33, 34]. However, the increasing knowledge on peptic ulcer disease, the causal connection to *Helicobacter pylori* infections and the role of tobacco use demands further elucidation.

Cardiovascular Effects

Acute Effects

The predominant acute effects of nicotine result from activation of the sympathetic nervous system [35], resulting in increases in heart rate (10–20 beats/min), systolic blood

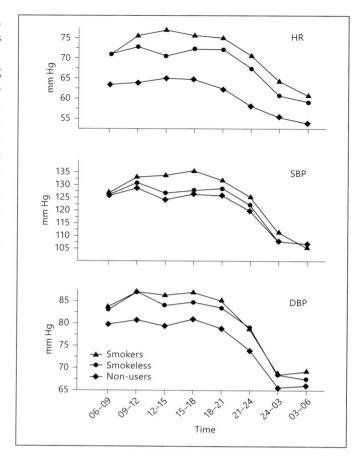

Fig. 3. Heart rate (HR) and systolic (SBP) and diastolic (DBP) blood pressure in subjects ≥45 years old (nonusers: n = 34; smokeless tobacco users: n = 23; smokers: n = 18). Mean values during 3-h periods of 24-h ambulatory blood pressure registration [39].

pressure (5–10 mm Hg) [9, 36], cardiac output, stroke volume and coronary blood flow, as well as cutaneous vasoconstriction and increased muscle blood flow [9, 37, 38]. The hemodynamic effects appear to be more pronounced immediately after cigarette smoking than after smokeless tobacco use, but, on the other hand, the increase in blood pressure and heart rate seems to persist for a longer period after the exposure to smokeless tobacco [9].

A study of the 24-hour ambulatory blood pressure and heart rate in normotensive middle-aged men showed significantly higher diurnal heart rates (5–10 beats/min) in both smokers and smokeless tobacco users compared with nonusers. Contradictory to most epidemiological findings, smokers exhibited significantly higher blood pressure levels during daytime, but not during nighttime, compared with nonusers. This was found also in smokeless tobacco users, but was only significant in those >45 years old (fig. 3) [39].

64 Bahrke MS, Baur TS, Poland DF, Connors DF: Tobacco use and performance on the US army physical fitness test. Mil Med 1988;153:229–235.

65 Bolinder G, Norén A, Wahren J, de Faire U: Long-term use of smokeless tobacco and physical performance in middle-aged men. Eur J Clin Invest 1997;27:427–433.

66 Conway TL, Cronan TA: Smoking and physical fitness among navy shipboard men. Mil Med 1988;153:589–594.

67 Milesis CA: Prediction of treadmill performance from clinical characteristics in healthy persons. J Cardiopulm Rehabil 1987;7:365–373.

68 Daniels WL, Patton JF, Vogel JA, Jones BH, Zoltic JM, Yaney SF: Aerobic fitness and smoking. Med Sci Sports Exerc 1986;16:195–196.

69 Krishna K: Tobacco chewing in pregnancy. Br J Obstet Gynaecol 1978;85:726–728.

70 Agrawal P, Chansoriya M, Kaul KK: Effect of tobacco chewing by mothers on placental morphology. Indian Pediatr 1983;20:561–565.

71 Krishnamurthy S, Joshi S: Gender differences and low birth weight with maternal smokeless tobacco use in pregnancy. J Trop Pediatr 1993;39:253–254.

72 Roquer JM, Figueras J, Botet F, Jiménez R: Influence on fetal growth of exposure to tobacco smoke during pregnancy. Acta Paediatr 1995;84:118–121.

73 Himmelberger DU, Brown BW, Cohen EN: Cigarette smoking during pregnancy and the occurrence of spontaneous abortion and congenital abnormality. Am J Epidemiol 1978;108:470–479.

74 Elenbogen A, Lipitz S, Mahiach S, Dor J, Levran D, Ben-Rafael Z: The effect of smoking on the outcome of in vitro fertilization-embryo transfer. Hum Reprod 1991;6:242–244.

75 Haste F, Brooke OG, Anderson HR, Bland JM: The effect of nutritional intake on outcome of pregnancy in smokers and non-smokers. Br J Nutr 1991;65:347–354.

76 Wikström AK, Cnattingius S, Stephansson O: Maternal use of Swedish snuff (snus) and risk of stillbirth. Epidemiology 2010;21:772–778.

77 Wikström AK, Cnattingius S, Galanti MR, Kieler H, Stephansson O: Effect of Swedish snuff (snus) on preterm birth. BJOG 2010;117:1005–1010.

78 Gunnerbeck A, Edstedt Bonamy AK, Wikström AK, Granath F, Wickström R, Cnattingius S: Maternal snuff use and smoking and the risk of oral cleft malformations – a population-based cohort study. PLoS One 2014;9:e84715.

79 Gunnerbeck A, Wikström AK, Bonamy AK, Wickström R, Cnattingius S: Relationship of maternal snuff use and cigarette smoking with neonatal apnea. Pediatrics 2011;128:503–509.

80 Neff RA, Simmens SJ, Evans C, Mendelowitz D: Prenatal nicotine exposure alters central cardiorespiratory responses to hypoxia in rats: implications for sudden infant death syndrome. J Neurosci 2004;24:9261–9268.

81 Wack JT, Rodin J: Smoking and its effects on body weight and the systems of caloric regulation. Am J Clin Nutr 1982;35:366–380.

82 Marti B, Tuomilehto J, Salomaa V, Kartovaara L, Korhonen H, Pietinen P: Body fat distribution in the Finnish population: environmental determinants and predictive power for cardiovascular risk factor levels. J Epidemiol Community Health 1991;45:131–137.

83 Benowitz NL: Pharmacologic aspects of cigarette smoking and nicotine addiction. N Engl J Med 1988;319:1318–1330.

84 Williamson DF, Madans J, Anda RF, Kleinman JC, Giovino GA, Byers T: Smoking cessation and severity of weight gain in a national cohort. N Engl J Med 1991;324:739–745.

85 Hofstetter A, Schutz Y, Jéquier E, Wahren J: Increased 24-hour energy expenditure in cigarette smokers. N Engl J Med 1986;314:79–82.

86 Clarke P, Quik M, Adlkofer F, Thurau K (eds): Effects of Nicotine on Biological Systems II. Basel, Birkhäuser, 1995.

87 Hansson J, Galanti MR, Magnusson C, Hergens MP: Weight gain and incident obesity among male snus users. BMC Public Health 2011;11:371.

88 Doherty K, Militello FS, Kinnunen T, Garvey AJ: Nicotine gum dose and weight gain after smoking cessation. J Consult Clin Psychol 1996;4:799–807.

89 Tønnesen P, Fryd V, Hansen M, Helsted J, Gunnersen AB, Forshammer H, et al: Effect of nicotine chewing gum in combination with group counseling on the cessation of smoking. N Engl J Med 1988;318:15–18.

90 Ashley DL, Burns D, Djordjevic M, Dybing E, Gray N, Hammond SK, Henningfield J, Jarvis M, Reddy KS, Robertson C, Zaatari G; WHO Study Group on Tobacco Product Regulation: The scientific basis of tobacco product regulation. World Health Organ Tech Rep Ser 2008;951:1–277.

91 German Cancer Research Center: Snus, a Harmful Tobacco Product. Heidelberg, German Cancer Research Center, 2010.

Prof. Hans Gilljam
Department of Public Health Sciences, Inst. för folkhälsovetenskap, Karolinska Institutet
Widerströmska huset, Tomtebodavägen 18A
SE–171 77 Stockholm (Sweden)
E-Mail hans.gilljam@ki.se

Loddenkemper R, Kreuter M (eds): The Tobacco Epidemic, ed 2, rev. and ext.
Prog Respir Res. Basel, Karger, 2015, vol 42, pp 252–257 (DOI: 10.1159/000369505)

Waterpipe Tobacco Smoking: A Less Harmful Alternative?

Mohammed Jawad

Department of Primary Care and Public Health, Imperial College London, London, UK

Abstract

Waterpipe smoking is a centuries-old method of inhaling tobacco after it has passed through a body of water. Cultural variations exist in its use; however, the West in particular has witnessed a surge in flavoured waterpipe tobacco use, known as *moassel*. This is typically shared among peers for 30–45 min, and is now the second most popular form of tobacco consumption after cigarettes in 20 out of 30 European countries. Contrary to the common belief that it is a safer method of tobacco intake than cigarettes, waterpipe tobacco smoke composition is known to contain significant quantities of harmful toxicants akin to cigarette smoke composition. Studies on the long-term health effects of waterpipe tobacco smoking, although of low quality in these early research stages, suggest significant morbidity and mortality is associated with its use. Cessation outcomes are promising although more work is needed to develop and test waterpipe-specific interventions. The waterpipe industry remains largely unregulated and threatens to undermine existing tobacco control policies. Government, policy makers and public health agents should consider waterpipe tobacco smoking as a growing public health concern that warrants attention, particularly in regions of high prevalence.   © 2015 S. Karger AG, Basel

History and Mechanisms of Its Use

Waterpipe tobacco smoking has been present for several centuries, likely originating in the Middle East or South Asia [1] (see also chapter 1). There are cultural variations in the names given to waterpipe smoking, such as narghile, shisha, qalyan and goza. Although several types of tobacco mixtures can be used in a waterpipe, the recent popularity surge in waterpipe tobacco smoking mainly uses *moassel* tobacco, which is a fruit-flavoured tobacco mixture laced in honey and treacle.

Figure 1 depicts a typical waterpipe apparatus. The user manually packs tobacco in the head of the apparatus, which is covered by pierced aluminium foil and has burning coal placed above it. The coal heats the underlying tobacco, and when the user inhales on the hose, smoke travels through the apparatus and into a water bowl prior to entering the user's lungs. One waterpipe session can last anywhere between several minutes to several hours [2]; however, users usually smoke for at least 30–45 min at a time [3]. Waterpipes are usually shared with peers and smoking is considered a social activity [4]. Waterpipes are manufactured in different shapes and sizes, with slight cultural variations in the type of tobacco and charcoal used.

Prevalence of Waterpipe Tobacco Smoking

The prevalence of waterpipe tobacco smoking has surged dramatically in all continents since the late 1990s, despite plateauing or decreasing cigarette prevalence [5]. This is most likely due to increased immigration as well as the mass industrialisation of waterpipe tobacco, resulting in at least 100 million daily smokers [1]. In the US, nationally representative data show that waterpipe smoking is now among the more popular forms of tobacco consumption among young people and college students, where current use is estimated at approximately 5–15%, just slightly lower than the current cigarette prevalence (16% for college students and 23% for high school students) [6, 7] (see also chapter 14). Among adults in the US, current use stands at 1.5%, but it is 10-fold higher among young adults and ethnic minorities

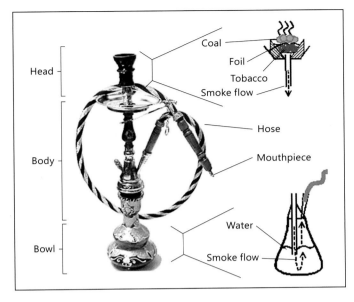

Fig. 1. Schematic image of a typical waterpipe apparatus (with permission from Jawad et al. [3]).

[8]. Among adults in Europe, nationally representative data show that waterpipe smoking is the second most popular form of tobacco use behind cigarettes in 20 out of 30 countries, with highest rates found in Latvia (11.5%), Lithuania (9.0%), Cyprus (8.5%) and Denmark (8.4%) [9]. A high prevalence among adults is also reported in Vietnam (6.4%), reaching as high as 13% among males [2]. Waterpipe tobacco smoking is traditionally highest in the Middle Eastern and South Asian regions. For example, school children in Lebanon and Egypt report a current prevalence of up to 30% [6]. In Pakistan, university students report a current prevalence of waterpipe smoking of 33% [10]. Adult Pakistani waterpipe smokers are known to be among the most frequent users, smoking a median 10 times per day [11], compared to Russia or Egypt, where a waterpipe is smoked on average 0.5 and 2.5 times a day, respectively [2].

Determinants of Waterpipe Tobacco Smoking

Nationally representative surveys show that in India, waterpipe tobacco smoking is associated with increased age, rural residence and low educational attainment. Importantly, in India, waterpipe is smoked equally between genders. These users are likely to be using non-flavoured tobacco in their waterpipe apparatus. While cigarette smoking in India is also associated with increased age, it is contrastingly associated with male gender, urban residence and high educational attain-

ment [2]. These disparities, in addition to the fact that only 5% of adult Indian cigarette smokers concurrently use waterpipe [2], show that waterpipe smokers are a unique nicotine-consuming group. However, Middle Eastern and European studies have hypothesised that waterpipe tobacco smoking may serve as a gateway to future cigarette use [12, 13].

In the West, determinants of waterpipe smoking slightly differ to those seen in South Asia, and this disparity is likely due to the fact that users almost exclusively use flavoured tobacco in their waterpipe apparatus. For example, adults in the United Kingdom are more than twice as likely to be waterpipe tobacco smokers if they are in a younger age group and in the highest socio-economic group compared to if they are in an older age group and in the lowest socio-economic group, respectively [14]. Similar patterns are seen in large US samples of waterpipe smokers [8]. In the West, waterpipe tobacco smokers also tend to be from ethnic minority backgrounds, particularly Middle Eastern and South Asian backgrounds [8, 14].

While prevalence may be high and increasing, many surveys lack information on the frequency of use. This is especially important among waterpipe tobacco smokers using *moassel* (flavoured) tobacco, considering it is a socially driven activity. Smokers tend to share a waterpipe in each session, mainly in waterpipe cafes, so the activity may be dictated more by availability of social outings rather than by nicotine [3]. In addition to the social aspect, another important motive for use is the false belief of reduced harm perception [15]. This is driven by unregulated and deceptive marketing of a product that is 'healthier than cigarettes' [16], and users believe the water in the apparatus safely filters the tobacco smoke [3]. Other common beliefs include waterpipe being attractive and safe because of fruit flavours, less addictive than cigarettes, and cool or fashionable [3, 15].

Health Effects

Despite the widespread belief that waterpipe tobacco smoking is a safer alternative to cigarette smoking [15], research has shown the contrary. The tobacco mixture itself contains significant levels of nicotine, known for its addictive properties, as well as volatile aldehydes, tobacco-specific nitrosamines, heavy metals and 'tar', which cause respiratory diseases and cancer [17, 18]. The charcoal used to heat the tobacco mixture emits high levels of carbon monoxide, and peak carboxyhaemoglobin blood levels among waterpipe smokers are as high as 4.5% compared to 1.2% for cigarette smokers [19]. The charcoal is also responsible for the release

Table 1. Toxicant yields assessed using smoking machines (orders of magnitudes greater than the amount found in the smoke of a single cigarette) of waterpipe moassel tobacco smoke (taken from Jawad et al. [3])

First author, year	Time, min	Toxicant yield, mg				
		TPM	tar	CO	nicotine	NO, ppm
Shihadeh [17], 2003	51	–	242 (25.7×)	–	2.25 (3.1×)	–
Shihadeh [18], 2005	56	1,380 (125.5×)	802 (27.1×)	143 (6.4×)	2.96 (1.2×)	–
Katurji [44], 2010	64	1,193 (108.5×)	602 (22.1×)	150 (6.7×)	4.82 (2.0×)	–
Schubert [45], 2011	57	2,710 (246.4×)	949 (101.0×)	367 (30.6×)	7.75 (10.6×)	–
Shihadeh [42], 2012						
Moassel	45	770 (70.0×)	464 (49.4×)	155 (12.9×)	1.04 (1.4×)	437 (2.0×)
Herbal	45	855 (77.7×)	513 (54.6×)	159 (13.3×)	<0.01 (0.0×)	386 (1.8×)

		Toxicant yield, ng					
		arsenic	beryllium	nickel	cobalt	chromium	lead
Shihadeh [17], 2003	51	165 (2.1×)	65 (0.2×)	990 (14.1×)	70 (411.8×)	1,340 (36.2×)	6,870 (114.5)

		Toxicant yield, µg					
		formaldehyde	acetaldehyde	acrolein	propionaldehyde	methacrolein	acetone
Al Rashidi [46], 2008	56	630 (27.5×)	2,520 (4.1×)	892 (18.9×)	403 (8.7×)	106 (4.5×)	–
Daher [47], 2010*	56	5,234 (14.7×)	5,084 (2.4×)	1,135 (7.9×)	441 (2.1×)	110 (1.1×)	–
Shihadeh [42], 2012							
Moassel	45	58.7 (2.8×)	383 (7.9×)	–	51.7 (1.1×)	12.2 (n.a.)	118 (0.4×)
Herbal	45	117.6 (5.7×)	566 (2.1×)	–	98.4 (2.0×)	20.4 (n.a.)	163 (0.6×)

		Toxicant exposure levels of smokers				
		blood carboxy-haemoglobin, %	blood nicotine, ng/ml	exhaled CO, ppm	exhaled NO, ppm	saliva cotinine, ng/ml
Bacha [48], 2007	60–90	–	–	22.4 (5.2×)	–	77.8 (0.9×)
Eissenberg [49], 2009	45	3.9 (3.0×)	10.2 (1.0×)	24.0 (8.9×)	–	–
Cobb [19], 2011	60	4.5 (3.8×)	9.8 (1.0×)	28.0 (4.4×)	23.2 (1.2×)	–
Maziak [50], 2011	33	–	15.7 (1.3×)	35.5 (5.3×)	–	–

Time = Mean smoking duration; TPM = total particulate matter; * data for sidestream smoke only.

of polycyclic aromatic hydrocarbons, which are known cancer-causing agents also found in cigarette smoke [20]. The evidence for these comes from laboratory studies using smoking machines, as well as in vivo studies looking at blood plasma levels of waterpipe smokers, which are well correlated with one another [21]. Table 1 presents a review of toxicant exposure related to waterpipe tobacco use.

Tobacco-like health effects from waterpipe tobacco smoking are therefore expected, and these are well documented. A recent systematic review showed that waterpipe tobacco smoking is associated with lung cancer, respiratory diseases, low birth weight and periodontal disease, although the quality of the studies was graded as low or very low [22]. Furthermore, a meta-analysis looking at the effect of smoking on lung function showed that the lung functions of waterpipe tobacco smokers were as bad as of cigarette smokers, and waterpipe smoking is likely to be a cause of chronic obstructive pulmonary disease [23]. One study showed that both active and passive smokers of the Chinese variant of waterpipe tobacco had ten and five times the odds of chronic obstructive pulmonary disease, respectively, compared to non-smokers; these odds were over twice as high than for cigarette versus never smokers and highlight the importance of not underestimating the adverse health outcomes of waterpipe tobacco smoking [24, 25]. As is seen with cigarettes, nicotine dependence is a key feature of regular waterpipe smokers, who exhibit cravings, withdrawal symptoms and other nicotine-modulated behaviours [26, 27]. However, the pattern of addiction among waterpipe tobacco smokers may differ to that seen in cigarette smokers. To address this problem, waterpipe-specific dependence scales have been created and validated for specific population groups [27, 28].

There are also unique waterpipe-specific health outcomes that are not documented among cigarette smokers. These include the threat of acute carbon monoxide poisoning [29] and risks of infection transmission from sharing the pipe with peers [30]. Due to the fact that waterpipe is self-assembled, there is an ability to experiment with substances used. Indeed, smokers may mix or replace the water in the apparatus with alcohol [4], and nearly half of US waterpipe smokers use marijuana instead of tobacco [31].

Waterpipe Smoking Cessation

The waterpipe tobacco smoking literature is bereft of information pertaining to cessation interventions. Most waterpipe tobacco smokers, especially those in Western countries, are not interested in quitting [15]. Among those who are interested in quitting, reasons for wanting to quit include health concerns, disinterest in waterpipe tobacco smoking, and smoking cigarettes or other tobacco products instead. Barriers to quitting are driven by the social nature of waterpipe tobacco smoking (peer pressure or boredom) as well as addiction [15].

To date, two known randomised controlled trials for waterpipe cessation have been conducted. One cluster randomised controlled trial was conducted in Pakistan between 2010 and 2011 and compared a control group receiving usual care to two interventions: a behavioural-only support group and a behavioural support group plus bupropion in a sample of cigarette-only (n = 1,255), waterpipe-only (n = 215) and dual cigarette and waterpipe smokers (n = 485). Compared to the control group, both the behavioural-only support group (relative risk, RR 2.2 and 95% confidence interval, CI 1.3–3.8) and behavioural support group plus bupropion (RR 2.5 and 95% CI 1.3–4.7) were effective in achieving 6-month abstinence among waterpipe-only smokers. The effect was not as pronounced as was observed among cigarette-only smokers (behavioural-only support group: RR 5.8 and 95% CI 4.0–8.5; behavioural support group plus bupropion: RR 6.6 and 95% CI 4.6–9.6). The differential effect size may have been due to the fact that interventions for this study were not originally intended for waterpipe tobacco smokers (only cigarette smokers), that sociodemographic characteristics differed between waterpipe and cigarette smokers, and that waterpipe tobacco smokers may have had higher nicotine dependence compared to cigarette smokers [11].

The second published randomised controlled trial for waterpipe cessation was a pilot study conducted in Syria between 2007 and 2008. This study compared a brief behavioural intervention (control group) with a more intensive behavioural intervention (intervention group), which both had similar adherence rates of around 30%. Between the two groups, there was no difference in efficacy, measured by 3-month smoking abstinence (30.4 vs. 44.4%); however, both rates are similar to a meta-analysis of behavioural cessation trials with cigarette smokers [32]. These studies demonstrate the need for further cessation interventions, particularly extending to Western waterpipe tobacco smoking populations.

Waterpipe Tobacco Industry Legislation

As waterpipe smoking primarily uses tobacco, the practice is enforceable under existing tobacco control laws. Recommendations of the World Health Organisation (WHO) Framework Convention on Tobacco Control (FCTC) are not exclusive to cigarettes [33], and countries who have ratified the Framework can apply these recommendations to the waterpipe tobacco industry (see chapter 13). However, the literature suggests waterpipe tobacco smoking policies are poorly enforced, and the industry remains largely unregulated without robust surveillance [34].

Several studies exemplify the lack of regulation within the waterpipe tobacco industry. Health warning label practices and general tobacco packaging have been found to be universally non-compliant with the recommendations of the WHO FCTC [35], which also display deceptive marketing techniques to give an impression of a healthy, harmless product [16]. In the United States, waterpipe premises (where waterpipe is served and consumed onsite) are largely exempt from smoke-free laws [36] despite the quality of air in these premises being worse than in many places where cigarette smoking was once allowed [37]. Furthermore, waterpipe tobacco is taxed at a lower rate than cigarette tobacco [38]; in Europe, waterpipe tobacco is exempt from bans on flavoured tobacco [39]. Underage sales are also commonplace in waterpipe premises and some evidence suggests the development of an underground culture, where waterpipe premises operate covertly and hence unsafely [34]. In Pakistan and India, waterpipe premises were recently outlawed due to overwhelming levels of anti-social behaviour associated therein, including using the waterpipe apparatus to smoke other substances of misuse [40]. Recently, the US Food and Drug Administration decided that waterpipe tobacco needs to be regulated in the same attention given other nicotine-containing products, such as smokeless tobacco and electronic cigarettes [41]. Officials in the United Kingdom have called for the waterpipe tobacco industry to be regulated much like the alcohol industry; that is, for waterpipe premises to hold a license to allow waterpipe tobacco consumption onsite [34].

The industry is still in the early phase of its life cycle, and new waterpipe tobacco and accessories are constantly being developed and industrialised for commercial use. One popular alternative to waterpipe tobacco is smoking a 'herbal' non-tobacco substitute, which is marketed as healthier than waterpipe tobacco but also contains similar levels of tar and carcinogens likely to induce disease [42]. Other alternatives include replacing the tobacco with 'steam stones' – porous stones filled with flavoured liquid [43]; however, the toxicology associated with these products is currently unknown. In principal, should they be heated with charcoal, at a minimum the user will be exposed to the carbon monoxide and carcinogens associated with charcoal combustion [20]. Anecdotal evidence suggests that the electronic cigarette industry is responsible for the development of electronic waterpipe devices, where the coal is replaced by an electric heating element and the tobacco is replaced by flavoured nicotine liquid similarly found in electronic cigarettes. However, the evidence surrounding the uptake of electronic waterpipe devices currently remains uncertain.

Conclusion

The recent resurgence of waterpipe tobacco smoking, in the light of its documented health effects, is a cause for public health concern. In some areas, its use may be typified by a unique nicotine-consuming population group with a potential gateway to cigarette use. Waterpipe tobacco smoking, therefore, has the ability to interact with and perhaps undermine ongoing cigarette cessation services. Epidemiological surveillance is improving, but more research is required to map the full burden of disease caused by waterpipe tobacco smoking. Meanwhile, countries experiencing a high prevalence of waterpipe tobacco smoking should take the lead in evaluating waterpipe health campaigns to prevent initiation and designing a tailored service to promote cessation. Governments should be aware of the regulatory challenges associated with the waterpipe tobacco industry and use guidance outlined by the WHO FCTC to enforce legislation on par with cigarettes.

Key Points

- Waterpipe tobacco smoking is growing in prevalence worldwide despite adverse health outcomes, including lung cancer, respiratory diseases, periodontal disease and low birth weight.
- Reduced harm perception is a key feature among users.
- Cessation interventions are scarce, but show that users may respond to typical cigarette cessation aids, including behavioural and pharmacological support.
- Several tobacco control challenges exist, including the exemption of waterpipe tobacco from cigarette tobacco legislation.
- As the research stands, waterpipe tobacco smoking is not a less harmful alternative to cigarette smoking.

References

1 Knishkowy B, Amitai Y: Water-pipe (narghile) smoking: an emerging health risk behavior. Pediatrics 2005;116:e113–e119.

2 Jawad M, Lee JT, Millett C: The relationship between waterpipe and cigarette smoking in low and middle income countries: cross-sectional analysis of the Global Adult Tobacco Survey. PLoS One 2014;9:e93097.

3 Jawad M, McEwen A, McNeill A, Shahab L: To what extent should waterpipe tobacco smoking become a public health priority? Addiction 2013; 108:1873–1884.

4 Jawad M, Jawad S, Mehdi A, et al: A qualitative analysis among regular waterpipe tobacco smokers in London universities. Int J Tuberc Lung Dis 2013;17:1364–1369.

5 Warren CW, Lea V, Lee J, et al: Change in tobacco use among 13–15 year olds between 1999 and 2008: findings from the Global Youth Tobacco Survey. Glob Health Promot 2009; 16(2 suppl):38–90.

6 Martinasek MP, McDermott RJ, Martini L: Waterpipe (hookah) tobacco smoking among youth. Curr Probl Pediatr Adolesc Health Care 2011;41:34–57.

7 Jarrett T, Blosnich J, Tworek C, Horn K: Hookah use among U.S. college students: results from the National College Health Assessment II. Nicotine Tob Res 2012;14:1145–1153.

8 King BA, Dube SR, Tynan MA: Current tobacco use among adults in the United States: findings from the National Adult Tobacco Survey. Am J Public Health 2012;102:e93–e100.

9 Agaku IT, Filippidis FT, Vardavas CI, et al: Poly-tobacco use among adults in 44 countries during 2008–2012: evidence for an integrative and comprehensive approach in tobacco control. Drug Alcohol Depend 2014;139:60–70.

10 Jawaid A, Zafar AM, Rehman TU, et al: Knowledge, attitudes and practice of university students regarding waterpipe smoking in Pakistan. Int J Tuberc Lung Dis 2008;12:1077–1084.

11 Dogar O, Jawad M, Shah SK, et al: Effect of cessation interventions on hookah smoking: post-hoc analysis of a cluster-randomized controlled trial. Nicotine Tob Res 2014;16:682–688.

12 Jensen PD, Cortes R, Engholm G, et al: Waterpipe use predicts progression to regular cigarette smoking among Danish youth. Subst Use Misuse 2010;45:1245–1261.

13 Mzayek F, Khader Y, Eissenberg T, et al: Patterns of water-pipe and cigarette smoking initiation in schoolchildren: Irbid longitudinal smoking study. Nicotine Tob Res 2012;14:448–454.

14 Grant A, Morrison R, Dockrell MJ: The prevalence of waterpipe (shisha, narghille, hookah) use among adults in Great Britain, and factors associated with waterpipe use: data from cross-sectional online surveys in 2012 and 2013. Nicotine Tob Res 2014;16:931–938.

15 Akl E, Jawad M, Lam W, et al: Motives, beliefs and attitudes towards waterpipe tobacco smoking: a systematic review. Harm Reduct J 2013;10:12.

16 Khalil J, Heath RL, Nakkash RT, et al: The tobacco health nexus? Health messages in narghile advertisements. Tob Control 2009;18:420–421.

17 Shihadeh A: Investigation of mainstream smoke aerosol of the argileh water pipe. Food Chem Toxicol 2003;41:143–152.

18 Shihadeh A, Saleh R: Polycyclic aromatic hydrocarbons, carbon monoxide, 'tar', and nicotine in the mainstream smoke aerosol of the narghile water pipe. Food Chem Toxicol 2005;43:655–661.

19 Cobb CO, Shihadeh A, Weaver MF, Eissenberg T: Waterpipe tobacco smoking and cigarette smoking: a direct comparison of toxicant exposure and subjective effects. Nicotine Tob Res 2011;13:78–87.

20 Sepetdjian E, Saliba N, Shihadeh A: Carcinogenic PAH in waterpipe charcoal products. Food Chem Toxicol 2010;48:3242–3245.

21 Shihadeh AL, Eissenberg TE: Significance of smoking machine toxicant yields to blood-level exposure in water pipe tobacco smokers. Cancer Epidemiol Biomarkers Prev 2011;20:2457–2460.

22 Akl EA, Gaddam S, Gunukula SK, et al: The effects of waterpipe tobacco smoking on health outcomes: a systematic review. Int J Epidemiol 2010; 39:834–857.

23 Raad D, Gaddam S, Schunemann HJ, et al: Effects of water-pipe smoking on lung function: a systematic review and meta-analysis. Chest 2011;139: 764–774.

24 She J, Yang P, Wang Y, et al. Chinese water-pipe smoking and the risk of COPD. Chest 2014;146: 924–931.

25 Leung JM, Sin DD: Smoke and mirrors: the perils of water-pipe smoking and implications for western countries. Chest 2014;146:875–876.

26 Maziak W, Eissenberg T, Ward KD: Patterns of waterpipe use and dependence: implications for intervention development. Pharmacol Biochem Behav 2005;80:173–179.

27 Salameh P, Waked M, Aoun Z: Waterpipe smoking: construction and validation of the Lebanon Waterpipe Dependence Scale (LWDS-11). Nicotine Tob Res 2008;10:149–158.

28 Kassim S, Al-Bakri A, al'Absi M, Croucher R: Waterpipe tobacco dependence in UK male adult residents: a cross-sectional study. Nicotine Tob Res 2014;16:316–325.

29 Clarke SFJ, Stephens C, Farhan M, et al: Multiple patients with carbon monoxide toxicity from water-pipe smoking. Prehosp Disaster Med 2012;27: 612–614.

30 Munckhof WJ, Konstantinos A, Wamsley M, et al: A cluster of tuberculosis associated with use of a marijuana water pipe. Int J Tuberc Lung Dis 2003; 7:860–865.

31 Sutfin EL, Song EY, Reboussin BA, Wolfson M: What are young adults smoking in their hookahs? A latent class analysis of substances smoked. Addict Behav 2014;39:1191–1196.

32 Asfar T, Al Ali R, Rastam S, et al: Behavioral cessation treatment of waterpipe smoking: the first pilot randomized controlled trial. Addict Behav 2014;39:1066–1074.

33 World Health Organisation Framework Convention on Tobacco Control. Geneva, WHO, 2003.

34 Jawad M: Legislation enforcement of the waterpipe tobacco industry: a qualitative analysis of the London experience. Nicotine Tob Res 2014;16: 1000–1008.

35 Nakkash R, Khalil J: Health warning labelling practices on narghile (shisha, hookah) waterpipe tobacco products and related accessories. Tob Control 2010;19:235–239.

36 Noonan D: Exemptions for hookah bars in clean indoor air legislation: a public health concern. Public Health Nurs 2010;27:49–53.

37 Cobb CO, Vansickel AR, Blank MD, et al: Indoor air quality in Virginia waterpipe cafes. Tob Control 2013;22:338–343.

38 Primack BA, Hopkins M, Hallet C, et al: US health policy related to hookah tobacco smoking. Am J Public Health 2012;102:e47–e51.

39 Jawad M, Millett C: Impact of EU flavoured tobacco ban on waterpipe smoking. BMJ 2014; 348:g2698.

40 Jawad M: Malaysia: Waterpipe tobacco smoking declared 'haram' in worldwide news and comment. Tob Control 2013;22:292.

41 McCarthy M: FDA moves to regulate e-cigarettes and pipe and hookah tobacco. BMJ 2014;348: g2952.

42 Shihadeh A, Salman R, Jaroudi E, et al: Does switching to a tobacco-free waterpipe product reduce toxicant intake? A crossover study comparing CO, NO, PAH, volatile aldehydes, 'tar' and nicotine yields. Food Chem Toxicol 2012;50: 1494–1498.

43 Lee YO, Mukherjea A, Grana R: Hookah steam stones: smoking vapour expands from electronic cigarettes to waterpipe. Tob Control 2013;22:136–137.

44 Katurji M, Daher N, Sheheitli H, et al: Direct measurement of toxicants inhaled by water pipe users in the natural environment using a real-time in situ sampling technique. Inhal Toxicol 2010;22: 1101–1109.

45 Schubert J, Hahn J, Dettbarn G, et al: Mainstream smoke of the waterpipe: does this environmental matrix reveal as significant source of toxic compounds? Toxicol Lett 2011;205:279–284.

46 Al Rashidi M, Shihadeh A, Saliba NA: Volatile aldehydes in the mainstream smoke of the narghile waterpipe. Food Chem Toxicol 2008;46: 3546–3549.

47 Daher N, Saleh R, Jaroudi E, et al: Comparison of carcinogen, carbon monoxide, and ultrafine particle emissions from narghile waterpipe and cigarette smoking: sidestream smoke measurements and assessment of second-hand smoke emission factors. Atmos Environ (1994) 2010;44: 8–14.

48 Bacha ZA, Salameh P, Waked M: Saliva cotinine and exhaled carbon monoxide levels in natural environment waterpipe smokers. Inhal Toxicol 2007;19:771–777.

49 Eissenberg T, Shihadeh A: Waterpipe tobacco and cigarette smoking. Direct comparison of toxicant exposure. Am J Prev Med 2009;37:518–523.

50 Maziak W, Rastam S, Shihadeh L, et al: Nicotine exposure in daily waterpipe smokers and its relation to puff topography. Addict Behav 2011;36: 397–399.

Dr. Mohammed Jawad
Department of Primary Care and Public Health, Imperial College London
Charing Cross Campus
Hammersmith, London W6 8RP (UK)
E-Mail mohammed.jawad06@imperial.ac.uk

Loddenkemper R, Kreuter M (eds): The Tobacco Epidemic, ed 2, rev. and ext.
Prog Respir Res. Basel, Karger, 2015, vol 42, pp 258–267 (DOI: 10.1159/000369506)

Electronic Cigarettes: The Issues behind the Moral Quandary

Constantine I. Vardavas[a, b] · Israel T. Agaku[a]

[a]Center for Global Tobacco Control, Department of Social and Behavioral Sciences, Harvard School of Public Health, Boston, Mass., USA; [b]Clinic of Social and Family Medicine, University of Crete, Crete, Greece

Abstract

Electronic cigarettes (e-cigarettes), along with other nicotine delivery systems which largely became commercially available in the late 2000s, represent the most recent products in the evolutionary trend of smoking habits and have been the subject of several arguments within the global public health community and beyond. This chapter undertakes a holistic examination of different issues raised by scientists and policy makers regarding e-cigarette design, manufacture, marketing and use, as well as their resultant impact on tobacco-related outcomes at individual and population level, including potential health hazards. Based on the predominant type of tobacco product used and the evolution of the global tobacco epidemic, three new, alternative stages of the tobacco epidemic are proposed: *stage 1* – predominant use of traditional tobacco products in countries that are still in the earlier stages of tobacco product use (South Eastern Asian countries, China, Middle Eastern countries and those in the African region); *stage 2* – combined use of traditional and modified-risk tobacco products in countries with developing tobacco control initiatives which are still at the apex of the mortality epidemic for males and females (Southern and Eastern European, certain Asian and South American countries), and *stage 3* – rapidly increasing use of modified-risk tobacco products in countries with relatively advanced tobacco control, steady reductions in cigarette sales and consumption, and a rapid increase in the popularity and application of harm reduction strategies (USA, Canada, Australia and countries in Northwest Europe). In stage 3 countries, the sudden exposure to e-cigarettes has created a moral quandary from a public health perspective. On the one hand, e-cigarettes may represent a potential game changer for smoking cessation efforts or be part of a harm reduction strategy. On the other hand, they are an untested product that could reinforce or renormalize nicotine addiction, and hence potentially undermine the effectiveness of evidence-based tobacco control activities which have contributed to declines in smoking rates over the past decades. Thus, a major public health concern regarding e-cigarettes is whether they serve as a potential gateway to nicotine addiction and subsequent tobacco use. Finally, the chapter summarizes the regulatory measures which are requested for the use of e-cigarettes as part of comprehensive tobacco control.

All is flux, nothing stays still
Heraclitus
(540-480 BC)

Change is an integral part of biological, planetary and social systems. Man-made products also evolve to keep up with changing technological and social climates. For example, the first telephone invented by Alexander Graham Bell in the 1870s was designed to convey voice – a crude device that evolved into the household phone, the cellular phones of the 1980s and now the sleek, multipurpose, newer-generation, digital phones that not only convey voice, but also have facilities for data, video, messaging and thousands of other software applications.

Tobacco products have similarly evolved greatly over the centuries – from being smoked in pipes for medicinal and ceremonial rituals in the pre-Columbian Americas, to industrially manufactured conventional cigarettes, to multiple newer and potentially more addictive products, each marketed as better – or potentially safer – than their predecessors (for details see chapter 1). Electronic cigarettes (e-cigarettes), along with other nicotine delivery systems which largely became commercially available in the late 2000s, represent the

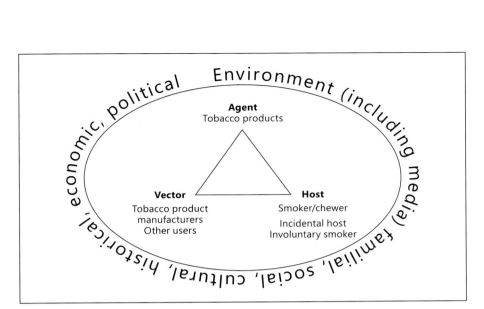

Fig. 1. Epidemic model of nicotine addiction and tobacco control (adapted from Orleans and Slade [68] , by permission of Oxford University Press, USA).

most recent products in the evolutionary trend and have been the subject of several arguments within the global public health community [1]. This chapter undertakes a holistic examination of different issues raised by scientists and policy makers regarding e-cigarette design, manufacture, marketing and use, as well as their resultant impact on tobacco-related outcomes at individual and population level.

Evolution of the Tobacco Epidemic: The Rise in the Electronic Cigarette

The traditional stages of the association between tobacco use and tobacco-attributable mortality were developed by Lopez et al. [2] in 1994; they outlined four stages based on the association between the prevalence of use among adults for both genders and the time frame when mortality attributable to tobacco would peak within both genders (see fig. 2 in chapter 2).

Based on the predominant type of tobacco product used and the evolution of the global tobacco epidemic, *we propose three new and alternative stages of the tobacco epidemic.* This theory is based on the hypothesis that tobacco use fits into the infectious disease paradigm (fig. 1) [3]. Just like the mutation of an infectious agent (e.g. a virus) might influence its infectivity, pathogenicity and transmissibility in a host, so the evolution (mutation) of tobacco products (infectious agent) induced by the tobacco industry (the vector) might influence the initiation and abuse potential (infectivity) of tobacco products in the host (adolescents and young adults). Subsequently, just as different viruses target different cells

and organs due to predisposition, evolving tobacco types may similarly affect different 'cells' (individuals) and 'organs' (societies).

A Novel Three-Stage Model of the Tobacco Epidemic
Stage 1: Predominant Use of Traditional Tobacco Products

Stage 1 countries of the global tobacco epidemic are those that are still in the earlier stages of tobacco product use. Within these countries, tobacco product use is still increasing in the population, either due to recent multinational tobacco industry infiltration or because of cultural use of traditional tobacco products, such as kreteks, waterpipes and oral/nasal smokeless tobacco products. Examples of such countries include South Eastern Asian countries, China, Middle Eastern countries and those in the African region.

Stage 2: Combined Use of Traditional and Modified-Risk Tobacco Products

Stage 2 countries of the global tobacco epidemic are those with developing tobacco control initiatives, but which are still at the apex of the mortality epidemic for males and females. As population awareness of the detrimental effects of tobacco use increases in these countries in concert with intensified tobacco control efforts, interest in and population use of harm reduction strategies might increase. Examples of such countries include Southern and Eastern European, certain Asian and South American countries.

Stage 3: Rapidly Increasing Use of Modified-Risk Tobacco Products

Stage 3 of the global tobacco epidemic is noticeable in relatively advanced tobacco control countries with steady reductions in cigarette sales and consumption, potentially attribut-

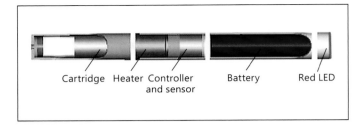

Fig. 2. Components of an e-cigarette [69].

able to greater population awareness of the harm caused by tobacco along with comprehensive tobacco control programs. A rapid increase in the popularity and application of harm reduction strategies has been observed in these countries (see chapters 1, 2, 3, 11, 21 and 22). Examples of such stage 3 countries include the USA, Canada, Australia and countries in Northwest Europe.

The sudden population exposure to e-cigarettes in stage 3 countries has created a moral quandary from a public health perspective. On the one hand, e-cigarettes may represent a potential game changer for smoking cessation efforts or as part of a harm reduction strategy; on the other hand, they are an untested product that could reinforce or renormalize nicotine addiction, and potentially undermine the effectiveness of evidence-based tobacco control activities which have contributed to declines in smoking rates over the past decades [4–6].

Electronic Cigarette Design

So what are e-cigarettes? e-cigarettes are a class of battery-powered devices (fig. 2) that aerolize a chemical mixture (e-liquid) that typically contains nicotine, flavorings and other functional constituents diluted within a humectant – most commonly propylene glycol or glycerine. This liquid is passed over an atomizer (the heating element), which transforms the e-liquid into a vapor which is subsequently inhaled by the user. While this basic aspect of design is incorporated into all e-cigarettes, they now encompass a wide variety of product types and brands available in different shapes, sizes and flavors – hence the definition of e-cigarettes as a composite 'class' of products. The three most common types of e-cigarettes on the EU and US market are disposable e-cigarettes, refillable/rechargeable e-cigarettes (including 'tank versions') and 'MODS' (from their ability to be modified by the user). Disposable e-cigarettes have a nonrechargeable battery and the entire unit is discarded af-

ter the liquid solution is depleted; rechargeable e-cigarettes have a rechargeable battery and changeable e-liquid cartridges or refillable tanks, while MODS are rechargeable e-cigarettes: the consumer can customize and/or regulate design features to suit their personal preferences. The latter are regarded as newer generation devices.

Electronic Cigarette Constituents

Nicotine

Nicotine delivery to the user is one of the most crucial aspects of e-cigarette design. The extent of nicotine delivery in e-cigarettes forms the biologic underpinning for either nicotine addiction (for details see chapter 5) in e-cigarette users or their potential use in nicotine addiction pharmacotherapy (for further details see chapter 20). The nicotine content of the e-liquid is only one of multiple factors that could influence nicotine delivery, other factors being the rate and area of absorption within the oral/pulmonary system – a factor directly linked to product topography and use. Peak nicotine levels with earlier generation e-cigarettes were demonstrated to be comparable to the low end of oral nicotine replacement therapy (NRT) products and significantly lower than conventional cigarettes [7]. Indeed, nicotine delivery through e-cigarettes currently may be more through mucosal absorption (which is slower and more like smokeless tobacco use) in comparison to the fast arterial absorption of nicotine noted during conventional cigarette use because of the deeper lung deposition following inhalation of cigarette smoke (the 'spike') [8, 9]. It is likely that in the near future, the e-cigarette will be engineered by the industry to mimic the uptake of conventional cigarettes and allow for faster nicotine absorption.

Consumer use characteristics and topography may also impact nicotine uptake, as the topography of smoking an e-cigarette substantially differs from conventional cigarette smoking due to a larger puff volume, duration and number needed to obtain a nicotine dose [10]. User experience also plays a role, with experienced e-cigarette users being shown to be more likely to obtain higher nicotine doses than naïve users [11].

Humectants

The most popular humectants used in e-cigarettes are propylene glycol and vegetable glycerine – either alone or mixed into different ratios. Humectants may not be safe for inhalation, especially among naïve e-cigarette users, who may inhale greater volumes of e-cigarette vapor to obtain the necessary nicotine 'kick' [12]. Notably, humectants have been shown to be precursors in the formation of secondary toxic compounds. During vaporization, humectants may undergo thermal decomposition with the atomizer, leading to the formation of low-molecular carbonyl compounds with well-established toxic properties, including formaldehyde, acetaldehyde and acrolein [12, 13]. The formation of these potentially harmful byproducts has been identified to be particularly increased with higher-voltage e-cigarettes (and thus higher temperature) and also with propylene glycol as the humectant [14].

Flavorings

It is well acknowledged through tobacco industry research that sensory characteristics maintain product appeal and ease of use, and are important in influencing smoking behavior independent of the direct effects of nicotine [15] (see also chapters 1 and 3). Flavors can act as secondary reinforcers of addiction, especially among adolescents and young adults (see also chapter 14). A plethora of characterizing flavors are available in e-cigarettes, and these may play a role in increasing ease of use, suppressing withdrawal and producing anticipatory reward perceptions [16].

Impurities

Studies have shown discordance between reported levels of constituents and those actually measured within the e-liquid or the produced vapor [17]. In addition, data suggest that earlier-generation e-cigarette cartridges, atomizers and vapors may contain trace amounts of a range of impurities. Previous research identified the existence of varying levels of carbonyls (e.g. formaldehyde, acetaldehyde and acrolein), volatile organic compounds (e.g. toluene) and tobacco-specific nitrosamines in the e-cigarette aerosol, with significant variations by brand [14, 17]. While being substantially lower than in the emissions of conventional cigarettes, they still pose a concern to consumer health. The discrepancy in the reporting as well as the potential harms from impurities can be reduced through the adoption of rigorous production quality assurance techniques, production modifications and the development of standardized measurement protocols.

Effect of Electronic Cigarettes on the Individual

Due to the lack of combustion and different emissions, e-cigarettes are most likely to be substantially less harmful to the pulmonary system than conventional cigarettes [12, 18]. However, the short- and long-term effects of prolonged inhalation of humectants and nicotine in e-cigarettes warrant further research [19, 20]. To date, research has indicated that in contrast to conventional cigarettes, acute e-cigarette use does not impact spirometry indices of pulmonary function, such as forced expiratory volume or forced vital capacity [21]. However, acute use of e-cigarettes in laboratory settings has been associated with a short-term increase in small-airway pulmonary resistance as assessed with impulse oscillometry (a technique unaffected by subject participation and more sensitive to slight changes than classical spirometry), a decrease in exhaled nitric oxide and a reduction in SpO$_2$ concentrations [22–24]. It must be noted though that while the aforementioned results all indicate statistically significant differences, the clinical implications in relation to the initiation or exacerbation of respiratory conditions remain largely unknown [22]. How e-cigarettes impact the pulmonary health of populations vulnerable to tobacco smoking is an area of significant debate. On the one hand, it may be argued that cigarette smokers who switch exclusively to e-cigarette use might reduce their risk of tobacco-attributable diseases. On the other hand, they may be more vulnerable than the general population to potential side effects of e-cigarette use. Animal models have indicated that the inhalation of e-cigarette solutions can exacerbate allergy-induced symptoms [25]. However, preliminary research assessing pulmonary resistance among human subjects with either chronic obstructive pulmonary disease or asthma found limited changes [23, 24].

The impact of e-cigarettes on cardiac function is an area which is relatively unexplored. e-cigarette use theoretically may impact cardiac function through its nicotine content (for details see chapter 8), its particulate matter (most below 100 nm) and nanoparticle content (more than half of the produced particles during e-cigarette use) [8, 11, 17]. To date, however, little if any research has investigated potential associations. In animal models, nicotine has been shown to trigger a wide range of physiological effects via nicotine acetylcholine receptors and to enhance the growth of atherosclerotic lesions. However, human studies using either NRT or oral tobacco product use have not indicated any such association. It is, however, possible that altering the route of exposure (oral/transdermal vs. inhaled) and the presence of nanoparticles and particulate matter may alter these noted associations. To date, only one study among healthy controls aged 20–45 years has assessed cardiovascular indices related to e-cigarette use and did not identify any significant alteration in any echocardiographic parameter – with the exception of a modest increase in one parameter [18]. Other clinical studies have identified that e-cigarettes do not impact circulating inflammatory markers, heart rate or complete blood indexes [26].

Studies assessing the cytotoxicity of e-cigarette refill fluid have shown inconsistent results. Bahl et al. [27] studied 40 samples of e-cigarette refill fluid using human embryo and mouse neural stem cells and adult human lung fibroblasts, with the first two found to be more sensitive to refill solutions than adult cell types. Within this study, cytotoxicity was significantly correlated with the number and concentration of flavor chemicals, but was not significantly associated with humectant type, while results were inconsistent with nicotine. Similarly, Romagna et al. [28] identified no cytotoxicity among most samples evaluated, with the exception of one with an elevated coffee flavor concentration. Another study indicated that some e-cigarette samples have cytotoxic properties on cultured cardiomyoblasts, which are associated with the production process and materials used in flavorings [29]. These findings are of interest due to the plethora of flavors within e-cigarettes – estimated to surpass 7,700 unique flavors within 466 brands [30]. Another study further highlighted the potential cytotoxicity of other trace impurities such as tin [31].

Impact of Electronic Cigarettes on the Population

Effect on Smokers: Harm Reduction

While the current chapter has focused so far on the risks of e-cigarette use, the discussion would be unbalanced if we omit the possible role e-cigarettes could play as part of a harm reduction strategy. Harm reduction in tobacco control is the process through which public policy regulatory actions focus on reducing the harmful consequences of tobacco consumption through the adoption and promotion of relatively less harmful nicotine-based products. The issue of harm reduction has always been controversial and a cause of significant debate within the tobacco control community, as it is also now in the case of e-cigarettes. Due to product design, e-cigarettes do not involve the combustion of tobacco, and hence are less likely than combustible tobacco products to pose a direct hazard to the user. Hence, when used exclusively instead of cigarettes, e-cigarettes could possibly lower an individual's risks of tobacco-related morbidity and mortality; it could thus be argued that they confer an individual benefit through a harm reduction strategy. Moreover, laboratory experiments have indicated significantly less exposure to toxic chemicals within e-cigarette vapor in comparison to conventional cigarette smoke [17, 32, 33]. However, to have a population effect, e-cigarettes should be regulated to ensure that their use will result in higher rates of complete quitting and a decrease in smoking intensity while not promoting dual use. As smoking-related cardiovascular and cancer risks are strongly dependent on the duration of tobacco use and not only on the intensity of use (cigarettes per day), there is debate on if dual users may have a significant health gain if they continue to smoke a few cigarettes per day [34, 35].

E-Cigarettes as a Smoking Cessation or Cigarette-Reducing Device

Several studies have demonstrated that e-cigarette use may lead to a reduction in the number of conventional cigarettes smoked daily [36, 37], while one randomized controlled trial to date has indicated that e-cigarettes may be at least as successful as NRT in helping smokers quit [38]. More recently, in a UK-based cross-sectional study, smokers who had used e-cigarettes were more likely to report continued abstinence than smokers who attempted to stop through unassisted NRT or without professional support [39]. Moreover, within our secondary analysis of the 2012 Eurobarometer data (the largest population-based study to our knowledge), we identified that after adjusting for sociodemographic characteristics, geographical region and cigarette preferences, current smokers who had made a quit attempt during the past year were twice more likely to have experimented with e-cigarettes in comparison to smokers who had not made a quit attempt [40]. In contrast, a recent meta-analysis of 5 other population-based studies indicated that current e-cigarette users were 39% less likely to quit smoking than smokers who did not use e-cigarettes [41]. This is in line with the US Institute of Medicine Report, which noted that the ability of other tobacco products may have a net negative impact on public health since smokers might delay or refrain from quitting, ex-smokers may relapse back to tobacco use while nonsmokers might be encouraged to initiate tobacco [42].

Taken together, these findings may suggest that e-cigarettes may have an equivocal effect, on one hand they may be potentially used as a smoking cessation aid among smokers already motivated sufficiently to quit (much like an NRT), but with the behavioral cues of smoking [43], while among smokers less motivated to quit it is possible that e-cigarettes may be used concurrently with conventional cigarettes (dual use) and hence may lead to a lower likelihood of quitting altogether.

Effect on Ex-Smokers

Currently, only hypotheses can be made on the potential effect of e-cigarette availability on relapse to conventional cigarette smoking. Few longitudinal studies have assessed this hypothesis, with some indicating that a percentage of ex-smokers may start to experiment with e-cigarettes; however, the sample size of these subgroups remains too small to lead to definitive conclusions [44]. Cross-sectional studies – which cannot attribute causality – note that a percentage of ex-smokers have tried e-cigarettes (i.e. 2.7% in the UK and 4% in the EU), but this study design is unable to determine if this percentage had tried e-cigarettes when they were smokers and subsequently quit (with or without the use of e-cigarettes), or whether this population of ex-smokers may be using e-cigarettes as a bridge or gateway back to nicotine addiction [40, 45].

Effect on Nonsmokers
A major public health concern regarding e-cigarettes is whether they serve as a potential gateway to nicotine addiction and subsequent tobacco use [41, 46]. To date, only cross-sectional studies have assessed the associations between e-cigarette use and susceptibility, experimentation or use of conventional cigarettes among nonsmokers. The prevalence of 'ever use' of e-cigarettes among adults has been estimated at 0.5% in the UK, 1.2% in the EU, 0.8–3.8% in US adults, and 0.9–4.4% in US and 1.4% in Korean teenagers [340, 45, 47–52]. While these numbers indicate a relatively low (although increasing) uptake of e-cigarettes among never smokers, the net population risk versus gain is still unknown, hence the overall impact of e-cigarette use on public health remains unclear and, as such, the precautionary principle remains a necessity [53–55].

Another hazard associated with the introduction of e-cigarettes is accidental poisonings of children. Recent research in the US has indicated an increase in the number of calls to poison control centers – increasing from 0.3% in September 2010 to 41.7% in February 2014 of combined e-cigarette and conventional cigarette calls [56]. In the US, the most common source of e-cigarette exposure was through the ingestion of e-liquid (69%), its inhalation (17%), or absorption through the eyes (9%) or skin (6%), indicating events that may take place either as an accident among children or potentially among e-cigarette users during the refill process [56, 57]. The 2014 US Surgeon General's Report notes that 'The evidence is sufficient to infer that at high-enough doses nicotine has acute toxicity', thus underscoring the need to prevent such accidental exposures through alterations in the design and refill process of e-cigarettes [58].

Exposure to Second- and Thirdhand Vapor
While the levels of toxicants in e-cigarette aerosol are significantly lower than the same volume of cigarette smoke, these concentrations nonetheless indicate that e-cigarettes

Table 1. Recommendations of the Forum of International Respiratory Societies regarding e-cigarettes [62]

(1) A ban on all advertising, promotion and sponsorship
(2) Prohibition of displays in retail stores
(3) Prohibition of sale to minors
(4) Regulation of Internet sales
(5) Taxation at rates similar to combustible cigarettes
(6) Prohibition of sales and refills with flavors that will appeal to children
(7) Requirement that packaging and labeling include a list of all ingredients and the quantity of nicotine
(8) Placement of appropriate warning labels (the same as required for tobacco products)
(9) Prohibition of their use in public places, workplaces and on public transportation

are not completely emission free nor are their aerosols entirely harmless [12, 14, 18, 32, 59]. More recently, in the first real-world environment study, e-cigarette use at home was related to elevated levels of airborne nicotine in homes of e-cigarette users that – while not as high as in cigarette smokers' homes – was significantly elevated over that observed in nonsmokers' homes [60]. Moreover, e-cigarette use was also associated with increased likelihood of thirdhand nicotine exposure from surfaces, with varying levels of exposure observed based on the surface type and e-cigarette brand [61]. Potentially harmful byproducts of e-cigarette use, including acrolein, polycyclic aromatic hydrocarbons, carbonyl compounds, heavy metals and particulate matter, could potentially be reduced through modifications in e-cigarette design or engineering.

The Regulatory Pathway of Electronic Cigarettes

Regulatory science research is imperatively needed to identify the ideal balance between over- and underregulation of e-cigarettes. To this end, more evidence base is needed on both the short- and the long-term effects of e-cigarettes, their potential in nicotine delivery and the specific assessment of how they may impact individual and public health possibly before definitive policies can be implemented. The Forum of International Respiratory Societies recommends that - if electronic nicotine delivery devices are not regulated as medicines - they should be regulated as tobacco products (table 1) [62]. Similar recommendations have been published in comprehensive position papers by the American Heart Association [63] and the American Association for

Cancer Research together with the American Society of Clinical Oncology [64].

e-cigarettes should be regulated to ensure that they do not lead to dual use and youth initiation, and also prevent undermining of tobacco control policies such as smoke-free laws. Taking into account that this rapidly evolving product is most likely going to have a significant impact on tobacco use and regulation, it is imperative to identify some regulatory measures that have already been implemented in varying measures by different countries with a view to strengthening them in the future. These measures may also be useful to countries intending to initiate e-cigarette regulation as part of comprehensive tobacco control [62–65]. These are summarized as follows:

(1) Regulation of Its Use in Public Areas
All electronic cigarettes should not be used in public areas where traditional tobacco products are not allowed so as not to undermine the benefits of smoke-free environments in promoting and supporting smoking cessation efforts. Permitting use of e-cigarettes in areas where tobacco smoking is not allowed would violate Articles 8 and 12 of the WHO Framework Convention on Tobacco Control (FCTC) since e-cigarettes may result in involuntary exposure of nonsmokers to secondhand smoke and also renormalize tobacco use (see chapter 13).

(2) Regulation of Its Marketing and Advertising
This also encompasses e-cigarette packaging, labeling, marketing and advertising. A recently released decision of the WHO obtained during the sixth Conference of the Parties 'urges Parties to consider banning or restricting advertising, promotion and sponsorship of electronic nicotine delivery systems (ENDS)' and 'prevent the initiation of ENDS/electronic non nicotine delivery systems (ENNDS) by nonsmokers and youth with special attention to vulnerable groups'. This is a key aspect of novel product regulation – especially if it is marketed for use only for smokers. Currently, health claims and smoking cessation are frequently used to sell e-cigarettes even in the absence of conclusive scientific evidence, as are the presence of doctors on Web sites and celebrity endorsements [66], with unknown consequences to consumers.

(3) Reporting and Regulating of Its Constituents with Standardized Protocols for Their Measurement and Reporting
Both the EU and the US are currently developing guidelines for the reporting of ingredients within e-cigarettes and their emissions. Should the constituents be regulated through a homogenous reporting format and through improvements in production and handling techniques, it would be possible to reduce harmful byproducts, including the constituents released from e-cigarette emissions. This process will be facilitated, at least within the EU, by the mandatory reporting of e-cigarette ingredients and emissions to Member State authorities and the European Commission, as outlined in Articles 7 and 20 of the EU Tobacco Products Directive (2014/40/EC) [67].

(4) Protection of Children and Vulnerable Populations from Accidental Exposures
e-cigarette packaging and its vials should be child and tamper proof so as to avoid accidental exposure or ingestion by children. This aspect may be easily regulated and enforced if it were incorporated into the aspects needed to market such a product. The EU Tobacco Products Directive paves the way for such handling in Article 20, an aspect which we are looking forward to [67].

(5) Protection of the Legislative Actions from Industry Interference
While the e-cigarette industry started off very small, by the end of 2012, the e-cigarette market was estimated to be worth approximately USD 2 billion globally. With the entry of transnational tobacco companies into the e-cigarette market, it is necessary to protect the regulatory process from industry interference (FCTC Article 5.3).

(6) Increased Funding from International and National Regulators to Investigate the Potential Harm versus Benefit of e-Cigarettes to Individual and Population Health
This would be necessary to provide the public and regulatory bodies with the science that would suggest in which way it would be ideal to handle e-cigarettes.

Focusing on the Forest, Not the Tree

Significant debate exists whether or not electronic cigarettes are a panacea or an additional menace to the largest cause of preventable death on the planet, tobacco use, and these debates will likely continue within the foreseeable future. However, the reality remains that combustible tobacco products such as cigarettes, cigars, pipes and waterpipes, which account for the overwhelming majority of tobacco-attributable morbidity and mortality, are not going to disappear from the face of the earth overnight even in the best-case scenarios. Even the best (bull) case industry projections indicate that by 2020 more than 80% of the revenue of the tobacco industry will still come from traditional smoked tobacco products, with less than 20% to arise from modified-risk tobacco products. Hence, while efforts should be made in addressing emerging tobacco products such as e-cigarettes in endgame strategies, we should maintain focused effort, funding and scientific interest primarily into how to reduce global exposure to combustible tobacco products and focus on the large forest, and not merely the fascinating tree.

Key Points

- Electronic cigarettes (e-cigarettes), along with other nicotine delivery systems, are the most recent smokeless tobacco products designed to deliver nicotine to the respiratory system.
- Besides varying amounts of nicotine, the liquid in e-cigarettes contains humectans (propylene glycol and/or glycerine) and flavorings (in order to maintain product appeal); some brands are often contaminated by toxic impurities. There are now more than 460 different brands and more than 7,700 different flavors on the market.
- The pros and cons of e-cigarettes are heavily debated from a public health perspective, as well in the public and scientific press.

- Because e-cigarettes generate less tar and carcinogens than combustible cigarettes, their use may reduce disease caused by those components.
- However, few data exist regarding the safety of the devices. A number of potentially acute harmful health effects have been reported, and results from long-term studies are still lacking.
- Likewise – up to now – there is only poor scientific evidence that e-cigarettes may be helpful in smoking cessation attempts.
- A major concern is the potential renormalization of smoking by the widespread use of e-cigarettes and that this may serve as a gateway to tobacco smoking, in particular in the youth.
- Regulatory measures of e-cigarettes should urgently be taken, including their regulation as tobacco products.

Acknowledgement

I.T.A. is currently affiliated with the Centers for Disease Control and Prevention's Office on Smoking and Health. The research in this report was completed and submitted outside of the official duties of his current position and does not reflect the official policies or positions of the Centers for Disease Control and Prevention.

Declaration of Interest

The authors have no competing interests to report.

References

1 e-cigarettes: a moral quandary. Lancet 2013;382: 914.
2 Lopez D, Collishaw NE, Piha T: A descriptive model of the cigarette epidemic in developed countries (editorial). Tob Control 1994;3:3.
3 Giovino GA: Epidemiology of tobacco use in the United States. Oncogene 2002;21:7326–7340.
4 Benowitz NL: Emerging nicotine delivery products. Implications for public health. Ann Am Thorac Soc 2014;11:231–235.
5 Drummond MB, Upson D: Electronic cigarettes – potential harms and benefits. Ann Am Thorac Soc 2014;11:236–242.
6 Berridge V: Electronic cigarettes and history. Lancet 2014;383:2204–2205.
7 Hajek P, Goniewicz ML, Phillips A, Myers Smith K, West O, McRobbie H: Nicotine intake from electronic cigarettes on initial use and after 4 weeks of regular use. Nicotine Tob Res 2014, Epub ahead of print.
8 Zhang Y, Sumner W, Chen DR: In vitro particle size distributions in electronic and conventional cigarette aerosols suggest comparable deposition patterns. Nicotine Tob Res 2013;15:501–508.
9 Goniewicz ML, Kuma T, Gawron M, Knysak J, Kosmider L: Nicotine levels in electronic cigarettes. Nicotine Tob Res 2013;15:158–166.

10 Trtchounian A, Williams M, Talbot P: Conventional and electronic cigarettes (e-cigarettes) have different smoking characteristics. Nicotine Tob Res 2010;12:905–912.
11 Vansickel AR, Eissenberg T: Electronic cigarettes: effective nicotine delivery after acute administration. Nicotine Tob Res 2013;15:267–270.
12 Schripp T, Markewitz D, Uhde E, Salthammer T: Does e-cigarette consumption cause passive vaping? Indoor Air 2013;23:25–31.
13 Uchiyama S, Ohta K, Inaba Y, Kunugita N: Determination of carbonyl compounds generated from the E-cigarette using coupled silica cartridges impregnated with hydroquinone and 2,4-dinitrophenylhydrazine, followed by high-performance liquid chromatography. Anal Sci 2013;29:1219–1222.
14 Kosmider L, Sobczak A, Fik M, Knysak J, Zaciera M, Kurek J, Goniewicz ML: Carbonyl compounds in electronic cigarette vapors: effects of nicotine solvent and battery output voltage. Nicotine Tob Res 2014;16:1319–1326.
15 Carpenter CM, Wayne GF, Connolly GN: The role of sensory perception in the development and targeting of tobacco products. Addiction 2007; 102:136–147.

16 Farsalinos KE, Romagna G, Tsiapras D, Kyrzopoulos S, Spyrou A, Voudris V: Impact of flavour variability on electronic cigarette use experience: an internet survey. Int J Environ Res Public Health 2013;10:7272–7282.
17 Trehy ML, Ye W, Hadwiger ME, Moore TW, Allgire JF, Woodruff JT, Ahadi SS, Black JC, Westenberger BJ: Analysis of electronic cigarette cartridges, refill solutions, and smoke for nicotine and nicotine related impurities. J Liq Chromatogr Relat Technol 2011;34:1442–1458.
18 Goniewicz ML, Knysak J, Gawron M, Kosmider L, Sobczak A, Kurek J, Prokopowicz A, Jablonska-Czapla M, Rosik-Dulewska C, Havel C, Jacob P 3rd, Benowitz N: Levels of selected carcinogens and toxicants in vapour from electronic cigarettes. Tob Control 2014;23:133–139.
19 Wieslander G, Norback D, Lindgren T: Experimental exposure to propylene glycol mist in aviation emergency training: acute ocular and respiratory effects. Occup Environ Med 2001;58: 649–655.
20 Chen IL: FDA summary of adverse events on electronic cigarettes. Nicotine Tob Res 2013;15: 615–616.

21 Flouris AD, Chorti MS, Poulianiti KP, Jamurtas AZ, Kostikas K, Tzatzarakis MN, Wallace Hayes A, Tsatsakis AM, Koutedakis Y: Acute impact of active and passive cigarette smoking on serum cotinine and lung function. Inhal Toxicol 2013;25:91–101.

22 Vardavas CI, Anagnostopoulos N, Kougias M, Evangelopoulou V, Connolly GN, Behrakis PK: Short-term pulmonary effects of using an electronic cigarette: impact on respiratory flow resistance, impedance, and exhaled nitric oxide. Chest 2012;141:1400–1406.

23 Vakali S, Tsikrika S, Gennimata S, Kaltsakas G, Palamidas A, Koulouris A, Gratziou C: E-Cigarette acute effect on symptoms and airway inflammation: comparison of nicotine with a non-nicotine cigarette. Tob Induc Dis 2014;12(suppl 1):A35.

24 Tsikrika S, Vakali S, Gennimata S, Palamidas A, Kaltsakas G, Koulouris N, Gratziou C: Short term use of an e-cig: influence on clinical symptoms, vital signs and eCO levels. Tob Induc Dis 2014;12(suppl 1):A30.

25 Lim HB, Kim SH: Inhalation of e-cigarette cartridge solution aggravates allergen-induced airway inflammation and hyper-responsiveness in mice. Toxicol Res 2014;30:13–18.

26 Flouris AD, Poulianiti KP, Chorti MS, Jamurtas AZ, Kouretas D, Owolabi EO, Tzatzarakis MN, Tsatsakis AM, Koutedakis Y: Acute effects of electronic and tobacco cigarette smoking on complete blood count. Food Chem Toxicol 2012;50:3600–3603.

27 Bahl V, Lin S, Xu N, Davis B, Wang YH, Talbot P: Comparison of electronic cigarette refill fluid cytotoxicity using embryonic and adult models. Reprod Toxicol 2012;34:529–537.

28 Romagna G, Allifranchini E, Bocchietto E, Todeschi S, Esposito M, Farsalinos KE: Cytotoxicity evaluation of electronic cigarette vapor extract on cultured mammalian fibroblasts (ClearStream-LIFE): comparison with tobacco cigarette smoke extract. Inhal Toxicol 2013;25:354–361.

29 Farsalinos KE, Romagna G, Allifranchini E, Ripamonti E, Bocchietto E, Todeschi S, Tsiapras D, Kyrzopoulos S, Voudris V: Comparison of the cytotoxic potential of cigarette smoke and electronic cigarette vapour extract on cultured myocardial cells. Int J Environ Res Public Health 2013;10:5146–5162.

30 Zhu SH, Sun JY, Bonnevie E, Cummins SE, Gamst A, Yin L, Lee M: Four hundred and sixty brands of e-cigarettes and counting: implications for product regulation. Tob Control 2014;23(suppl 3):iii3–iii9.

31 Williams M, Villarreal A, Bozhilov K, Lin S, Talbot P: Metal and silicate particles including nanoparticles are present in electronic cigarette cartomizer fluid and aerosol. PLoS One 2013;8:e57987.

32 Czogala J, Goniewicz ML, Fidelus B, Zielinska-Danch W, Travers MJ, Sobczak A: Secondhand exposure to vapors from electronic cigarettes. Nicotine Tob Res 2014;16:655–662.

33 Hutzler C, Paschke M, Kruschinski S, Henkler F, Hahn J, Luch A: Chemical hazards present in liquids and vapors of electronic cigarettes. Arch Toxicol 2014;88:1295–1308.

34 Bjartveit K, Tverdal A: Health consequences of smoking 1–4 cigarettes per day. Tob Control 2005;14:315–320.

35 Frost-Pineda K, Appleton S, Fisher M, Fox K, Gaworski CL: Does dual use jeopardize the potential role of smokeless tobacco in harm reduction? Nicotine Tob Res 2010;12:1055–1067.

36 Caponnetto P, Campagna D, Cibella F, Morjaria JB, Caruso M, Russo C, Polosa R: EffiCiency and Safety of an eLectronic cigAreTte (ECLAT) as tobacco cigarettes substitute: a prospective 12-month randomized control design study. PLoS One 2013;8:e66317.

37 Orr KK, Asal NJ: Efficacy of electronic cigarettes for smoking cessation. Ann Pharmacother 2014;48:1502–1506.

38 Bullen C, Howe C, Laugesen M, McRobbie H, Parag V, Williman J, Walker N: Electronic cigarettes for smoking cessation: a randomised controlled trial. Lancet 2013;382:1629–1637.

39 Brown J, Beard E, Kotz D, Michie S, West R: Real-world effectiveness of e-cigarettes when used to aid smoking cessation: a cross-sectional population study. Addiction 2014;109:1531–1540.

40 Vardavas CI, Filippidis FT, Agaku IT: Determinants and prevalence of e-cigarette use throughout the European Union: a secondary analysis of 26 566 youth and adults from 27 countries. Tob Control 2014, Epub ahead of print.

41 Grana R, Benowitz N, Glantz SA: E-cigarettes: a scientific review. Circulation 2014;129:1972–1986.

42 IOM (Institute of Medicine): Scientific Standards for Studies on Modified Risk Tobacco Products. Washington, The National Academies Press, 2012.

43 Pokhrel P, Fagan P, Little MA, Kawamoto CT, Herzog TA: Smokers who try e-cigarettes to quit smoking: findings from a multiethnic study in Hawaii. Am J Public Health 2013;103:e57–e62.

44 Choi K, Forster JL: Beliefs and experimentation with electronic cigarettes: a prospective analysis among young adults. Am J Prev Med 2014;46:175–178.

45 Dockrell M, Morrison R, Bauld L, McNeill A: E-cigarettes: prevalence and attitudes in Great Britain. Nicotine Tob Res 2013;15:1737–1744.

46 Kandel ER, Kandel DB: Shattuck Lecture. A molecular basis for nicotine as a gateway drug. N Engl J Med 2014;371:932–943.

47 Bunnell RE, Agaku IT, Arrazola RA, Apelberg BJ, Caraballo RS, Corey CG, Coleman BN, Dube SR, King BA: Intentions to smoke cigarettes among never-smoking U.S. middle and high school electronic cigarette users, National Youth Tobacco Survey, 2011–2013. Nicotine Tob Res 2014, Epub ahead of print.

48 Pearson JL, Richardson A, Niaura RS, Vallone DM, Abrams DB: e-cigarette awareness, use, and harm perceptions in US adults. Am J Public Health 2012;102:1758–1766.

49 Regan AK, Promoff G, Dube SR, Arrazola R: Electronic nicotine delivery systems: adult use and awareness of the 'e-cigarette' in the USA. Tob Control 2013;22:19–23.

50 Dutra LM, Glantz SA: Electronic cigarettes and conventional cigarette use among U.S. adolescents: a cross-sectional study. JAMA Pediatr 2014;168:610–617.

51 King BA, Alam S, Promoff G, Arrazola R, Dube SR: Awareness and ever-use of electronic cigarettes among U.S. adults, 2010–2011. Nicotine Tob Res 2013;15:1623–1627.

52 Lee S, Grana RA, Glantz SA: Electronic cigarette use among Korean adolescents: a cross-sectional study of market penetration, dual use, and relationship to quit attempts and former smoking. J Adolesc Health 2014;54:684–690.

53 Frieden T: E-Cigarette Use More than Doubles among U.S. Middle and High School Students from 2011–2012. Atlanta, Centers for Disease Control and Prevention, 2013, http://www.cdc.gov/media/releases/2013/p0905-ecigarette-use.html.

54 Blasi F, Ward B: Electronic nicotine delivery systems (ENDS): the beginning of the end or the end of the beginning? Eur Respir J 2014;44:585–588.

55 King AC, Smith LJ, McNamara PJ, Matthews AK, Fridberg DJ: Passive exposure to electronic cigarette (e-cigarette) use increases desire for combustible and e-cigarettes in young adult smokers. Tob Control 2014, Epub ahead of print.

56 Vakkalanka JP, Hardison LS Jr, Holstege CP: Epidemiological trends in electronic cigarette exposures reported to U.S. Poison Centers. Clin Toxicol (Phila) 2014;52:542–548.

57 Chatham-Stephens K, Law R, Taylor E, Melstrom P, Bunnell R, Wang B, Apelberg B, Schier JG; Centers for Disease Control and Prevention (CDC): Notes from the field: calls to poison centers for exposures to electronic cigarettes – United States, September 2010-February 2014. MMWR Morb Mortal Wkly Rep 2014;63:292–293.

58 US Department of Health and Human Services: The Health Consequences of Smoking – 50 Years of Progress: A Report of the Surgeon General. Atlanta, US Department of Health and Human Services, Centers for Disease Control and Prevention, National Center for Chronic Disease Prevention and Health Promotion, Office on Smoking and Health, 2014.

59 Schober W, Szendrei K, Matzen W, Osiander-Fuchs H, Heitmann D, Schettgen T, Jorres RA, Fromme H: Use of electronic cigarettes (e-cigarettes) impairs indoor air quality and increases FeNO levels of e-cigarette consumers. Int J Hyg Environ Health 2014;217:628–637.

60 Ballbè M, Martínez-Sánchez JM, Sureda X, Fu M, Pérez-Ortuño R, Pascual JA, Saltó E, Fernández E: Cigarettes vs e-cigarettes: passive exposure at home measured by means of airborne marker and biomarkers. Environ Res 2014;135C:76–80.

61 Goniewicz ML, Lee L: Electronic cigarettes are a source of thirdhand exposure to nicotine. Nicotine Tob Res 2014, Epub ahead of print.

62 Schraufnagel DE, Blasi F, Drummond MB, Lam DC, Latif E, Rosen MJ, Sansores R, Van Zyl-Smit R; Forum of International Respiratory Societies: Electronic cigarettes. A position statement of the Forum of International Respiratory Societies. Am J Respir Crit Care Med 2014;190:611–618.

63 Bhatnagar A, Whitsel LP, Ribisl KM, Bullen C, Chaloupka F, Piano MR, Robertson RM, McAuley T, Goff D, Benowitz N; American Heart Association Advocacy Coordinating Committee, Council on Cardiovascular and Stroke Nursing, Council on Clinical Cardiology, Council on Quality of Care and Outcomes Research: Electronic cigarettes: a policy statement from the American Heart Association. Circulation 2014;130:1418–1436.

64 Brandon TH, Goniewicz ML, Hanna NH, Hatsukami DK, Herbst RS, Hobin JA, Ostroff JS, Shields PG, Toll BA, Tyne CA, Viswanath K, Warren GW: Electronic nicotine delivery systems: a policy statement from the American Association for Cancer Research and the American Society of Clinical Oncology. J Clin Oncol 2015; pii:JCO.2014.59.4465. [Epub ahead of print].

65 WHO Framework Convention on Tobacco Control: Sixth Session. Moscow, Russian Federation, 13–18 October 2014. Decision: Electronic Nicotine Delivery Systems and Electronic Non-Nicotine Delivery Systems. http://apps.who.int/gb/fctc/PDF/cop6/FCTC_COP6(9)-en.pdf.

66 Grana RA, Ling PM: 'Smoking revolution': a content analysis of electronic cigarette retail websites. Am J Prev Med 2014;46:395–403.

67 Directive 2014/40/EU of the European Parliament and of the Council of 3 April 2014 on the approximation of the laws, regulations and administrative provisions of the Member States concerning the manufacture, presentation and sale of tobacco and related products and repealing Directive 2001/37/EC Text with EEA relevance. http://eur-lex.europa.eu/legal-content/EN/TXT/?qid=13987613 79066&uri=OJ:JOL_2014_127_R_0001.

68 Orleans CT, Slade J: Nicotine Addiction: Principles and Management. New York, Oxford University Press, 2002.

69 Bertholon JF, Becquemin MH, Annesi-Maesano I, Dautzenberg B: Electronic cigarettes: a short review. Respiration 2013;86:433–438.

Constantine I. Vardavas
Center for Global Tobacco Control, Department of Social and Behavioral Sciences, Harvard School of Public Health
401 Park Drive, 4th West
Boston, 02215 MA (USA)
E-Mail vardavas@tobcontrol.eu

Author Index

Subject Index

Addendum